The Book of
Oriental Medicine

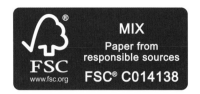

The Book of Oriental Medicine

A Complete Self-Treatment Guide

Clive Witham, LicAc. MBAcC

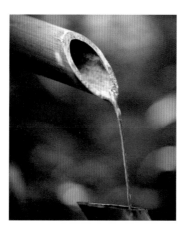

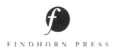

FINDHORN PRESS

Published in 2012 by Findhorn Press, Scotland

ISBN 978-1-84409-604-6

Illustrations © Clive Witham
except for pp. 6/7 © Martimaniac

Photographs: p. 2 © jojobob; p. 42 © Alex Chared; p. 50 © Julien Grondin;
p. 70 Dong Jiu Wang; p. 88 © Kre_geg; p. 116 © Sweet Oasis

Edited by Nicky Leach
Cover design by Richard Crookes
Designed in Shaker by Geoff Green Book Design, CB34 4RA
Printed and bound in the EU

1 2 3 4 5 6 7 8 9 17 16 15 14 13 12

Published by
Findhorn Press
117-121 High Street
Forres IV36 1AB
Scotland, UK

t +44 (0)1309 690582
f +44 (0)131 777 2711

e info@findhornpress.com
www.findhornpress.com

氣 Contents

氣 Introduction

The idea for this book stems from the sense of helplessness that some of us feel when things start going wrong with our bodies.

I could have done with a book like this when I was around eight years old and developed small blue bruises all over my arms and legs. I remember counting them on just one arm, and the number reached to well over 40. With the other limbs covered in even more bruises, it was quite clear to me and my parents that I was sick.

I was admitted as a patient at Great Ormond Street Hospital (formerly the Hospital for Sick Children) in London, and while I did bumper word searches, read Dandy comics, and listened to my mono radio through a mushroom-shaped earpiece, the cream of Britain's paediatricians spent the best part of a week doing a series of inconclusive tests on what was going on inside my body.

In the absence of any better solution (I think they needed the hospital bed for someone really sick), it was decided that since I had had an aspirin a few days before the appearance of the bruises, it was very probably an allergic reaction to this. As with most families at the time, aspirin was always the first port of call when any member showed the slightest sign of sickness, and we had all grown up with the familiar foil packets and the fizzy sound as the flat white pills dissolved in water.

It was, therefore, a surprise that one of us was allergic, but when a man with lots of letters after his name, wearing a white coat, and grasping a clipboard with scribbled numbers, tells you you are allergic to aspirin – well, you are allergic to aspirin. And with that, I was promptly discharged and sent home.

The bruises gradually disappeared, and as flared trousers and polo neck sweaters changed to skin-tight jeans and leg warmers, they ceased to appear. I grew up and continued proclaiming to any nurse with a sharp needle that I had an allergy to aspirin. Other than that, the whole bruising incident was forgotten for many years.

That is, until I began studying to be an acupuncturist and one day, after reading a section on nutrition, the bruise penny dropped.

How a little knowledge could have saved a lot of worry and wasted time.

This is what I now think happened.

I was part of Britain's school milk generation. Because my birthday hit during the summer holidays and I was at the little runt end of my academic year group, I was obliged, along with the other late birthday people, to pop a mini plastic straw through the foil top and sip a bottle of milk a day. Either that or I could not go to playtime and waste a quarter of an hour trying to play football with a tennis ball.

My dairy consumption then continued at home with a glass of fresh pasteurized milk and a pile of ginger snaps and this, added to the milk-soaked Frosties for breakfast and milky hot chocolate later on, meant that with just milk alone I was drinking like a newborn calf. Add to this my daily buttery sandwiches, my liking for potato chips, bananas, peanuts, large glasses of fresh orange juice, chocolate, and all things sweet, and it was no wonder I had developed into a barrel with chubby cheeks.

What I know now but what my mother (who like any mother had only the best intentions) did not know then was that the food I was eating was proving too much for me to digest. It was getting stuck and being processed very slowly through my steadily expanding body. This was quite literal, as I had chronic constipation and was subjected to the torture of sennacot suppositories, which meant that the other functions of the digestive organs (actually the Spleen, but that will be explained later) stopped working well.

According to Oriental medicine, one of these functions involves keeping the blood in the blood vessels. If digestion gets too weak, the Spleen does not send out enough "holding energy" to stop the blood from spilling out from veins and capillaries, many of which are almost too small to see, thereby causing bruises.

This is what was happening to me. I had bruises all over my arms and legs because my Spleen could not send enough energy around my body to control my blood. According to Oriental medicine, the Spleen specifically affects the four limbs. This was why the bruises appeared only on my arms and legs and not on my body.

If we had had this information back in the hot summer of 1977, the solution would have been simple. Stop the milk. And stop the orange juice, the bananas, the potato chips, the peanuts, and all of the other food that was grinding my digestion to a halt.

If we had had this book back then, my mother could have dug her thumb into some key points on my body to help strengthen my Spleen. I could also have done some stretches to help harmonize the balance of my organs. We could have borrowed a soup spoon from the local Chinese takeaway restaurant, spread vapour rub on my back, and Scraped just below the shoulder blades to help digestion. We also could have Tapped my muscles and released the tension that had manifested from my body imbalance. I would also have been forced to stop playing war with mini toy soldiers and to get outside in the fresh air for some exercise.

But, alas, we did not have this book. Instead, we had panic, powerlessness, and confusion, and we were forced to rely on a form of allopathic medicine that, despite the shiny scalpels and the long Latin names, is ultimately flawed.

Far too much of the medicine we see and experience, whether at the local doctor's office or clinic or in a hospital bed, is antithetical to how we would want it to be if we were the people in charge.

If I designed a system of health care, I would not entrust my well-being to an overworked practitioner who is running late with a waiting room full of people and has barely five minutes to scribble an unpronounceable drug on a stamped piece of paper and send me off to the pharmacy.

Surely, in an ideal world, any one of us can come up with a better plan than that. I do not want to spend a fortnight blindly taking an antibiotic "just in case," then have to return for another prescription when it turns out that I have something completely different wrong with me. I want someone to investigate. But to investigate properly, find the problem, and fix it.

But we do not live in an ideal world, and for many of us the current state of confusion is where we find ourselves, our children, our partners, and the people we care most about in the world. We have to follow a system, not because it is right but because it is there and alternatives are not often easily available.

One of the curious and incredibly frustrating things about acupuncture is that many people come to be treated at the end of a long medical journey. They have seen a doctor, a specialist, a surgeon, a physiotherapist, a chiropractor. They have had a blood test, a urine test, an x-ray, an ultrasound, a CT scan, an MRI. They have travelled great distances for a second opinion with another doctor and another specialist, then had a new round of x-rays, ultrasounds, CTs, and MRIs. They have tried every medication the doctors have thrown at them – antibiotics, anti-inflammatories, painkillers, sleeping tablets, even valium. And then, and only then, do they finally step over my clinic threshold and beg me to fix them, as I am their last hope before a desperate operation to remove some important part of their anatomy.

I am usually left bemoaning these harrowing stories and muttering just below earshot, "Why, oh, why, didn't you come to me at the beginning?" This is not to claim that I would have had the answer, but the problem may have been a lot easier to treat if they had.

This was as true for my practice in the UK as it is in my present practice in Africa. More often than not, I am the afterthought, the "let's just see what happens now that those pills don't work" man or the "why not? What have we possibly got to lose?" guy.

It would be nice to be the first in the treatment queue before the symptoms get worse, but here that place is reserved for doctors, surgeons, and specialists. These things take time. Ideas do not change overnight, nor do they change cheaply. You have to pay for them in time and effort. You have to nurture them like precious seedlings, especially entrenched ideas of health and medicine. And so, here I find myself, on the shores of North Africa, watering these seedlings and trying to make big changes in a wonderfully strange little piece of the world.

I have to admit that this is not the most obvious destination to set up a clinic nor, to be sure, is it the easiest. A quirk of history has created a fenced-in Spanish city in northeastern Morocco, where Europe and Africa meet in the most dramatic of ways. The resulting melting pot of cultures, languages, and religions means that it is not unusual to have several languages at play during treatments and an inexhaustible supply of almost childlike curiosity and goodwill.

This whole project has its seeds in my experiences as a fledgling Non-Governmental Organization (NGO) worker in Uganda in the early 90s, and the sheer impotence I felt in trying to meet large-scale illness and poverty with nothing more than a notepad and vague promises.

The key here, as with health anywhere else in the world, is education. Ignorance is a cloud that darkens our view on the world. The simple solution is to lighten that darkness whenever you can. If we are properly informed, we can make decisions that are right for us,

and then we are less likely to blindly accept what we are told. There are, after all, more choices than the seemingly endless (and often very expensive) pharmaceutical merry-go-round that most of us get shoved into when we show the slightest signs of illness.

There are not many acupuncturists in this part of the world. In fact, I am the only one that I know of from here to the Sahara Desert. And many people just do not have the means or the opportunity to visit an Oriental medicine health practitioner on a regular basis.

This lack of access does not have to be such a major disadvantage if you avail yourself of a little common-sense knowledge – knowledge that has been passed down generation to generation, almost unchanged, for thousands of years; knowledge that is based on practice, testing, and refining, and that has matured like a fine wine in a dusty cellar. Just a fraction of this knowledge is included in this book.

This book is not designed to replace an in-person visit to your local Oriental medical doctor for a professional diagnosis and treatment. Far from it. The human element is one of the things missing from modern medicine, and the last thing I want to do is remove it from the process. Indeed, another person can sometimes piece together things about you that are too obvious for you to see. So please do go and visit a qualified Oriental health practitioner, get your diagnosis, and follow the professional advice you are given. Use this book to help you in working with your doctor.

The techniques and advice I have included in this book are what I generally tell my patients and what I encourage them to do in addition to their clinical visits. We all need to keep our bodies working properly, and there are a variety of ways of doing that at home that help prevent disease and ill health.

For those of you who, for whatever reason, do not have access to an Oriental health practitioner, this book offers valuable information and tools that can help you bring back balance to the body. My goal with this book is to help you regain control of your health. I want you to realize that your health destiny does not have to be totally in the hands of a white-coated, pill-toting medical industry. The knowledge of the ancients is still as relevant today as it has always been and when used correctly can transform lives. After all, true knowledge is power, and in this day and age there is not enough of it about.

Power to the people.

– Clive Witham LicAc. MBAcC

氣 How to use this book

How to use this book

This book is not designed to replace a health practitioner. Oriental medicine can be extremely complex, and diagnosing even more so. However, if you use due care and attention, the information in this book can provide valuable help, as it is designed to empower you by educating you about how the body works and what to do when it goes wrong.

The book is divided into six parts.

Part One offers an introduction to how the body functions and explores how we become ill, according to Oriental medical theory. As well as trying to make the world of Oriental medicine more accessible and understandable for those of you without specialized knowledge, this is designed to get you to look at how you are living and see how the things you do on a daily basis affect your body.

Part Two lists the visible signs of ill health – obvious if you know where to look but easily missed if not. These signs of ill health offer a guideline only and are not designed to be used in isolation; they must be reviewed alongside the conditions of imbalance or health conditions that are discussed later in the book. For example, a bluish nose tip does not have to mean intestinal pain, if you do not have any; or if, on close examination, you look yellowish, you do not automatically have jaundice. They are merely clues that should be added to other clues, which together should find the cause.

Part Three explains the techniques that can be used to treat the conditions that can cause illness. They have been separated into six categories:

DIET: Proper nutrition is one of the most important categories when treating yourself. We all have to eat, so why not eat foods that will prevent ill health rather than cause it?

ACUPRESSURE AND MASSAGE: Healing touch, whether performed on yourself or by another person, has a special healing quality. Knowing which places to touch, press, and manipulate on your body can direct this healing to where it is needed most.

SCRAPING: Once the bizarre idea of performing this ancient technique has worn off, you will find it offers a simple and effective preventative treatment.

TAPPING: Gently hitting the body with a small wooden peg can sometimes be a lot faster and less effort than trying to manipulate or massage an area, it can also be extremely effective.

STRETCHING EXERCISES: Along with diet, these exercises are essential in preventing ill health. They do not take up much time, are very repetitive, and can be done by almost anyone.

LIFESTYLE ADVICE: Old habits die hard. Sometimes it is these very habits that are contributing to ill health and it may be time to kill them off for good.

You do not have to do each of these therapies simultaneously; I have included them all so that you have choices, as sometimes a therapy may be inappropriate or impractical to do. A combination of three or four of these therapies, performed regularly, can make all the difference when trying to rebalance inside.

Part Four helps you locate the various acupressure points suggested in the book – on the body, hand, foot, and ear. These points can sometimes be tricky to find: the key is to follow the description given and find a point that feels a little sore when pressed. This may be exactly where described in the book, or it may be nearby.

Part Five introduces the most common imbalances that can occur in the body and explains how to treat them. These imbalances are independent of any disease or illness: even someone who appears fit and healthy will have some kind of imbalance. One of the keys to remaining strong and healthy is to make sure that these imbalances do not become too extreme.

Part Six lists common health conditions, chosen on the basis of how often I see patients presenting with these conditions in my clinic. Of course, there are many conditions that could have been included in this book. I did not do so, purely because I do not see them very often.

For the hypochondriacs among us, it can be easy to read through the list of symptoms and believe that you have the lot. Indeed, most of us have several basic imbalances going on at the same time, and fixing them can mean a mixture of treatment choices.

It is common to note presenting symptoms that fit with several different health conditions. In that case, the way you proceed is very similar to the way an acupuncturist diagnosing a patient would proceed: decide which of the symptoms are the key symptoms and which may be secondary. The key symptoms are the ones that bother you the most – those that, if you were to go to the doctor to explain your problems, would be first on the list.

Like life, medicine is about trial and error. As long as you listen to your body, and do not force it to do anything based on, for example, a fad diet or a random magazine article, little harm is done. If you do make mistakes – following the wrong diet, for example – you may find that this leads to a worsening of your symptoms. But as long as you recognize that you've made a mistake, and avoid doggedly following the same damaging diet like some kind of food fundamentalist, negative side effects can usually be reversed, allowing you to find the right type of diet for you.

Take salads, for example. If you tend towards heat in the Stomach, have a yin imbalance, or live in a hot climate, the coolness of a salad can be really beneficial. If however you tend towards cold in the Stomach, have a yang imbalance, and are tired and run down, a salad would be somewhere near the bottom of the dietary list. Salads are indeed healthy – but not for all of us, all of the time.

My most important prescription is to use a large dose of common sense while using this book. Use your head as well as how you feel, and do not continue to do anything that could harm your body. If it feels wrong in your body, it probably is wrong. If it feels right in your body, then it is probably doing some good. Either way, stay in control of your own destiny, and use a little self-help to weave through the obstacles that life throws at you.

Part One

What Makes Us Ill?

A great deal can be gleaned from Oriental medicine about what makes us ill. There are often clear patterns to illnesses that connect seemingly disparate and random symptoms. A little of this knowledge goes a long way in managing health, and especially in preventing any future problems.

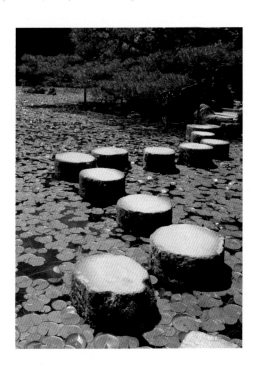

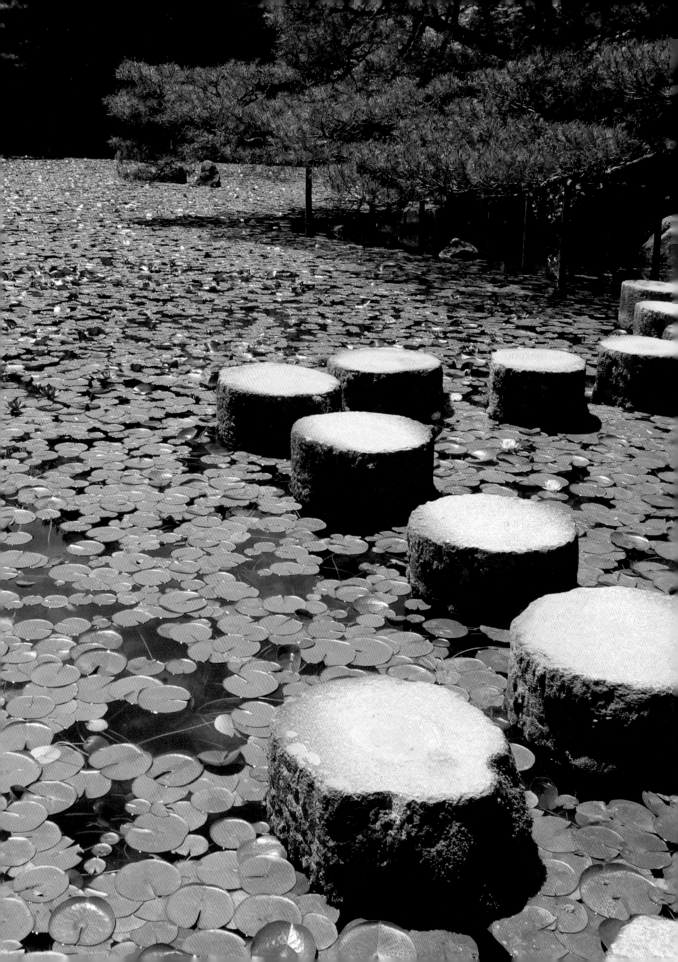

Chapter 1
氣 **The State of the Body's Qi**

We take it as fact that beneath our skin lie muscles, tendons, nerves, blood vessels, organs, cartilage, bones, and so on. What is less commonly understood, especially among those of us in Western cultures, is that within this complex system lies something harder to quantify – something equally real and just as essential to good health: the concept of **qi** (chee).

Qi is defined in many different ways, but it is commonly referred to as "energy." While this is technically correct, as **qi** is certainly energetic, it is much more than just energy.

The Chinese character for qi looks like this 氣, and therein lies the problem – there is not an English translation for 氣 that encapsulates its true meaning. The Japanese recognize the character as **ki**, the Chinese read **chi**, the Koreans call it **gi**, and Thais refer to it as **ghi**. But without any explanation in English, 氣 is nothing but half mathematical equation and half doodle. We do not see it as a meaningful Chinese character representing steam rising above boiling rice, and even if we did, it would not enlighten us much further.

The concept of qi is used to explain all forms of what we might call energy, but essentially it is not energy at all. It exists in all living things, no matter how big or small. It is solid like a rock, and therefore material; yet it is also like vapour, and is therefore immaterial, too.

It is the universe, and at the same time it is you and it is me.

It is the very breath you take, the life you have, or your very existence.

It flows around the body in an intricate network of channels, much as the blood does through the blood vessels, and without it breath would never reach our lungs and our hearts would cease to beat.

It does not show up on conventional medical tests, and for this reason its existence is sometimes scoffed at. But something does not have to be visible to the eye for us to know that it exists. We can feel a breeze on our cheeks, see the gentle swaying of the trees, and hear the whistle of tall buildings but, although we do not see it, we know the wind must be there. We know because we can clearly see the effects on the world around us.

Qi is not something to be believed in or not. In order for Oriental medicine to work, no belief system needs to be in place to help it along. Qi exists independent of what we think about it. An apple will fall down from the tree whether we believe in the theory of gravity or not. It just is, whether we like it or not.

Qi is not something we usually feel on a day-to-day basis, although we could if we knew what to look for and how to practise looking for it.

We do, however, feel it when something goes wrong. If qi gets stuck on its journey around the body,

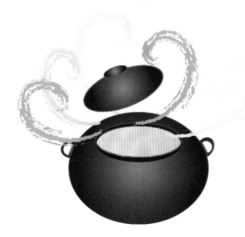

Qi: Steam rising above boiling rice

the body lets us know by triggering pain or discomfort. If it weakens, we feel exhausted. Sometimes we know something is wrong but cannot quite put a finger on it. Or exhaustive medical tests come up short of any clear diagnosis. Simply changing your viewpoint can sometimes be the answer and recognizing that qi has a role to play in regaining your health.

Chapter 2
氣 **The Balance of Yin and Yang**

Within this concept of qi is a balancing system so perfectly simple that it can be applied to absolutely everything, from the limitless universe to the tiniest known molecule. This is the theory of yin and yang.

Volumes of works dating back thousands of years have been devoted to the theory of yin and yang. The original concept came from a careful observation of nature and the environment. This established a dynamic thought process that is hugely relevant when it comes to staying healthy.

For many people, the common understanding of yin and yang is a slight oversimplification. Yin and yang are seen as representing opposites: black versus white, night versus day, good versus evil, Luke Skywalker versus Darth Vader, and so on. But while this idea of opposites is true, there is much more to understand about yin and yang than merely this, and it can be challenging not to overcomplicate explanations.

The obvious place to start an understanding of yin and yang is in its common pictorial representation.

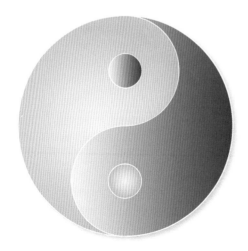

This tennis ball–like symbol is instantly recognizable and adorns countless keyrings, T-shirts, earrings, and martial arts studios. The lighter colour is usually associated with yang and the darker one with yin. Both yin and yang take up equal parts and symmetrically match each other perfectly.

Despite the common belief about the relative merits of one versus the other, neither yin nor yang is implicitly good or bad. Think of them as the two sides of a coin: heads on one side and tails on the other. Without either side being present, a coin would no longer be a coin but a rounded piece of metal. Both must be present in order for it to exist. The symbol shows this in a deceptively simple way.

Yin and yang are not just opposites; they are not mutually exclusive, either. Yin can actually change into yang, and vice versa. Much as a high fever sometimes creates chills, an excited toddler can suddenly fall asleep or contact with ice can burn, so the extreme end of one is the extreme end of the other.

Perhaps the easiest way to understand yin and yang is to see them in terms of something else. And what better something else than a puffer fish.

I gleaned this from my time as a fisherman working the deck of a Japanese flying fish boat in the East China Sea. This whole episode was based on the flawed premise that in order to truly understand treating with the concepts of nature, you first have to truly live them. So, against my better judgement, I became a rural Japanese fisherman for six months and battled all the elements nature and the captain could throw at me.

For anyone not familiar with fishing for flying fish, there is very little to do when waiting for the nets to

Yin and yang symbol

fill up other than flop in the only bit of shade the mast provides and let the sway of the ocean drift your thoughts. The nature of the job meant there were bursts of extreme exertion followed by extended periods of waiting. I suppose it was inevitable that at some point yin and yang would pop up somewhere along the horizon.

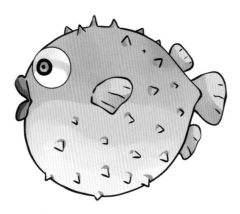

Fugu when agitated and fully expanded

The nets used to bring up all kinds of flying fish, dolphin fish (not the mammal), dart fish, mackerel, the odd sea horse, and, every now and then, what appeared to be a bouncing, spiky ball.

This perfectly rounded yellow ball had two large eyes and a pinched mouth, which gave it a permanently surprised expression. It was known as fugu, a fish so ugly that it is actually very cute, and so dangerous that, second only to the golden poison frog of the Amazon rainforest, it is the most poisonous vertebrate in the world.

The reason why fugu is helpful in understanding yin and yang is that it does not always look like this.

Fugu is normally small, blue, smooth, and rather unassuming (if you discount the mounted bug eyes). Like yin and yang, it has appearances that are virtual opposites: one – aggressive, bloated and spiky (yang); the other – calm, short, and flat (yin).

It is, however, what is inside that really counts. When our slow-moving, spiked friend is relaxed and mulling around in the depths, darting here and there at the sight of microscopic food, it has the contracted appearance of yin. When it expands, however, with all the heat and energy required to pump water into its stomach and bend its spine into an almost impossible shape, it appears the complete opposite, yang.

After expanding, the sheer concentration of energy it needed to enlarge itself has all been used up, so it is actually yin inside while being yang outside. And when it is inert and blue, all that power for ballooning itself up is still sitting there waiting, so in that case, it is yang inside and yin outside. Even when lying lifeless on the deck in the most yin of states, it has enough neurotoxin to kill 30 people.

So within yin there is yang, and within yang there is yin. Hence, in the symbol, there is a dark- or light-coloured dot representing one within the other.

This idea is essential in trying to figure out how the human body functions, as it is not only yin or only yang. As with the fugu, there is a lot going on beneath the surface.

In the body as a whole, yin and yang can be balanced, but the act of living ensures that this is only for a short time. The norm is that the balance of the body swings more towards one or the other. If yang is weak,

Fugu at rest

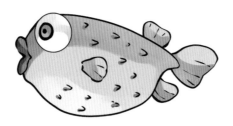

(right) Balanced yin

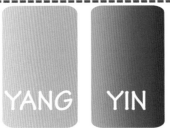

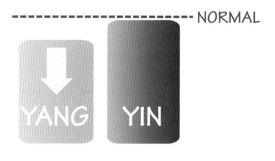

NORMAL

there may be symptoms of coldness and tiredness, and, if yin is weak, signs of heat and agitation.

If yang is too strong, there may be signs of heat rising upwards to the head, and if yin is too strong, signs of coldness and water retention.

This balance is not as stable as you may think and is more like a pendulum continuously swaying from one side to the other. It is only when the difference between the two becomes pronounced, either through weakness or through illness, that the signs of one of them predominate.

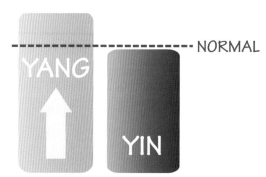

NORMAL

The same patterns of rising and falling of yin and yang exist when we venture deeper within the body. Blood, qi, vessels, and organs all have their own yin-yang balance, which may or may not be contributing to the balance of the whole body.

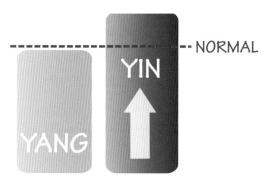

NORMAL

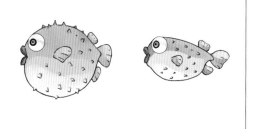

YANG	YIN
Warm body	Cool body
Dry skin	Moist skin
Outgoing	Introverted
Active	Passive
Masculine	Feminine
Positive	Negative
Aggressive	Timid
Angry, impatient	Fearful, insecure
Loud voice	Soft voice
Logical	Intuitive
Desire-filled	Complacent
Strong body	Weak body
Tense	Flaccid
Red complexion	Pale complexion

NORMAL

For example, an exhausted person may suffer from lower back pain due to weak yang in the Kidney. They may also have headaches in the temples from too much stress at work, causing weak yin in the Liver. In this way, both yin and yang can be imbalanced at the same time within different parts of the body. The application of yin-yang theory means that it would be possible to follow this pattern all the way down to a microscopic cellular level and still find yin and yang imbalances.

The body is therefore in a constant state of yin-yang balance, on many different levels from one moment to the next. As the balances become more skewed one way or the other, physical signs often appear that give us clues about where the yin-yang imbalances are, and also how severe they may be.

This theme of balance runs throughout the whole book, but for now take note of some common useful associations of yin and yang in the table provided on the previous page.

Chapter 3
氣 The Balance of the Five Elements

In the ancient Oriental medical system that was developed long ago, both yin and yang and the theory of the five elements were integrated as a way of better understanding the dynamics of the human body.

As in nature, the five elements–Earth, Metal, Water, Wood, and Fire – were noted to interact with each other within the body and to form an intricate relationship in maintaining good health.

Each of the elements is associated with organs in the body, as well as a whole host of other categories. Note: It is important to remember that the elements are representations of processes and functions in the body and not supposed to be taken literally. So, for example, the Lungs and Large Intestine are categorized as being within the Metal element, even though there is nothing physically metallic about them. It is merely the case of using the principles of nature and applying them to other areas. Sometimes this makes logical sense – the Bladder is within the Water element, for example. Sometimes not – the Liver is categorized as Wood.

To maintain good health, all five elements must be in balance with each other. When they are not, signs and symptoms appear that can tell us which of the elements may be weak.

For example, an aggressive, tense person with a curt voice and a slight green tinge around their mouth could very well have an imbalance in Wood. This would probably mean that the two organs associated with Wood – the Liver and Gall Bladder – have developed their own imbalances.

Of course, the real situation is usually much more complicated than this, but these serve as very useful clues as to what is happening in the body.

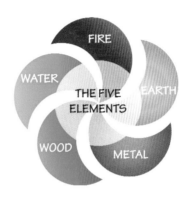

The five elements

The following is a summary of how the body may react when one of the elements is out of balance. This information can be of great help in understanding some of our tendencies and where they come from.

When Wood is balanced it allows us to be calm, unaffected by stress, and have good decision-making and leadership skills. When imbalanced we can become frustrated, angry, impatient, aggressive,

WOOD	
Organs	Liver and Gall Bladder
Colour	green
Sound	shouting
Emotion	anger
Odour	rancid
Season	spring
Climate	wind
Taste	sour
Fluid	tears
Orifice	eyes
Sense	sight
Residue	nails

FIRE	
Organs	Heart, Pericardium, Small Intestine, and Triple Burner.
Colour	red
Sound	laughing
Emotion	joy
Odour	scorched
Season	summer
Climate	heat
Taste	bitter
Fluid	sweat
Orifice	tongue
Sense	taste
Residue	hair

EARTH	
Organs	Spleen and Stomach
Colour	yellow
Sound	singing
Emotion	sympathy
Odour	fragrant
Season	late summer
Climate	damp
Taste	sweet
Fluid	saliva
Orifice	mouth
Sense	touch
Residue	fat

METAL	
Organs	Lungs and Large Intestine
Colour	white
Sound	weeping
Emotion	grief
Odour	rotten
Season	autumn/fall
Climate	dryness
Taste	pungent
Fluid	nasal mucous
Orifice	nose
Sense	smell
Residue	body hair

WATER	
Organs	Kidneys and Bladder
Colour	blue
Sound	groaning
Emotion	fear
Odour	putrid
Season	winter
Climate	cold
Taste	salty
Fluid	sputum
Orifice	ears
Sense	hearing
Residue	teeth

explosive, depressed, moody, unable to structure our lives appropriately, and prone to headaches, eye problems, and swellings.

A tendency towards having any of these characteristics or symptoms could mean that the strength of the Wood element holds an important place in keeping you healthy.

When Fire is balanced it is easy to be open-minded, genuinely friendly, enthusiastic, humble, to think clearly, and be a problem-solver. When Fire is imbal-

anced, however, we can have depression, mood swings, memory problems, confusion, a pale or red complexion, and be inappropriately open and vulnerable. A predominance of these characteristics or symptoms could mean that the state of the Fire element holds the key to your good health.

When Earth is balanced we can have a strong appetite, smooth digestion, strong arm and leg muscles, and can be responsible, stable, creative, and imaginative. When it is imbalanced we can have a poor appetite and digestion, stuck feelings, put on weight, and be tired, overly concerned, and worried. If these characteristics feel more familiar to you, the Earth element may be the most important to keep in balance for your health.

When Metal is balanced we can be principled, consistent, ordered, good at prioritizing, and have well-conditioned skin and hair. When Metal is imbalanced we are more likely to be confused, dissatisfied, disordered, unable to let go, have an inappropriate view of own worth, and have dull skin and hair. Should any of these symptoms or characteristics ring true, the Metal element may be the one that most needs to be balanced.

When Water is balanced we can be calm, consistent, wise, easygoing, and flexible. When Water is imbalanced we can become fearful and insecure, take inappropriate risks, have joint, bone and teeth problems, problems with hearing, and urinary and reproductive problems.

A tendency towards having these characteristics or symptoms suggests that the Water element may hold sway inside our system and be the one most in need of balance.

Chapter 4
氣 **The State of the 12 Organs, Channels and Points**

Within this idea of yin and yang and the five elements, the internal functioning of the body is dominated by an intricate and finely balanced network of "channels" or "meridians." When seen on a chart or illustration, this network resembles a subway map, with colourful lines criss-crossing the body. These lines represent the relationships among the 12 main organs and their channels, and what look like stations on the map are actually acupuncture points.

This idea that there are points along these channels, and that you stimulate the point by pressing, poking, hitting, or zapping, is fundamental to Oriental medicine. The points are places that have been tested and refined over thousands of years, so that each one has its own specific set of functions, a combination of which can be used to treat different kinds of illness.

Proper stimulation of a point can set off a chain reaction, often along the channel where the point sits. It is rather like throwing a pebble into a pond and watching the ripples go steadily farther away until they lap at its grassy edges. Stimulating the point along the channel sends ripples like this, except more focused to a particular destination in the body. A particularly strong headache at the temples, for example, might be relieved by stimulating Liv-3, a Liver point all the way at the foot not far from the big toe.

The 12 organs and channels (Lungs, Large Intestine, Stomach, Spleen, Heart, Small Intestine, Kidneys, Bladder, Pericardium, Triple Burner, Gall Bladder, and Liver) are neatly organized and paired within the five-element system, and each has a specific physical and mental function in Oriental medicine.

(left) The main channels: Front

(middle) The main channels: Side

(right) The main channels: Back

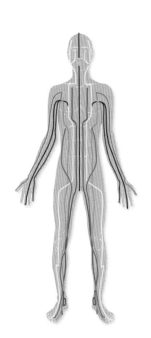
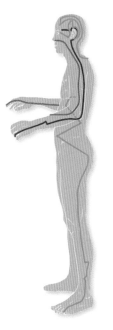
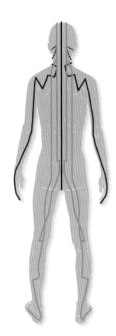

This organization often clarifies things, but it can also be a major source of misunderstanding. Most of us are familiar with the names of the main organs and roughly what they do in the body. The heart, as we all know, is a big muscle that pumps blood around the body; if it stops, you probably have quite a serious problem. The lungs are those two large balloon-type organs that allow us to breathe and help to oxygenize blood. If I then say, however, that your Lung qi is weak, or that there is imbalance in your Heart, you would not be the first to go pale and rush out for a chest x-ray.

Here's the problem: in Oriental medicine, the English words are the same but the meaning is different. When referring to the Lungs or the Heart (or any other of the main organs), it is not the actual organ, as in the anatomical organ that you studied in biology class, that is being referred to, but its overall function.

To try to avoid this, I am following the custom often followed in books about Oriental medicine of capitalizing the organ when referring to the Oriental meaning of the word (e.g., Liver) and lower-casing the word for the biological term (e.g., liver).

So, weak Lung or Heart qi does not mean that you should put your name down for a double transplant just yet. It means that, energetically speaking, the Lungs or the Heart are not performing their functions well. This is why clinical medical tests of the actual biological organ sometimes show no obvious signs of any problem, despite symptoms. The problem is usually there alright, but the search is in the wrong place.

The organs in Oriental medicine are roughly in the same anatomical place and follow the same general ideas as in Western medicine, but the theories of illness differ greatly. For example, ill health might be caused by a yin-yang imbalance within the organ or a blockage in the channel that is connected to that organ. In order to find out where the cause of any blockage or imbalance is, there are often tell-tale symptoms hinting at the source.

The following is a general summary of each organ and its channel and some of these common associated symptoms.

The metal organs
Lungs

The Lung channel begins at the chest near the shoulder. It then follows the front of the arm, over the inside of the elbow, then straight across the forearm to the outside of the thumb.

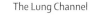

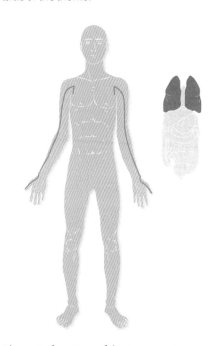

The Lung Channel

The main functions of the Lungs are to:

- ensure your skin is nourished with enough moisture and blood;
- regulate your breathing and the passage of qi from the Lungs downwards to the rest of the body;
- generate grief to allow us to let go and move on with our lives.

Common symptoms of imbalanced Lungs include: respiratory disorders such as asthma, coughs, and shortness of breath; skin problems such as eczema and dry skin; tiredness; and hand, arm, and shoulder pain.

Large Intestine

The Large Intestine channel is not where you would think it should be based on its name. It begins at the index finger and follows the side of the arm up to the shoulder. It then crosses the shoulder, goes up the side of the neck, and ends at the flare of the nostrils.

The earth organs
Stomach

The Stomach channel crosses the body from just under the eyeball, down the neck, chest, abdomen, thigh, and leg, finally reaching the end of the second toe.

(left) The Large Intestine Channel

(right) The Stomach Channel

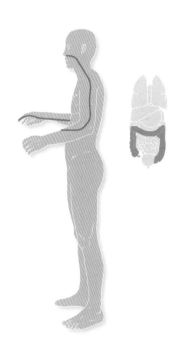

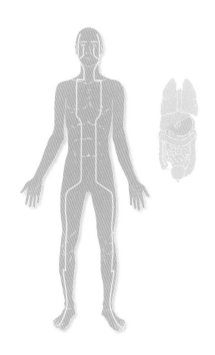

The main functions of the Large Intestine are to:

- control the transformation of digestive wastes from liquid to solid and then transport them out of the body;
- absorb fluid to keep blood volume steady;
- help the Lungs control the pores of the skin.

Common symptoms of an imbalanced Large Intestine include: abdominal pain; diarrhoea; fever; sweating; cold symptoms like a sore throat; skin problems like dry skin and runny nose.

The main functions of the Stomach are to:

- digest food and send qi to the rest of your body and the four limbs;
- ensure that there are sufficient fluid levels in your body;
- maintain a downwards motion with food and qi.

Common symptoms of an imbalanced Stomach are: anxiousness; worry; depression; eye problems; nosebleeds; swelling of the neck; facial pain; weak legs and arms; abdominal pain; diarrhoea; lack of appetite and taste; and thirst.

Spleen

The Spleen channel begins at the side of the big toe and runs up the inside of the foot, ankle, and leg. It continues up through the groin to the chest, then finishes at the side of the chest, below the arm.

The main functions of the Spleen are to:

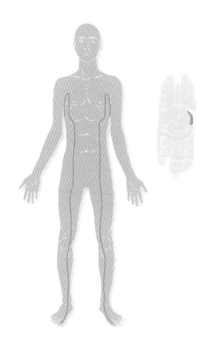

The fire organs
Heart

The Heart channel begins in the chest and comes from the armpit down the inside of the arm and on to the end of the little finger.

The main functions of the Heart are to:

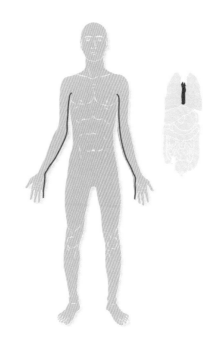

(left) The Spleen Channel

(right) The Heart Channel

- extract qi from digested food and transport it to your four limbs;
- keep your blood in the blood vessels to prevent bruising;
- bring colour to your lips;
- regulate bodily rhythms like periods;
- help you think clearly.

Common symptoms of an imbalanced Spleen include: tiredness; weak limbs and muscle atrophy; dizziness; pale lips; numb limbs; a heavy feeling; headaches; low appetite; and over-worrying.

- control blood and the blood vessels throughout your body;
- affect your complexion by controlling the blood supply to your face;
- balance your emotions, as healthy blood allows your mind to rest.

Common symptoms of an imbalanced Heart include: a pale complexion; anxiety; palpitations; sweating easily; tiredness; poor memory; disturbing dreams; insomnia;, agitation; and rash behaviour.

Small Intestine

Like the Large Intestine channel, the Small Intestine channel is not where you would think it should be. It begins at the tip of the little finger and heads up the back of the arm, zigzagging over the shoulder blade, and up to the cheek via the side of the neck. It then ends in front of the ear. Because of its positioning, the state of the Small Intestine channel can easily affect the upper back, the shoulder and the neck, and is often

abdominal pain; bloating; and being unable to understand and work through ideas easily.

Pericardium

The Pericardium channel begins in the chest not far from the nipple and flows down the inside of the arm to the middle finger. Interestingly, this is often the reported path of the pain associated with a heart attack.

(left) The Small Intestine Channel

(right) The Pericardium Channel

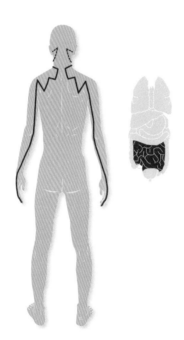
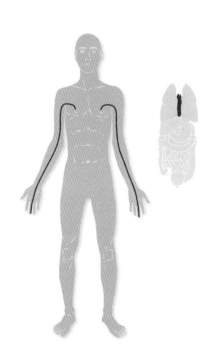

the first port of call in any neck problem.

The main functions of the Small Intestine are to:

*   process food from your Stomach (the pure fluids head to the large intestine to be reabsorbed, and the impure fluids are sent to the bladder to be excreted);
*   help you think clearly by separating out your thought processes.

Common symptoms of imbalanced Small Intestine include: chest tightness and pain; elbow, arm, shoulder and neck pain; problems with hearing; depression;

It is closely related to the Heart and its main functions are to:

*   protect and guide your emotions and relationships;
*   cool and move the blood in your body;
*   calm your Stomach.

Common symptoms of an imbalanced Pericardium include: heart problems; arrhythmias; pain and swelling in the breasts; uterine fibroids; depression; phobias; hiccups; and gas.

Triple Burner

The Triple Burner channel has a name that does not sound as familiar as many of the others. This is because it is not one of the solid organs you may have studied in biology class but refers to a separation of the torso into three clear sections: the upper, middle, and lower. It is often connected to physical symptoms along its channel. The channel starts at the tip of the ring finger and crosses the outside of the forearm to the tip of the

The Water organs
Kidneys

The Kidney channel starts at the soles of the feet, then meanders around the ankle and up the inside of the leg. It then comes through the groin area and up the abdomen and chest, until just below the collar bone.

The main functions of the Kidneys are to:

* store qi;
* produce marrow and keep your bones strong;

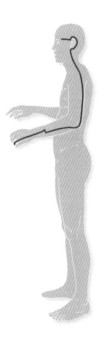

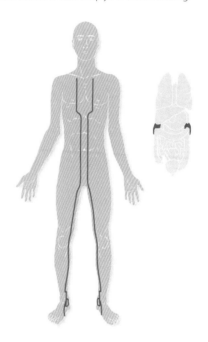

(left) The Triple Burner Channel

(right) The Kidney Channel

elbow. It then goes up the back of the arm, across the shoulder, around the outside of the ear, and ends at the temple.

The main functions of the Triple Burner are to:

* regulate the separate parts of the torso and ensure that qi, fluids, and blood are correctly distributed among them.

Common symptoms of an imbalanced Triple Burner include: hearing problems, including deafness and tinnitus; dizziness; constipation; arm; chest; shoulder and neck pain; headaches; and eye problems.

* keep your hearing in good condition;
* maintain the strength and colour of your hair;
* regulate your sexual organs and the uterus.

Common symptoms of imbalanced Kidneys include: urinary problems; hearing loss and ear infections; knee and lower back problems; problems with teeth; respiratory problems, especially difficulty inhaling; and an excess of sexual energy.

Bladder

The Bladder channel encompasses the whole body. It starts next to the eyeballs, in between the eyes, then zigzags over the head. It then flows straight down the back twice, then goes over the buttocks and down the midline of the back of the legs. It finishes at the outside of the foot, at the little toe.

The wood organs
Liver

The Liver channel begins at the big toe and twists up the inside of the leg, through the groin area, and ends near the bottom of the ribcage.

(left) The Bladder Channel

(right) The Liver Channel

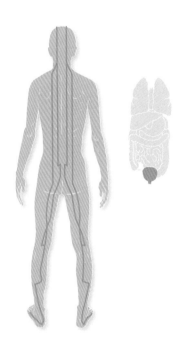

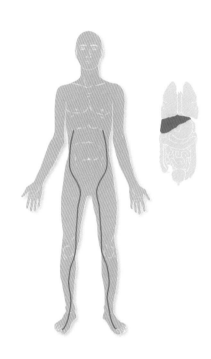

The main functions of the Bladder are to:

- store and release body fluids sent to it by the Kidneys;
- stabilize the tissues and organs in the body.

Common symptoms of an imbalanced Bladder include: lower back pain; sciatica; urinary problems like cystitis; eye problems; and genital and reproductive problems.

The main functions of the Liver are to:

- move and store blood;
- ensure that qi smoothly flows around the body;
- nourish your tendons, to prevent weakness and cramp.

Common symptoms of an imbalanced Liver include: headaches (especially at the temples and behind the eyes); neck and shoulder pain; bloating; eye problems; depression; irritability; nausea; gas; a lump in the throat; problems in swallowing; brittle nails; and painful, irregular periods.

Gall Bladder

The Gall Bladder channel begins at the temple, close to the corner of the eye. It then criss-crosses the top of the head, the neck, and the shoulder, and then runs down the side of the body until it reaches the groin. Here it moves around the hip and heads down the side of the leg until it reaches the second from last toe.

The extra channels

In addition to the 12 channels connected to organs, there are several additional channels which are not. The most important of these, in terms of this book, are the Conception, or Ren, channel and the Governing, or Du, channel. They are both easy to spot on any Oriental medicine chart. The Ren channel goes up the

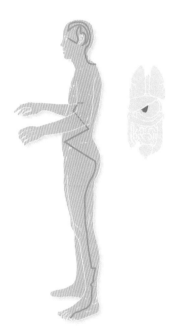

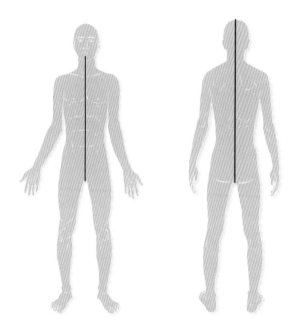

(left) The Gall Bladder Channel

The main functions of the Gall Bladder are to:

- store and excrete bile to help digestion;
- ensure your tendons are nourished;
- help you make decisions.

Common symptoms of an imbalanced Gall Bladder include: sciatica; chest pain; neck and shoulder pain; headaches (especially one-sided); an inability to digest fats; dizziness; sighing; and a lack of courage.

centre line of the body, over the neck, and into the mouth. The Du channel goes up the centre line of the back, over the head, down the nose, and finishes above the top lip.

They are both hugely important in treating imbalances and ill health, in general, but the Du channel is heavily implicated in back-related problems, and the Ren channel is invariably involved in abdominal, gynecological, and chest problems.

(middle) The Ren Channel

(right) The Du Channel

Chapter 5
氣 **The Emotions We Feel**

One of the most important aspects of the five elements when it comes to our health is our emotions – what we feel can actually make us ill.

Each element and associated organ can be strongly affected by a particular emotion. This is normally short term in healthy people, but if the emotion remains unexpressed for any length of time, it can result in a whole range of health conditions.

It is common for people to complain of a condition that began soon after a strong emotional issue. A skin condition soon after the death of a loved one. Intestinal problems after a much-loved only daughter left home for university. A stiff neck and shoulder after a particularly stressful, frustrating week at work. The connection between these events and the resultant health problems is not always acknowledged or, if it is, can often be dismissed as coincidence since it cannot easily be explained in conventional terms.

For many people, it seems easier to treat the eczema with steroid cream than it is to see it as a representation of grief. That the grief has destroyed the balance in the Metal element and its two organs, the Lungs and the Large Intestine. That the imbalance in the Lungs has spilled out into the skin because, in Oriental medicine, the Lungs have the function of controlling the skin. That one of the key parts of eczema treatment would be to strengthen Metal, so that the grief can then be worked through and the skin can improve.

Likewise, a few pills may take away a mother's anxiety and worry for a while, but the root of her anxiety problem is a weak Earth element, and strengthening her Stomach and Spleen through diet and treatment

is far preferable to the damage that might be caused to the stomach lining by medication.

A stiff neck and shoulder can also be medicated or injected for temporary relief. However, unless there is an acknowledgement that frustration at work is causing qi in the neck and shoulder channels to slow down and become blocked, due to an imbalanced Liver, and then the appropriate Oriental medical treatment is given, the problem may never really go away.

For many people emotions come and go, and there are no long-standing emotional issues; for others, though, especially when one of the elements is weaker than the rest in a person, the emotion is harder to let go of.

The longer an emotion remains unresolved in the body, the greater the potential for internal disruption and ill health. The problem is that by this time any connection between the health condition and the emotion that caused it can all too easily be forgotten.

What follows is a short summary of key emotions and how they can affect the body:

Anger: frustration, irritability, and resentment

These emotions affect the Wood element and cause the qi in the Liver to both rise up and then stagnate.

When we get angry we often "erupt," "burst," "blow a fuse," "go through the roof," or "see red." These common words and phrases describe the dramatic rising of qi that can quite literally bring heat up to the face and head.

Angry emotions can suddenly stop the smooth flow of qi from circulating throughout the body but, all things being well, normal functioning is resumed soon afterwards. It is rather like taking the Underground in London or the Subway in New York: sometimes the train has to temporarily stop between stations. Of course, this only ever seems to happen when your very life depends on rushing across the city to make an appointment on time. The windows show only the dirty, black walls of the tunnel, and your eyes dart from window to door to window to insurance advert to window to the nearest passenger in a desperate attempt to will the train along.

A short while later, just after you have given up on telepathically moving the train, it creaks off again. The journey continues with a slight but all-important delay.

When you finally step onto the platform, en route to your destination, the frustration dies down and emotions return to normal. That is until you squeeze on to the escalators and try to elbow your way through chattering tourists who do not know their left from their right. Doing this once in a while is going to cause stress and frustration but only on a temporary basis. Doing this day in, day out, every week, means that the potential is there for problems.

What sometimes happens is that the emotion of anger or frustration does not totally disappear. It can linger, especially if it is repressed and part of long-running emotional issues, and can easily "fester" inside. This is because if qi stagnates in the body, it literally gets stuck. More qi will build up behind it, and the pressure will eventually cause physical pain or discomfort or emotional stagnation.

Common related conditions include: mood swings, depression, timidity, over-controlling, inflexibility, and also very physical symptoms, such as intestinal conditions like irritable bowel syndrome (IBS), internal growths, and uterine fibroids.

Worry: anxiety, over-thinking, and fretfulness

When we are particularly worried or anxious, a tightening feeling can be felt in the stomach, which is often described as being "tied in knots."

In Oriental medicine, worry-type emotions are said to tangle up or bind Spleen qi. The Spleen is paired with the Stomach within the Earth element, so the physiological feelings in the stomach when we are worried reflect the sudden changes in qi in the Stomach or Spleen.

These organs are responsible for digestion and extracting qi and nutrients from the food we eat. Weakness in the Stomach and Spleen can make someone more susceptible to worrying, then a vicious circle can develop whereby continued worrying weakens the Stomach and Spleen.

Common related conditions include: ulcers, nausea, digestive problems, constipation, diarrhoea, frontal headaches, and a tendency towards repetitive thinking, a lack of clarity, and obsessiveness.

Grief: sadness, loss, regret, and separation

The sudden experience of grief and loss can cause temporary breathlessness and a struggle to "catch your breath." This is often felt because the emotion of grief goes straight to the Lungs, where it disperses and stagnates qi. Grief does not have to be due to events like the death of a loved one but can be felt in less obvious situations, such as when something changes in your life. It can also come from looking back on how things used to be.

If the emotion is expressed and worked through, grief can be strengthening for the Lungs and your general health, but when it is repressed it can lead to health problems.

The paired organ of the Lungs within the Metal element is the Large Intestine, hence there are often intestinal symptoms connected with this emotion.

Common related conditions include: lung congestion, asthma, recurrent lung infections or colds, skin conditions, and intestinal problems such as IBS and colitis. There may also be a tendency to be detached, critical, arrogant, and stubborn.

Shock: fright and distress

Shock can seem to almost freeze time. When shocked we cannot speak, cannot think, and cannot move. It is only when the emotion sinks in that time appears to start up again and the body responds.

This physiological response is because shock quite literally scatters qi. Stamp your feet near a flock of feeding pigeons and they fly off in all directions to temporary safety. When they think you are no longer a threat, they will fly back and continue their pecking at the scattered breadcrumbs on the ground. The same thing happens to qi after a shock. It shoots off in all directions, and normal functioning is resumed only when it returns to its natural ordered state some time later.

Sometimes this ordered state is not the same as it was before, and an imbalance can develop. This could result in a general feeling that things have never been the same since. Shock can take many forms, from a difficult birth or an accident to a marriage breakup, and the Heart is the main organ affected. Qi and blood are drained from the Heart to compensate for the sudden loss of qi and blood around the body. This can lead to a weakening of yin in the Heart and a weakness in the circulation of blood and qi around the body.

Common related conditions include: chronic pain, sleep disturbances, chronic fatigue, and fibromyalgia.

Fear: panic, anxiety, and apprehension

Fear is part of the Water element. It is also part of an essential natural response to dangerous situations. We perceive a danger, recognize it, and respond to it, usu-ally by reducing the threat in some way. When we feel fear, Kidney qi is sent rapidly downwards. For this reason, it can sometimes feel as if our insides have sunk and there is an urgent need to visit the toilet.

Weakness in Kidney qi can often feed or be the cause of some fears and anxieties. Any strong imbalance can lead to a state of general fear and anxiety, where the actual threat is undefined.

Common related conditions include: on a mental level, symptoms such as panic attacks, paranoia, suspicion, phobias, and a sense of anxiety about life; on a physical level, symptoms like backache and urinary problems.

Joy: mania, overexcitement, and vulnerability

Joy is placed firmly in the Fire element and is very much about love, laughter, and enjoyment. When we feel these, the organ most affected is the Heart.

The qi of the Heart slackens with these emotions, and we can then experience the normal range of happy feelings, often to the benefit of Heart qi and the release of stagnation in the body. This can affect not only our own happiness but those around us. According to a heart study in the USA,[1] feelings of joy increase the likelihood of partners, siblings, and neighbours being happy by up to a third. The study also found that the relationship between people's happiness can extend much farther – up to three degrees of separation in fact (to the friend of one's friends' friend) and that people who are surrounded by many happy people are themselves likely to become happy.

When, however, an imbalance in the Heart develops, people can find it very difficult to deal with feelings of joy and happiness. Sometimes their reactions are inappropriate – too much at the wrong time or in the wrong place, or even a total absence of happiness. An insatiable desire for joy, pursued relentlessly through work or play, can put much stress on the Heart and sometimes be the cause of this imbalance.

The Heart and the mind are part of the same continuum in Oriental medicine, hence an excess in the Heart can rise up and disturb the mind. For this reason, many of the symptoms connected to imbalances in the Heart and the effects of joy come under familiar psychological names.

Common related conditions include: palpitations, insomnia, manic behaviour, heart problems, and a tendency to be defensive, overly sensitive, and paranoid and uncommunicative.

Chapter 6
氣 **The Natural World Around Us**

"Don't go to bed with wet hair or you'll catch a cold."

"Tuck your shirt in at the back."

"Pull your shoulders back."

Wisdom does not get passed down generation to generation without good reason. The sayings my grandmother would quote, and my over-confident teenage mind used to scoff at in my youth, contain truths that make a great deal of sense in terms of Oriental medicine.

External factors have an influence on what happens internally much more directly than many people think.

Damp

Wearing wet clothes, living in a damp house, sitting on damp grass, wading through water, going to bed with wet hair – all of these activities can introduce damp into the body. Once inside, it is extremely difficult to remove. It is slow, sticky, and heavy and is notorious for its lingering, hard-to-budge quality.

The usual way dampness enters the body is via the legs, and it makes it up to the pelvic area. In women, this could mean in the genital system and the beginning of unpleasant discharges, or it could be the intestine causing bowel problems or urinary "infections" in the bladder.

Damp can get almost anywhere and there are generally tell-tale symptoms to indicate that it has. A feeling of heaviness in your arms, legs, or head is a classic symptom, and it can feel as if someone has wrapped you in a giant piece of cotton wool.

The reason for this is that the dampness is weighing down yang and preventing it from rising up to the head to clear the brain. The cotton wool feeling is the damp getting between you and your brain and often leads to a lack of concentration and clarity in thought.

Wind

On windy days, many people have a strange inability to concentrate. Teachers often complain about the behaviour of their students when the wind blows hard, as they are often overexcitable and unable to sit still. There is a simple reason for this and one that is not widely known.

The reason is that wind penetrates the body through the skin. In the narrow space between skin and muscle, something called "defensive qi" circulates through the body and acts as the first line of defence against the natural environment. Imagine a human version of the deflector shields of the Starship Enterprise (as in Star Trek) and you would be close – except the body's shields do not always run on full power and, when they weaken, wind rushes in and lodges just beneath the skin.

People are most vulnerable where the skin is normally exposed, and the typical area for wind to enter is through the neck. Indeed, many of the most important points located around the neck area have "wind" in their names, such as Wind Screen, Wind Treasury, and Wind Pond.

To know what wind does when it enters the body, we only need look to the natural world and see how wind normally behaves on a day-to-day basis. A still day rarely stays that way for very long: wind often appears out of nowhere and blows in the clouds. Changes are fast – a gentle breeze can turn into a gust in seconds and then back to being perfectly still. By its very nature, it is inconsistent and intermittent.

In the body we can therefore expect wind to bring on symptoms fast and for them to change just as quickly and to move these symptoms around from place to place. It is not uncommon to have a roaming ache, which may begin as a sore shoulder and end up with backache. Wind also affects the top part of the body, causing stiffness, and it also affects the skin and tends to cause itching.

The first sign of wind could be a chilly feeling and a strong desire to avoid actually going outside in the wind. The Lungs are in control of defensive qi, so if there is wind interfering with its flow, the normal pushing-down function that the Lungs perform gets blocked.

This inability to keep qi going in a downwards direction causes sneezing or coughing. Not only that but the Lungs cannot send fluids down either and so the nose starts running.

The sore neck so often accompanying exposure to wind is connected to the depth the wind reaches in the body. As it enters the body through the skin, it reaches the channels closest to the surface of the skin. These are the Small Intestine channel and the Bladder channel (together known as the Greater Yang channels, the most superficial of all channels). As the wind begins to wreak havoc with the smooth flow of qi along these channels, pain and stiffness appear.

Cold

Cold normally enters the body with wind via the nose or mouth. Usually this results in a runny nose, sneezing, an itchy throat, and a stiff neck, which are clear signs of wind in the Lungs. When cold is also present, there is a tendency to shiver and to be unable to sweat. Sweat does not come because the skin pores have contracted owing to the cold.

Cold also enters through outside exposure to it. This could be walking barefoot, sitting on a cold step, or not wearing appropriate clothing. The exposed area allows the cold to penetrate the body's normal defenses. The most common places cold can lodge itself are in the hands and feet, arms, knees, lower back, and shoulders. Of these, it can often be found in the joints.

When cold is present, it contracts body tissues and causes pain. This commonly consists of stiff, aching joints that get worse in cold weather.

Heat and fire

Fire is different from the other environmental factors as, rather than invading the body, it is generated from within, usually from long-standing wind, cold, or damp.

Take wind, for example. It affects the Liver more than any other organ. It is yang in nature, so when it gets in the body it damages yin and blood in the Liver. The greater the damage, the more severe the condition. Weak yin may send yang spiraling upwards out of control to cause headaches and dizziness, but if too much heat has been created in the process, much more intense heat can go blazing up.

Heat of this intensity is going to show with a fever, intense thirst, and a bitter taste. In severe conditions, the fire will also disturb the mind, and the afflicted person will appear quite mad. They could be shouting and screaming in the street, laughing uncontrollably, or becoming violent.

Dryness

As an external factor, dryness is not as common as the others. Living or working in a centrally heated building, you may notice how dry it feels from your skin or lips. Should you be anywhere near a desert, much more so. But dryness of the skin, mouth, bowel movements, and lack of urine are usually the result of dryness that comes from the inside, not the outside.

The Stomach is the key organ here. The Stomach

is the origin of all fluids in the body. A sure way to dry up this fluid is to have bad eating habits such as eating in a hurry, eating late at night, or rushing back to work immediately after a meal. If we do this frequently enough, the stomach fluids evaporate, leading to weak yin, dryness, and a whole host of associated problems.

Chapter 7
氣 **The Food and Drink We Consume**

Most people are familiar with the idea that foods can be broken down into separate categories according to what they contain. For example, food can contain various combinations of protein, carbohydrates, fats, minerals, and vitamins.

If in doubt, the food can be tested scientifically with simple chemical solutions to see in which category it lies. This is how we know, for example, that potatoes are carbohydrates, meat is protein, and folic acid is a vitamin. They have been broken down, analyzed, and clearly categorized.

If we eat any of those foods, the body then contains more of that category than it had previously. So, for example, after lunching on a steak, the body very probably has more proteins and fats than it did beforehand.

This way of looking at the body and food is to see both in terms of their chemical constituencies. The body needs protein, carbohydrates, and fats to create its calorific energy. So in order to maintain our stores of energy, the appropriate requirement of calories should be consumed every day. Again, this can be measured and quantified down to the last ounce.

There is, however, something missing from this mechanical picture of the body and nutrition – the relationship between the two is much more than the nuts and bolts of nutritional theory. There is no simple chemical test to see how the body actually reacts to the food that it consumes. During the digestive process, when food is transformed into energy, different foods will cause different reactions in the body's energetic structure.

In a laboratory, a carbohydrate is a carbohydrate, but when that carbohydrate arrives in the warmth of the stomach, along with a cocktail of other foods, it will do something to the body around it that could be completely unrelated to the fact that it is a carbohydrate. It could heat or cool things down, speed them up or slow them down, or even strengthen or weaken an organ.

It is here, after the food has reached the stomach not before, that the ancient Oriental masters began their classification of food.

They developed a theory that all food can be categorized according to its temperature and taste. This is defined according to the effect the food has on the body *after* digesting it and not in the actual taste or temperature the food is eaten at.

Being aware of this categorization can be of great benefit in understanding how food fits in with the overall picture of maintaining health and balance in the body.

For example, for someone who is suffering from heat rising to the head, as is often the case with migraines, menopausal hot flushes, or trigeminal neuralgia, eating food classified as hot or warm, such as coffee or rich meat, can easily exacerbate the problem.

At the other end of the spectrum, someone who feels exhausted, chilly, and has a sore lower back should avoid eating too many cold-natured foods, such as salad and uncooked fruit.

With just a little of this knowledge, you can make changes to eating habits to keep yourself healthy, and even find yourself able to transform long-standing medical conditions.

The following is a list of foods and their temperatures. It is not exhaustive nor is it exclusive. Sometimes food can be more than one category at the same time: for some foods, I have simplified this by keeping it in just one. Inevitably there will be some individual differences with this list and others that may be found on Chinese food classification and should be seen as a set of guidelines rather than rules.

Foods that cool down the body
Cold-natured foods

Cold foods cool the body down by directing energy inwards and downwards. They will also slow digestion and the flow of qi and blood around the body. Too many cold foods can weaken the digestion and cause weight gain. For anyone with weak yang or a cold condition, too many of these foods can worsen the condition.

FRUIT: bananas, cranberries, grapefruit, persimmons, limes, melons, mangos, tomatoes, and watermelons.

VEGETABLES: bean sprouts, celery, cucumbers, lettuce, and seaweed.

HERBS AND SPICES: salt.

LEGUMES, SEEDS, AND NUTS: tofu, mung beans, and bamboo shoots.

MEAT, FISH, AND SEAFOOD: crab, clams, and octopus.

DRINKS: milkshakes and yogurt drinks.

OTHER: Ice cream or ice lollies (popsicles), cottage cheese, spreads, and yogurt.

Cool-natured foods

Cool foods also have a cooling effect on the body but less so than cold foods, and they can also help to strengthen the blood. Consuming too many cool foods may weaken digestion and the level of yang in the body. Any long-standing cold condition may also worsen.

FRUIT: apples, avocados, blackcurrants, lemons, pears, prunes, mandarins, oranges, strawberries, tangerines, kiwi, and mulberries.

VEGETABLES: artichokes, aubergines (eggplants), broccoli, cauliflower, chicory, button mushrooms, radishes, rhubarb, spinach, and watercress.

HERBS AND SPICES: marjoram, peppermint, and also nettle.

LEGUMES, SEEDS, AND NUTS: almonds and soya beans.

MEAT, FISH, AND SEAFOOD: oysters, pork, rabbit, frog, and snails.

DRINKS: beer, milk, soya milk, black tea, green tea, chamomile tea, oolong tea, and mint tea.

GRAINS: barley, green lentils, millet, buckwheat, wheat, and wheat bran.

OTHER: cheese (the harder the cheese, the less cooling it is), sesame oil, sunflower oil, soy sauce, tofu, and miso soup.

Foods that warm the body
Warm-natured foods

Warm foods create warmth in the body by moving qi upwards and outwards from the centre. They also strengthen yang and qi. For anyone with a hot or weak yin condition, consuming too many of these foods will exacerbate the heat.

FRUIT: cherries, coconuts, dates, pomegranates, peaches, raspberries, blackberries, tomatoes (cooked), hawthorn fruit, and nectarines.

VEGETABLES: asparagus, onions, garlic, kale, leeks, parsnips, green peppers, squash, and fennel.

HERBS AND SPICES: basil, cardamom, caraway, chamomile, chives, coriander, fresh ginger, parsley, sage, turmeric, cumin, cloves, nutmeg, oregano, thyme, and rosemary.

LEGUMES, SEEDS, AND NUTS: almonds, black-eyed peas, chestnuts, sunflower seeds, sesame seeds, walnuts, and pine nuts.

MEAT, FISH, AND SEAFOOD: chicken, turkey, mutton, ham, venison, lobster, mussels, anchovies, prawns, shrimps, eel, and most freshwater fish.

DRINKS: coffee, wine, and goat's milk.

GRAINS: oats, quinoa, and glutinous rice.

OTHER: chocolate, cocoa, egg yolk, miso, brown sugar, vinegar, soy oil, and butter.

Hot-natured foods

Hot foods speed up yang in the body and encourage a rising and outwards movement of qi. Anyone with a hot condition or with weak yin should be very cautious with these foods, as they are likely to increase the heat and worsen the condition.

HERBS AND SPICES: black and white pepper, chillies, cayenne pepper, cinnamon, dried ginger, Tabasco, mustard, and horseradish.
MEAT, FISH, AND SEAFOOD: lamb, smoked fish, and trout.
DRINKS: whisky and strong alcohol.
OTHER: peanut butter.

Foods without heating or cooling qualities

Neutral foods are those that have no particular leaning towards heat or cold. They tend to strengthen qi and keep it moving steadily around the body.

FRUIT: apricots, cherries, figs, grapes, pineapples, and plums.
VEGETABLES: green beans, beetroot, cabbage, carrots, celery, corn, olives, peas, potatoes, pumpkins, turnips, Brussels sprouts, and sweet potatoes.
HERBS AND SPICES: rosehip and coriander.
LEGUMES, SEEDS, AND NUTS: aduki beans, chickpeas (garbanzo), lentils, and kidney beans.
MEAT, FISH, AND SEAFOOD: whitefish, beef, duck, pigeon, salmon, mackerel, sardines, and abalone.
DRINKS: water.
GRAINS: buckwheat, bread, rice, and rye.
OTHER: honey, olive oil, peanut oil, raisins, white sugar, and eggs.

Temperatures and cooking styles

The temperature of food can also be heavily influenced by how it is cooked. Fruit can be very cooling when eaten raw, but by cooking lightly before eating it loses this cooling quality. Bananas, for example, become less cooling when baked or when eaten with cinnamon or brandy added. The same is true for other cooling foods like tea, which changes with the addition of cardamom or ginger. Note, however, that cold foods cannot actually be made into hot foods with cooking – only less cool or less cold.

The following are the effects on the heating or cooling qualities of foods subject to different cooking styles.

COOL: Juiced or raw food tends to be cooling.
NEUTRAL: Steaming or boiling are neutral and normally have no effect either way.
WARM: Stir-frying, stews, and baking create warmth.
HOT: Barbecues, grilling, roasting and deep-frying can be very heating.

The logic of this information is simple yet unfortunately seems not to be widely known. For someone suffering from migraines, for example, with a red face and a hot head, it would not be a great idea to have a barbecue. Equally, someone who is weak and pale should probably not eat raw salads every day.

The flavours of food

In addition to heat and cold, all foods can be classified according to their taste. As each taste corresponds to an element, and each element corresponds to organs, food can be directly related to imbalances within the body. Choosing the right combination of foods can, therefore, help remove an imbalance, and choosing the wrong combination can worsen it.

Here follows a list of the tastes and their corresponding foods:

Bitter

The bitter taste is considered part of the Fire element. This means that it can directly affect the condition of the Heart and Small Intestine. It is drying and cooling and has the effect of pushing qi downwards in the body. It helps digestion, helps to cool fevers, can help to open your bowels, and can help clear away congestion when taken in small amounts. When large amounts are eaten habitually, however, too much moisture is dried and yin can then be damaged. It can also overload the digestive system, causing a swollen sensation in the abdomen.

The following foods are considered bitter:

FRUIT: grapefruit rind.

VEGETABLES: asparagus, broccoli, celery, lettuce, turnips, radishes, watercress, and bamboo shoots.

GRAINS: hops, oats, and rye.

HERBS AND SPICES: chicory, chamomile, basil, and parsley.

LEGUMES, SEEDS, AND NUTS: alfalfa sprouts.

DRINKS: beer, black tea, and coffee.

OTHER: vinegar.

Sweet

The sweet taste is part of the Earth element and can directly affect the Stomach and Spleen. It is the most common taste in a standard diet and can be found in almost all naturally grown food no matter what other tastes they may have. It is usually warming and helps digestion when taken in small amounts. It also builds up tissues and fluids (yin) and strengthens qi and blood.

Too much sweet food (usually in the form of processed sugary food like chocolate, cookies, and cakes) can have the opposite effect and weaken the Stomach and Spleen. When weak, the Stomach and Spleen begin to crave sweetness, as this is the taste that will strengthen them. This craving is usually fed by more concentrated sugar-based sweet foods leading to a cyclical destructive cycle. The more concentrated sweet foods consumed, the weaker the Stomach and Spleen become, and the weaker they become, the more sweetness they crave.

The following foods are considered sweet:

FRUIT: apples, apricots, dates, figs, grapes, grapefruit, mandarin oranges, papayas, oranges, peaches, pears, pineapples, plums, raspberries, strawberries, and tomatoes.

VEGETABLES: almost all vegetables, but especially beetroot, cabbage, carrots, celery, cherries, courgettes (zucchini), corn, cucumbers, lettuce, button mushrooms, peas, potatoes, pumpkins, radishes, spinach, and sweet potatoes.

GRAINS: almost all, but especially barley, wheat, oats, malt, and rice.

LEGUMES, SEEDS, AND NUTS: aduki beans, almonds, chestnuts, chickpeas (garbanzos), kidney beans, mung beans, peanuts, walnuts, sunflower seeds, and pine nuts.

MEAT: most meats, but especially beef, chicken, lamb, pork and rabbit.

DRINKS: milk and wine.

OTHER: olive oil, cheese, butter, honey, and sugar.

Pungent

The pungent taste is in the Metal element and affects the Lungs and Large Intestine directly. It has a warming effect, helps to move qi and blood around the body, and helps to expel phlegm, especially from the Lungs. If taken in large quantities, pungent foods will dry the Lungs and Stomach and create weakness in qi and yin. This can lead to flabby muscles and lack of drive or spirit.

The following foods are considered pungent:

VEGETABLES: cabbage, chillies, garlic, leeks, turnips, onions, radishes and watercress.

HERBS AND SPICES: black pepper, cayenne pepper, basil, cloves, cinnamon, cumin, peppermint, rosemary, marjoram, nutmeg, and chamomile.

OTHER: mustard and horseradish.

NOTE: The degree of pungency can be reduced through cooking.

Salty

The salty taste is in the Water element and affects the Kidneys and Bladder directly. It cools and moistens the body and can often have a detoxifying effect. It also acts as a diuretic, has a downwards effect on qi, and can soften any hard masses. Too much salty food can worsen dampness, damage yin, and weaken the bones and blood.

The following foods are considered salty.

VEGETABLES: garlic, kelp, and seaweed.

HERBS AND SPICES: salt and parsley.

GRAINS: barley and millet.

MEAT, FISH, AND SEAFOOD: crab, duck, ham, lobster, mussels, octopus, oysters, pork, pigeon, and sardines.

OTHER: miso, soy sauce, and pickles.

Sour

The sour taste is in the Wood element and affects the Liver and Gall Bladder directly. It has a contracting, shrinking effect and controls the release of fluids by closing the pores to stop sweating and constricting the urinary system to stop urination. For this reason, sour foods are often recommended in cases when body fluids are leaking, as in diarrhoea and bleeding. Too much sour food can cause the body to contract too much and keep in too much fluid. This can slow down the digestive system, damage yin, and weaken the tendons.

The following foods are considered sour:

FRUIT: apples, apricots, blackberries, blackcurrants, gooseberries, grapes, grapefruits, hawthorn berries, lemons, limes, lychees, mandarin oranges, mangoes, peaches, pears, pineapples, plums, pomegranates, raspberries, sour plums, strawberries, tangerines, and tomatoes.

VEGETABLES: leafy greens, olives, and sauerkraut.

LEGUMES, SEEDS, AND NUTS: aduki beans.

MEAT, FISH, AND SEAFOOD: trout.

DRINKS: green tea and wine.

OTHER: vinegar, pickles, yogurt, and cream cheese.

Adjusting diet

When it comes to the body, knowledge is power, but at the same time too much knowledge can sometimes be confusing. It is important, therefore, not to get too distracted with the classifications of temperature and taste.

They are guidelines to empower changes in diet that will improve health and are not designed as restrictive recipe lists.

If after reading through this book, it is clear there is an imbalance somewhere inside with heat and cold, the lists can be used to identify any foods in your diet that may be adding to the problem. You can then reduce or remove some of these foods, and by trial and error adjust your diet appropriately.

Likewise, if there is an obvious organ imbalance, food of a particular taste can be added or taken away to adjust the diet. It is never too late to change, according to some experts. Even those over 65 years old who change to a diet high in fruit and vegetables (and accompanied by regular exercise) can decrease their chances of developing chronic conditions like hypertension, cancer, and osteoporosis. [2]

An important principle to remember is that too much of anything, no matter how good it is supposed to be for you, can be bad for you. Be skeptical of claims made in commercials for "probiotic" yogurts that improve digestion or morning cereals that protect your heart. There may be some truth in their claims, if seen in the context of a healthy lifestyle with regular exercise and a carefully adjusted diet, but alone, and seen in terms of the relationship between a weak Stomach and damp, they can do more harm than good.

Chapter 8
氣 **How We Eat**

It is not only what we eat that has a great impact on health but also how we eat. Food that has been gulped down, or eaten mindlessly when under stress at work or in front of the television while engrossed in watching a programme, is often not processed properly by the body.

Our eating habits directly affect the digestion process and the ability of the body to extract the qi it needs from the food. If those eating habits are good, the whole process is optimized and runs like a well-oiled machine. If they are bad, no matter how healthy your diet is, food you consume will get caught up in a slow, sluggish process that will either add to or cause a series of blockages and imbalances and ultimately ill health.

The following are general guidelines for maintaining good eating habits.

Enjoy your food

Eating should be a pleasurable experience, not only in how it tastes but how it affects the senses. In the Far East, professional and home chefs take great pains to ensure that food is presented in an appealing way, based on the knowledge that digestion begins with the eye, the nose, the ear, and the texture of the food.

Staying present while you eat is a very important concept – one that is connected to this idea of appreciating your food. At the risk of stating the obvious, in order to really enjoy your food, you have to be aware of the fact that you are eating.

It is easy to be distracted by a whole variety of things during meal times, from a television programme to screaming children, but, unless you realize

and acknowledge what you are actually doing, eating can become just another routine, similar to other daily tasks such as driving a car. Few people have to think much when behind a wheel; the body generally does it all automatically. Sometimes you can drive for many miles thinking or daydreaming before suddenly realizing where you are and what you are doing.

Focusing on the eating experience, the tastes, the colours, the sounds, the smells, the textures, and the people, if only for a short time, can remove the automatic behaviour from the dinner table and can subsequently help strengthen the digestive organs.

This idea of enjoyment of food is also relevant when it comes to restrictive diets that force people to eat certain types of food that they may or may not like, all in the hope of losing weight. In situations like this, it is sometimes important to also eat "enjoyable" food and, when eating, to really appreciate it. This can often provide nourishment for the "spirit" as well as the body.

Chew well

Chewing breaks down the food, so that the Stomach has to use less energy in the digestive process. It can also serve to relax the body and ease stress at meal times. The actual chewing action is essential for some types of food to break down. Whole grains, for example, do not reach their optimal nutritional state unless broken down with saliva in the mouth first.

I am fortunate to have a father-in-law who is the epitome of good chewing. He is always the last to leave the table: when everyone else just has pools of sauce where the food once was, he is invariably still crunching on his pre-meal fermented pickles!

This camel-like ability to chew just would not be practical for most of us, so unless you share the same Ishizuka ancestral genes, ideally food should be chewed for long enough to put down any eating implements during each mouthful.

Chewing well is especially important for anyone wanting to lose weight, as the more you chew the less you end up eating. According to recent research in China, those who chew food 40 times consume about 12 percent less calories than those who chew the same food but only 15 times.[3]

Observe regular eating habits

The natural cycle of the body usually requires several meals a day at regular intervals (for most people this means three main meals), and this is important to maintain strength in the digestive organs.

Regularly missing meals can cause a range of problems:

- Miss breakfast and the qi of the Spleen can become weak. Traditionally this was the main meal of the day and served to fuel the body to go out and work. If the Spleen becomes weak, digestion slows down and damp can accumulate. What this means in real terms is that if you miss breakfast – or any meal, for that matter – you are more likely to put on more weight at the times when you do choose to eat. For anyone wanting to lose weight, missing breakfast is, therefore, somewhat self-defeating.
- Miss lunch and heat can develop in the Stomach, as it prepares for food but none is delivered. The heat can damage the stomach lining, moisture levels, and yin. This can result in a burning, uncomfortable sensation in the stomach, constant hunger, thirst, and weak gums.
- Miss dinner and the yin of the Stomach weakens further, causing a lack of appetite, stomach discomfort, and a dry mouth.

- Eating between meals and snacking can cause qi to stagnate and damp to accumulate. This is another cause of weight gain, as well as pain and discomfort, wind, and bloating.
- Frequent changes of diet, such as when travelling or dieting, can also weaken the Stomach.

Regulate the speed of eating and drinking

Eating too quickly can damage the Stomach and Spleen and put a burden on the process of digestion. It can lead to stagnation of qi and the production of damp. This is confirmed by recent Japanese research that studied the habit of eating quickly at meal times. It concluded that people who eat quickly are three times more likely to become overweight than those who eat at a normal speed.[4]

Drinking too much can flood the stomach and should be avoided during meal times so as not to put a strain on the Stomach and Spleen. Meal times should be accompanied by sipping rather than gulping.

Eat without distractions

Avoid eating during an emotionally charged situation, an argument, a discussion, or in front of the television or a computer screen, while working or studying, or generally when stressed. All of these activities can weaken digestion.

If stressed, the circulation of qi can become blocked and the delicate relationship between the Liver and the Spleen and Stomach can become damaged. This can cause indigestion, stomach pain, and bloating.

Regulate the quantity of food

Overeating is such a part of everyday life that most of us do not even realize how often it happens. The extreme symptoms of overeating, including indigestion, bloating, and wind, are no longer extreme. In fact, they are now so commonplace that people put up with them on a daily basis without realizing that it is not their body at fault but their eating habits.

Eating too much at once can cause food to stagnate, as there is literally not enough room to pass it all through. This can cause pain and discomfort in the stomach, bad breath, bloating, constipation, and tiredness. Damp-heat can also develop in the Stomach, as the stagnation starts to build up heat and accumulate fluids. This can cause frontal headaches; nausea; a sense of heaviness; pain, and discomfort in the stomach; and diarrhoea.

The ideal time to stop eating is before you feel full, when the stomach is around two-thirds full.

Be cautious about dieting

Weight-loss diets that require undereating also can weaken the Stomach by generating heat and damaging yin. Following this type of diet will probably shed fat, but the effect on the Stomach and Spleen often means that, once you are off the diet, it all returns again. Diets that require eating a lot of one type of food can also create a Stomach or Spleen imbalance and often lead to the accumulation of damp.

Be cautious about how you combine foods

With a weak Stomach, it is best to avoid the combination of hot (cooked) and cold (refrigerated) foods together. The reason for this is simple: your stomach has to work harder to process them.

Also combining too many different types, tastes, and qualities of food in a short space of time can prove too much for a weak Stomach to process and lead to stagnation or damp. In this case, it is best to keep meals simple.

Fruit can be very moistening for the body, easy for the Stomach to digest, and can help to keep bowel movements regular. If eaten during meal times, however, in combination with other foods, many of these benefits get diluted. To receive the greatest benefits from fruit, it should be eaten alone outside of main meals, if possible.

An ideal diet

A Greek study published in 2009 found that many of the features of a traditional Mediterranean diet contribute substantially to a long life. These include moderate consumption of alcohol, low consumption of meat and meat products, high consumption of vegetables, fruits, nuts, and legumes, and a high ratio of monounsaturated to saturated fats.[5]

The Mediterranean diet promotes dietary habits that have much in common with those considered beneficial for strengthening the Stomach and Spleen. If the two digestive organs are strong and receiving food that will enhance the production of qi and blood, the whole body will benefit.

According to Oriental medicine, an ideal diet is one that includes all five tastes: bitter, sweet, pungent, sour, and salty (see the previous chapter). But since we are all individuals, with different bodies, imbalances, preoccupations, and lives, the exact combination of tastes and temperatures is going to vary from person to person. What may be healthy for one person may make another person sick. People with weak qi, for instance, can easily feel bloated with dairy produce but those with weak yin can thrive from its moisturizing effect.

A balanced diet for most people may consist of the following:

AROUND 35 PERCENT: whole grains such as rice, millet, barley, wheat, oats, corn, rye, quinoa, and amaranth.

AROUND 35 PERCENT: fresh seasonal fruits and vegetables.

20 PERCENT: legumes, seeds, or nuts, including beans, lentils, sunflower seeds, almonds, and walnuts.

10 PERCENT OR LESS: animal proteins, including dairy foods, meat, fish, poultry, and eggs.

As much food as possible should be of the highest quality and organically grown, as commercial animal products may contain growth hormones, antibiotics, and steroids, none of which we want to enter our bodies with any great frequency.

This is the basis of a balanced diet and should be adjusted according to individual needs.

Fats

Conventional ideas about healthy and unhealthy foods seem to be dominated by ideas about fats and how the quality of these fats can make us ill.

The logic is that overconsumption of saturated fats and trans fats (sometimes known as "bad fats") is notorious for increasing your susceptibility to all kinds of serious conditions, such as heart disease and elevated levels of cholesterol. Saturated fats are found in many kinds of meat, dairy products, ice cream, and some oils like palm and coconut. Trans fats, or hydrogenated fats, are in most packaged and processed foods and include cookies, potato chips, donuts, cakes, fried junk foods, and most chocolate or candy bars.

People are often encouraged to reduce these fats and consume more "good fats" (monounsaturated fats and polyunsaturated fats) because they are believed to have a generally beneficial effect on the state of your heart and your cholesterol levels. Monounsaturated fats (including omega 9 fatty acids) are contained in foods such as olive oil, sunflower oil, peanut oil, sesame oil, avocados, olives, almonds, peanuts, macadamia nuts, hazelnuts, pecans, and cashews. Polyunsaturated fats (including omega 3 and 6 fatty acids) contain "essential fatty acids" and include soybean oil, corn oil, safflower oil, walnuts, sunflower, sesame, and pumpkin seeds, flaxseed, fatty fish (salmon, tuna, mackerel, herring, trout, sardines), dark green vegetables, soymilk, and tofu.

There is a strong correlation between conventional and Oriental medicine in much of this, especially the avoidance of the "bad fats," which will damage digestion and lead to an accumulation of damp and phlegm in the body. The trouble with this view of nutrition, however, is that many of these foods contain other constituents apart from fatty acids, or sometimes have a slightly different classification in traditional Oriental medicine nutrition.

Also, while it is true that many people chronically overconsume "bad fats" in their diets – fats that are a major source of damp and phlegm in the body – these fats are not bad for everyone, all the time. Thin people with very weak yin, for example, can greatly benefit from foods high in saturated fats, providing they are of good quality and in moderation.

Overconsumption of "good fats" can also be problematic. Many of these seem to have a beneficial effect on the movement of qi and the reduction of phlegm and damp, but if you eat too much, the picture becomes more complicated. Too many walnuts, for example, can aggravate phlegm in the Lungs and heat in the Heart. Tofu can weaken Spleen yang because it is too cooling. The saltiness of anchovies can weaken Kidney qi and bones. Sardines can actually increase phlegm, and peanuts and avocados are sources of damp and can damage Spleen qi. A better view of fats, therefore, would be to stand back and see them in the wider context of diet and eating habits.

Vegetarians

As animal products should ideally be no more than ten percent of a normal healthy diet, vegetarians should not be overly concerned that they lack the nutritional benefits of meat. Legumes, grains, and nuts can more than compensate for meat in the diet when eaten regularly. It is important, however, to avoid relying on concentrated high-fat protein foods like nuts and seeds and focus more on whole grains.

A common problem is that because meat generally has a warming quality, without it there can sometimes be a lack of balance. Many vegetarians eat a lot of cold, raw foods, such as salads, which can weaken digestion and cause weak yang. This can be redressed with the addition of warming foods, such as ginger, cinnamon, and other spices.

It is also common for vegetarians to develop a weakness in their blood, not because they are not eating meat but because of the combinations and the quality of the food that they do eat. To redress this imbalance, see Weak Blood for more details on diet.

Allergies

Some people suffer reactions to certain types of foods, like nuts for example. If this is the case with you, please listen to your body rather than strictly following a diet or list of foods. If you have an "allergic" reaction after eating what should be beneficial foods, then those foods are probably not beneficial for you and should find alternatives. Remember, common sense is the key.

Chapter 9
氣 **The Lifestyle We Lead**

The lifestyle we lead has a direct bearing on how long we live. A recent American study, for example, reported that more than half the deaths in women from chronic conditions like cancer and heart disease could have been avoided if they had exercised, refrained from smoking, and eaten a diet consisting of large quantities of vegetables, fruits and nuts, legumes, fish and seafood, and cereals, and a low intake of meat and meat products and bad fats.[6]

The balance of how we lead our lives can all too often become either too yang or too yin and, therefore, a potential cause of ill health. Signs that our lives are either too yang or too yin include:

TOO YANG: Working long hours, stressed, eating late in the evening, sleeping in the early hours, rushing from place to place, and doing too much.

TOO YIN: Seated at a desk for most of the day, watching television, playing computer games, surfing the Internet, driving instead of walking, and snacking.

A useful indicator about lifestyle is the meridian clock. This was developed in ancient times within the theories of yin and yang and the five elements. It assigned a time of day to each of the 12 organs, based on when qi was thought to flow most strongly. The following are the meridian times for each of our organs:

Lungs: 3.00–5.00

The Lungs control our breathing, our skin, and its ability to sweat, and the state of our defensive qi, which protects us from catching illnesses. During this time, it needs to recharge itself to protect the body for the day that is coming. For monks, the early-morning hours are a time of reflection and prayer, and they traditionally meditate at this time as the Lungs are thought to be the organs most connected with heaven.

As the Lungs control breathing and qi, some lung conditions and coughs can worsen at this time. Also, an imbalance in the Lungs could feature if regularly waking early, although this is more likely to be connected to feelings of grief or detachment, the emotions that can affect the Lungs the most.

The 24-hour Meridian Clock

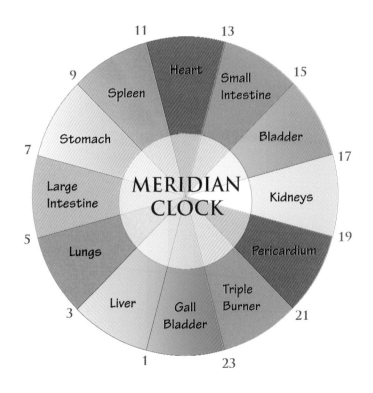

Large Intestine: 5.00–7.00

The Large Intestine is not in charge of transforming digestive wastes from fluid to solid and transporting them out of the body. As qi is concentrated here at this time, logic dictates that it is the best time to open your bowels. Like the Lungs, the Large Intestine can also be affected by grief, detachment, and also a general feeling of being stuck in life. This can often manifest in a very physical form as constipation or as a more general malaise at this time of day.

Stomach: 7.00–9.00

The Stomach is at its most efficient at this time, so it is the optimal time to eat and digest food. This is one of the reasons why breakfast is such an important meal. If there is an imbalance here there may be a lack of appetite or difficulty in waking or getting out of bed.

Spleen: 9.00–11.00

Breakfast is processed by the Spleen at this time, and it sends freshly extracted qi into circulation around the body. This allows much better concentration and clarity of thought, so this period is by far the best time to study.

Heart: 11.00–13.00

The Heart is like an engine room that powers the mechanics of the rest of the body. For this reason, lunch time is not a good time for strenuous exercise that may push that engine too far. This is especially so for those with any history of heart problems, as circulation and heart-related conditions often appear more pronounced at this time.

Small Intestine: 13.00–15.00

The food that enters the Small Intestine via the Stomach is broken down, separated, and absorbed during this time. This idea of separation in the Small Intestine allows us to think clearly, make judgements, and gives us powers of discernment. The ability to see with clarity before an important decision is heightened in this time period.

Bladder: 15.00–17.00

The Bladder has a stabilizing effect on the nervous supply to all tissues and organs of the body during this time. This means that it is usually the least productive time of day and so it is a good time to rest.

Kidneys: 17.00–19.00

The Kidneys store the energy reserves that we draw on during the day. During the early evening hours, the Kidneys replenish what has been used, and it is a good time to continue to relax and allow them to do so.

NOTE: the two Water organs above are squeezed between the four Fire organs, the Heart and Small Intestine before, and the Pericardium and Triple Burner after them. For this reason, they act as water does in nature and dampen the fire around them by soothing and calming the body.

Pericardium: 19.00–21.00

The body becomes more active again at this time, and the Pericardium is associated with greater mental functioning and increased brain activity. This is, therefore, a good time to try to come up with ideas and solutions.

Triple Burner: 21.00–23.00

The Triple Burner distributes heat among three areas of the body: the chest, the abdomen, and the pelvic area. Fevers and body temperature have a tendency to stabilize at this time, as the heat is redistributed. If you are slightly under the weather or recovering from an illness, this is a very beneficial time to go to bed.

Gall Bladder: 23.00–1.00

The Gall Bladder secretes bile at this time to help digest fats and oils, and along with the Liver ensures that qi flows smoothly around the body. If there is an imbalance here, sometimes it is difficult to switch off and fall asleep. This time has the additional quality of helping us sort through problems and reach decisions. This is why sometimes we wake up in the morning with the solution to something that the night before seemed quite intractable.

Liver: 1.00–3.00

During this time, the Liver is very busy filtering and replenishing blood, and the body needs to rest while the Liver detoxifies the excesses of the previous day. Sleep-related problems during this time period suggest a Liver imbalance. As the Liver is easily affected by strong emotions like anger, frustration, and resentment – and stress, in general - this imbalance is quite often due to emotional factors.

Specific lifestyle habits

The following are areas of lifestyle that can often affect health:

Sleep

Yin and yang are a reflection of the natural order of things, so it should come as no surprise that sleep should come during yin time (night) and our waking hours during yang time (day). Consistently breaking this rule by staying up late or working the nightshift can create an imbalance in yin and yang.

Sleeping is rejuvenating for the body, but too much can damage Lung qi. Like all things, sleep should be in moderation and regular extended periods of sleep should be avoided.

A 2010 study has shown that the ideal sleeping time for most people is 7–8 hours. Sleeping for less than 6 hours can lead to a 12 percent increase in the chance of dying prematurely, while conversely, sleeping for more than 9 hours can lead to a 30 percent increase in the chance of dying prematurely.[7]

Work, exercise, and rest

The correct balance between work and rest is essential for the maintenance of good health. Long periods of standing are traditionally thought to harm the Kidneys and, therefore, the bones, and are often linked to lower back pain. On the other hand, long periods of sitting can weaken the Spleen and Heart. They can slacken the muscles and stagnate qi, leading to aches and pains.

Australian researchers who monitored the waist sizes, blood pressure, and cholesterol levels of several thousand people found that prolonged sitting periods actually lead to larger waist sizes and higher cholesterol levels, even in people who exercised regularly. Their recommendation was that even short breaks in sitting time, which could be as little as standing up for one minute, can help to lower this health risk.[8]

As well as the above effects of being seated for too long, extended periods of watching television or sitting in front of a computer screen can weaken yin and damage the strength of the blood. This is because prolonged use of the eyes can damage Heart and Liver qi.

Overthinking can cause damage to the Heart and Spleen. Too much concentration and thinking can lead to heart palpitations, absent-mindedness, insomnia, dream-disturbed sleep, anorexia, bloating, and loose stools.

Regular exercise is essential to keep qi smoothly circulating, but too much exercise can weaken the Liver and cause weak tendons or weaken the Kidneys and cause damage to the bones. People who overexercised as children often have joint or bone conditions causing discomfort and pain well before old age.

The seasons

Following the rhythms of the seasons can help to keep the balance of good health:

SPRING: This corresponds to the Wood element. It involves the idea of qi moving upwards and outwards, growth, and the start of something new. It is a time to be active and outside, doing gentle exercise such as yoga, tai chi, walking, hiking, and swimming. It is about reinvention and seeing people and situations in a new light. It is important not to under-dress, especially during early spring, as the winter cold can still be present.

SUMMER: This corresponds to Fire and is a time of blossoming, flourishing, and cultivating yang. It is a time for lots of activity, fun, and to live your passion whatever it may be. The days are drawn out and more active, so late nights and early starts are much more tolerable than the rest of the year.

LATE SUMMER: This corresponds to Earth and the idea of transformation. It is a time of gathering and slowing down. There is often an Indian Summer at this time of year, when the days are hotter, damper, and more humid. It is harvest time, and it is time to enjoy the fruits of your labour. Within this is the idea of nourishing yourself and others. Listening and attending to the needs of others and them to you.

AUTUMN/FALL: This corresponds to Metal and is the time of harvesting, sorting, and preparing for the winter. A time when deciduous trees and plants shed their leaves, this season symbolizes not holding on to things, of letting go of old attachments and emotional baggage, of rummaging through the possessions you have collected throughout the year and clearing out the junk. It is important not to wrap up too warmly too quickly as temperatures begin to drop in autumn/fall. Ideally, the body should gradually adapt to the change in temperature.

WINTER: This corresponds to Water and the idea of storage and containment. Like the rest of nature during the winter months, the focus is on slowing down, rest, and conserving energy. It is a time for reflection and thoughtfulness, and for being more aware of your senses, dreams, and goals in life. Shorter days also mean going to bed earlier than during the rest of the year.

Part Two

What are the Signs of Ill Health?

Signs of health and ill health are often right under your nose and obvious if you know what to look for. This section is designed to point you in the right direction.

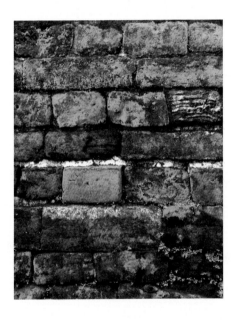

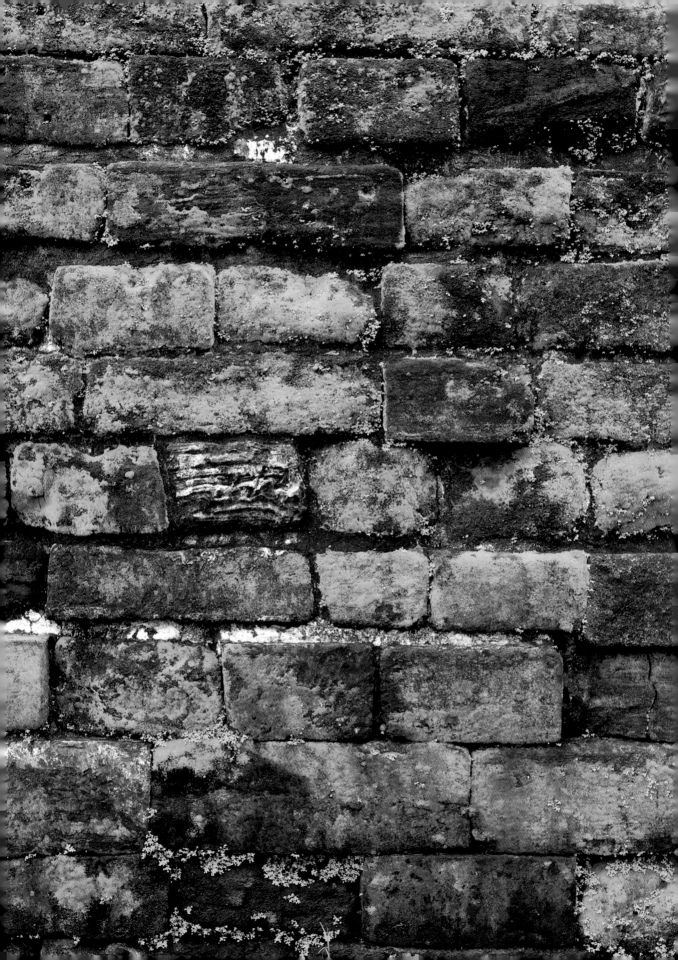

Chapter 10
氣 **Physical Characteristics to Look Out For**

You can tell a lot by "reading the body." The following are some physical characteristics to look out for that are a tipoff to certain health conditions, according to Oriental medicine.

The body, in general

Someone who is overweight normally has too much damp and phlegm in their bodies. If there are any health problems, the obvious place to start would, of course, be to reduce the sources of damp and phlegm.

People who remain very thin, despite eating well, can often have a weakness in yin that burns up the fluids that would normally increase weight.

Those who persistently under-dress in cold weather – shorts or a T-shirt instead of a fleece jacket and woolly hat – probably have a condition of heat or yin weakness. This makes their bodies feel warm despite the low temperatures.

And those who over-dress in the heat probably have the opposite condition. If cold or yang weakness is predominant in the body, you can feel chilly whatever the weather.

Habitual posture can reveal a lot about how someone feels or where problems may lie. Someone who is usually hunched over their desk at work can often have weakness in their chest organs (Heart and Lungs), perhaps owing to some unresolved emotional issue.

Hair

Hair or the lack of it can of give us clues about the state of qi or blood.

Going grey early can look rather distinguished on some people, but in fact it reveals a weakness in Kidney qi. This is because the Kidneys store the original qi we were born with and uses this with energized blood to maintain our bones, teeth, and hair.

Baldness can also mean weak Kidney qi, but it often depends on where the baldness is located. If, for example, it is on the upper forehead and upper part of the temples, a very common site for hair loss, it is considered the realm of the Stomach and Large Intestine. If there is excessive heat in either of these organs, the greater the likelihood of a receding hairline in this area. The simple logic to this is that, whereas the body grows hair in particular areas to protect from the cold, it will lose hair in areas it needs to cool down.

Dull, lifeless hair means that qi is not getting to the skin and nourishing the roots. It suggests a weakness of qi in the Kidneys and Lungs.

Dry, brittle hair and dandruff can mean blood and yin weakness. The blood at the roots is not being nourished, the low heat from weak yin burns up body fluids.

Complexion

The face is a very obvious place to look for an imbalance, and this can often be found in the colouring of the complexion. When seen in natural light, red, yellow, green, white and black hues can sometimes clearly be seen that stand out from the person's normal shade. These colours may generally signify the following:

RED: heat.
YELLOW: a weak Spleen or Stomach and the accumulation of damp.

GREEN: a Liver imbalance.

WHITE: a weakness in blood or yang.

BLUE: when found at the temples, this can mean shock.

BLACK: a Kidney imbalance or cold and pain.

Nose

The colour of the tip of the nose can sometimes be quite revealing.

GREEN OR BLUE: may accompany abdominal pain.

YELLOW: damp heat somewhere in the body.

WHITE: may mean a weakness of blood.

RED: suggests heat in the Lungs and Spleen.

Eyes

Different colours found in the whites of the eyes and around the eyes themselves may reveal several health conditions:

RED: suggests heat in the Heart.

YELLOW: suggests damp and heat.

BLUISH TINGE: may mean an imbalanced Liver.

RED, SWOLLEN EYES: normally means Liver qi is rising or wind-heat has entered the body.

DARK RINGS OR SWELLING UNDER THE EYES: suggests weak Kidney qi.

SWOLLEN EYELIDS: may mean weak Spleen or Stomach qi.

Ears

Ear characteristics are also useful in diagnosing body conditions:

SWOLLEN EARS: signifies that wind, damp, heat, or cold has entered the ear and is blocking it.

THIN EARS: Suggest weak qi and blood.

DARK, DRY, AND WORN EARS: suggest weak Kidney qi.

Mouth and Lips

Lip colour and mouth positions are useful for body reading:

PALE LIPS: may mean weak blood, as there is not enough nutritive blood to give the lips a full colour.

OVERLY RED, DRY LIPS: often means heat in the Stomach. The lips reflect the state of the Stomach and, when there is heat and, therefore, less body fluid in the Stomach, this then manifests with redness and dryness of the lips.

BLUE OR PURPLE LIPS: mean stagnation of blood. This can accompany serious conditions, such as a cardiac arrest. Appropriate measures should be taken immediately, if present.

MOUTH OPEN: Absently leaving the mouth open can often signify weak qi. This is rather like leaving the door open because nobody has the strength to get up and shut it.

Teeth and Gums

WEAK TEETH: may mean weak Kidney qi. The Kidneys control the state of teeth and bones by producing marrow from its stores of qi.

DRY, GREY TEETH: suggest weak Kidney yin. The yin has dried up body fluids both in the Kidneys, causing discoloration, and in the mouth to make them dry.

PALE GUMS: normally means weak blood. There is not enough enriched blood in the body to reach them to make them a healthy pink.

BLEEDING GUMS: suggests heat in the Stomach. The state of the Stomach directly affects the strength of the gums and, when the heat rises up, the gums can no longer contain the blood.

Hands

PALE, BRITTLE NAILS: suggests weak blood. Not enough nutritive blood can reach the nail beds to strengthen them.

BLUE TINGE TO THE NAILS: may mean stagnation of qi or blood restricting circulation.

TINY BLUISH OR RED VESSELS ON THEMAR EMINENCE: The themar eminence (the fleshy muscle on the palm below the thumb) can sometimes have tiny bluish or red blood vessels: this usually signifies cold (blue) or heat (red) in the Stomach.

Skin

DRY SKIN: often caused by weak blood.

VISIBLE SMALL BLOOD VESSELS: Small blood vessels and capillaries on the skin anywhere on the body can mean the following: red – heat; blue – cold; and purple – stagnation.

Taste

BITTER TASTE: usually caused by heat, rising from the Liver and Gall bladder.

SWEET TASTE: may be caused by damp-heat in the Spleen or Stomach.

SOUR TASTE: may signify an accumulation of heat in the Liver and Stomach.

LACK OF TASTE: usually due to the dysfunction of the digestive organs: the Stomach or Spleen.

Voice

The five elements and their associated sounds can reveal the strength or weakness of a particular element or set of organs:

- A shouting or clipped voice, as if someone is annoyed or angry, indicates an imbalance in the Wood element.
- A voice that sounds like laughter suggests the Fire element.
- A voice that goes up and down as if singing indicates Earth.
- A whimpering, weeping voice that sounds as if the person is about to burst into tears is Metal.
- A groaning or moaning tone suggests Water.
- Someone who sighs a lot can have stagnation of qi in the Liver. We often get stagnation of qi due to emotional stress, and it causes muscles to tighten. The body then tries to release pent-up emotion by expanding the chest muscles and sighing.
- A weak voice suggests a cold pattern or a weakness of yang.
- A forceful voice suggests heat from within.

Odours

STRONG ODOURS: In general, these are due to heat in the body.

LACK OF BODY ODOUR: This is a sign of cold and applies to the breath, urine, stools, vomit, sweat, and any discharges that should have an odour and do not.

BAD BREATH: often means that there is heat in the Stomach. This can often be due to poor dietary habits and overeating, which can cause stagnation of food in the Stomach.

A SWEET SMELL: linked to an imbalance in the Stomach or Spleen and can sometimes be connected to diabetes.

A URINE-LIKE SMELL: associated with a Kidney problem.

Tongue

The tongue can reveal some very useful indicators about what is happening in the body. I grew up noticing that my tongue sometimes had a coating with random circular bare patches and sometimes a coating on just one side. I knew that it had to mean something but, in the dark days before the Internet, information was so much more difficult to find.

If someone had told me that it was not just disorganized tongue fur but my body informing me to stop damaging Liver or Gall bladder qi, I would have perhaps listened and gone to bed earlier or done a bit more exercise.

The tongue has traditionally been divided into areas corresponding to the key organs in the body:

FRONT: the chest organs – the Heart and Lungs;
MIDDLE: the digestive organs – the Stomach and Spleen;
SIDES: the circulatory organs – the Liver and Gall bladder;
BACK: the lower organs – the Large and Small Intestine, Kidneys, and Bladder.

Marks, discolorations, and spots on particular areas of the tongue can give us information about the corresponding organ. For example, a line or groove in the middle of the tongue indicates that body fluids have been damaged in the Stomach and Spleen area, which usually signifies that Stomach yin is weak. This is commonly caused by a poor diet; if it continues over a long period of time it can lead to heat in the Stomach and digestive complaints. This could cause a correspondingly deeper groove in the midline of the tongue.

When examining your tongue, keep in mind the following:

- Look at the tongue in clear daylight; otherwise, the variations in artificial light can make you believe you have all kinds of imaginary disorders.
- Some types of food and drink, such as coffee, beetroot, chewing gum, and lollipops (popsicles), can change the colour of the tongue coating.

Some common features of balance and imbalance seen on the tongue are as follows:

- A NORMAL HEALTHY TONGUE: is considered to be pale red, with a thin, white coating. It should be neither thin nor swollen. It should be moist but not wet, and should not tremble when stuck out.
- A PALE TONGUE: often means weak qi and yang and means that there is not enough nutritive energy to bring sufficient amounts of qi and blood up to the tongue. It would usually be accompanied by weak qi symptoms.
- A RED TONGUE: often means weak yin. Heat rises from an agitated yang, dries up the fluids on the tongue, and removes its coating.
- A THICK WHITE COATING: suggests a lot of cold inside the body.
- A THICK YELLOW COATING: suggests a lot of heat inside the body.
- PALE SIDES: usually means a weakness in the blood. The Liver moves and stores blood, so it is logical that a weakness in this can be seen on this area of the tongue.
- A SWOLLEN TONGUE: can mean that too much body fluid has expanded the tongue and usually reflects the amount of damp in the body.

Organ areas on the tongue

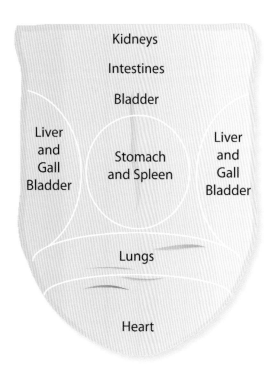

Kidneys

Intestines

Bladder

Liver and Gall Bladder

Stomach and Spleen

Liver and Gall Bladder

Lungs

Heart

- TEETH MARKS ON THE SIDES OF THE TONGUE: can mean weak Spleen qi and also the buildup of damp as a byproduct of this. The tongue has expanded so much that the only available space is being squeezed into the gaps of the teeth.
- A PURPLE TONGUE: suggests stagnation of qi and blood and can sometimes be a warning sign of a serious condition.
- CRACKS ON THE TONGUE: these appear because of a lack of moisture and body fluids and usually signify that yin levels in the body are weak.

- PATCHES ON THE TONGUE COATING: can mean weak yin, which burns off the moisture on the tongue. This can be caused by some medications, in particular antibiotics.
- MOUTH ULCERS: signifies heat rising from the body. If they are under the tongue, the heat could be from the Spleen or Kidneys; if they are actually on the tongue, it could be from the Heart; or if they are on the gums, it may be Stomach heat.

Part Three

How Can You Treat Yourself?

In the following chapters, there are lists of conditions and corresponding massage techniques, points, dietary changes and exercises. These are quite specific and may not be fully understood without a clear explanation of what is happening and why. In this section each of the techniques is explained.

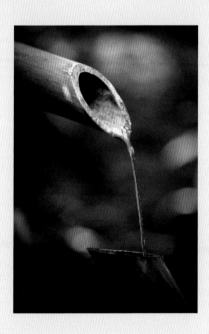

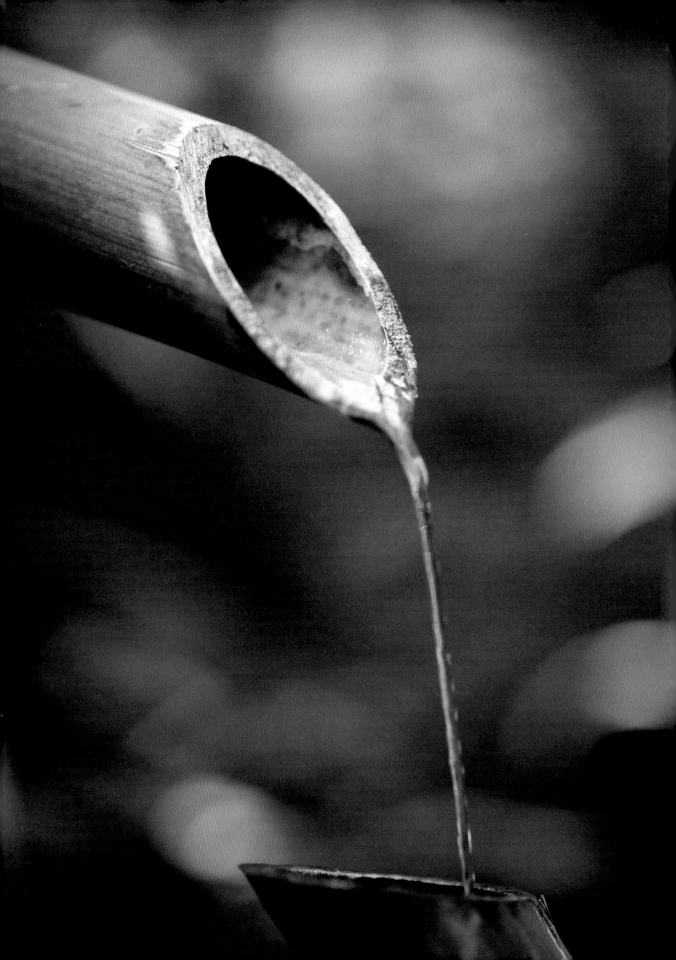

Chapter 11
氣 **Acupressure and Massage**

One of the most important healing techniques of all is touch, and most of the treatments in this book begin here. Massage techniques along the 14 channels mentioned earlier in the book, and on their individual points, can be very beneficial. Pain and muscular tightness often reflect internal imbalances via the channel of a particular organ.

For example, muscle soreness in the middle of the trapezius muscle on the shoulder is often a reflection of disturbance in the Gall Bladder channel – usually due to stress or emotional factors affecting both the Liver and Gall Bladder organs. Loosening up any tight muscles and tendons in this area will usually positively affect the imbalance of these organs.

Each channel has an exact trajectory, and each point has an exact location, but sometimes the place to treat is not so precise. It depends on if and where any soreness is felt. If there is no soreness at a particular point, but it is sore close-by, then this is the point to treat. The descriptions of points are like home addresses: once there it is necessary to look around for the right postbox.

Techniques

The techniques of Acupressure and massage in this book have been drawn from Thai massage, Chinese tuina, and Japanese shiatsu. They follow no one tradition exclusively and have been chosen according to what works and what is feasible. The following is a brief summary of the techniques involved.

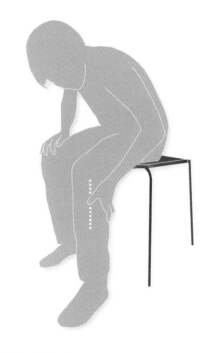

Self body massage

Individual point massage

PRESS = an exploratory press with the thumb or finger to see if there is any soreness.

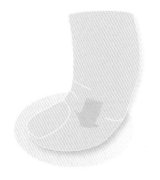

Press Technique

HARD-PRESS = pressing with the thumb with your body weight behind it and keeping it in place for several seconds.

(left) Hard press
Technique

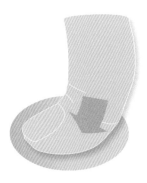

Note that if you are using these massage techniques on yourself there are some points, on the back for example, which can be difficult to treat effectively. In this case it is usually better to use the knuckles of a closed fist to apply pressure instead of your fingers or thumb.

Channel massage

THUMB-PRESS – pressing in a forwards motion with your thumb(s) and continually moving along a channel or muscle.

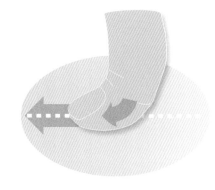

KNEAD = pressing with the thumb while slightly rotating it in a circular motion. Make sure both that the thumb stays on the point and that pressure is maintained.

(left) Knead
Technique

(right) Thumb press
Technique

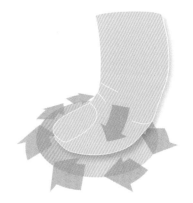

FINGER-PRESS – pressing in a forwards motion as above, but with the tips of the fingers.

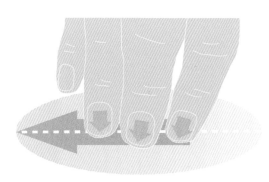

(left) Knuckle press
Technique

(right) Finger press
Technique

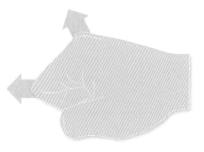

THUMB-CIRCLE – circling in a forwards motion with firm pressure, usually on the face, hands, or feet.

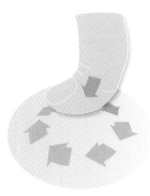

FINGER-CIRCLE – circling in a forwards motion with firm pressure, usually on the breastbone.

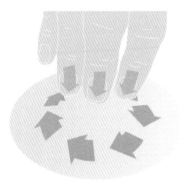

Wide area massage

PALM-CIRCLE – circling with the full palm of the hand, so as to cover a wide area. Usually on the abdomen.

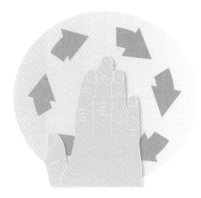

Precautions

Massage is generally safe, but use caution in the following situations:

- When massaging frail or weak people, be careful not to massage too strongly or for too long.
- Avoid the following points on pregnant women, as they can affect the uterus: LI-4 on the hand, Sp-6 on the inside leg, Bl-67 on the little toe, Bl-60 at the outside ankle, GB-21 at the top of the shoulder muscles and points on the abdominal area (look at the point location section for how to find them).
- Do not massage or press on or around open wounds, varicose veins, tumours, inflamed or infected skin, sites of recent surgery, or areas where a broken bone is suspected.

Acupressure and massage of specific parts of the body
The hand

Although performed since ancient times, hand acupressure as a microsystem of treating the whole body has only fairly recently become popular for the treatment of health conditions.

The system is based upon the idea that, like many other parts of the body, the hand contains the same basic information as the body as a whole. It is, in essence, the body in miniature and will reflect any imbalances that exist there. This means that, if you know where each part of the body, organ, and channel is reflected on the hand, you can treat it directly via the hand.

As is so common with theories that have existed for millennia and been used by diverse cultures speaking different languages and with ideas about the world, there are conflicting ideas about how the body is set out on the hand. This does not mean that one is right and the other is wrong, merely that there is more choice.

Thumb circle Technique

Finger circle Technique

Palm circle Technique

Techniques

The techniques of hand massage are almost identical to those for the body: press, knead, and hard-press to focus on one point, and thumb-press and finger- or thumb-circle to follow along a line.

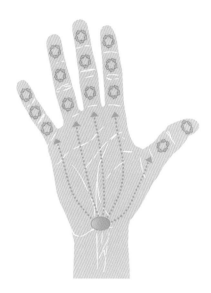

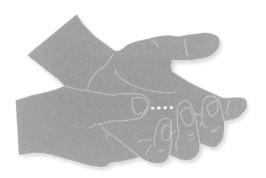

Precautions

- A key point to avoid in pregnancy is on the hand: LI-4 is in the muscle between the thumb and index finger on the back of the hand.
- Do not massage or press on or around open wounds, growths, nodules, inflamed or infected skin, sites of recent surgery or areas where a broken bone is suspected.

Healthy hand massage

The following massage covers many of the main areas on the hand and can be very beneficial, both locally to the hand and also generally for the body.

PALM MASSAGE: Hard-press at the centre of the wrist crease at the base of the palm. Thumb-press from here up to the base of the little finger and then thumb-circle up to the finger tip. At the tip, pull the finger to stretch it. Repeat with all five digits.

BACK-OF-THE-HAND MASSAGE: Hard-press at the centre of the wrist at the back of the hand. Thumb-circle from here all the way up to the base of the

little finger, then thumb-circle again up to the finger tip. At the tip, pull the finger to stretch it. Repeat with all five digits.

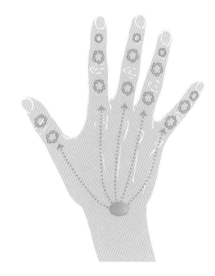

The foot

The foot is another ancient Oriental microsystem, whereby treating points on the feet can have a direct effect on the body as a whole. It became well known after it was championed by an American doctor called William Fitzgerald, who developed a system known as

Zone Therapy in the early 20th century, which later became known as Reflexology.

Reflexology theory holds that the shape of the foot roughly resembles the shape of the body with the head at the toes, the chest at the ball of the foot, the spine on the arch of the foot, and the abdomen and main organs in the centre of the foot; many of the lower-positioned organs, such as the bladder and intestine, are on the heel of the foot. There are also many points on the main channels located in the feet that are often considered to be very potent in terms of treatment. Indeed, the foot is seen by some as the root of qi and is very closely connected with the 12 organs of the body.

Many of the suggested treatment areas and points are a combination of reflexology areas, Chinese foot-point research, and the main channel points. Massaging these can effect a change in the balance of the channels and organs connected to the foot area, thereby treating the whole body via the feet.

Techniques

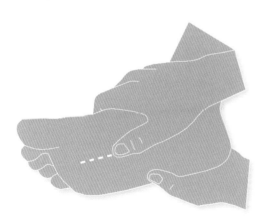

The techniques of foot massage are almost identical to those for the hand: press, knead, and hard-press to focus on one point, and thumb-press and finger- or thumb-circle to follow along a line.

Precautions

- Some of the key points to avoid in pregnancy are on the foot: Bl-67 is just before the outside corner of the nail bed of the little toe and Bl-60 is between the Achilles tendon and the outside ankle bone.
- Do not massage or press on or around open wounds, growths, nodules, inflamed or infected skin, sites of recent surgery or areas where a broken bone is suspected.

Healthy foot massage

The following massage covers many of the main areas on the foot and can be very beneficial both locally to the foot and also generally for the body.

SOLE MASSAGE: Hard-press at a central point just before the ball of the heel. Thumb-press from here up to the base of the little toe, then thumb-circle up to its tip. At the tip, pull the toe to stretch it. Repeat with all five toes.

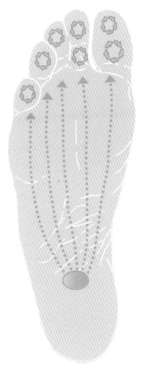

(left) Self-foot massage

(right) Healthy Foot massage: Sole

TOP FOOT MASSAGE: Hard-press at the centre of the ankle at the front of the foot. Thumb-circle from here down to the base of the little toe, then thumb-circle again up to its tip. At the tip, pull the toe to stretch it. Repeat with all five toes.

(left) Healthy Foot massage: Top

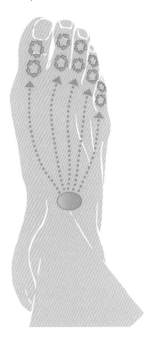

The ear

There is a long and distinguished history of treatment on the ear dating from over two millennia ago, when a classic medical text called The Yellow Emperor's Classic of Medicine mentioned bleeding points on the ear to treat headaches and period pain. It was revived in the 1950s by a French neurologist called Paul Nogier, who mapped the ear in terms of treatment. In his map, and in subsequent Chinese maps, the ear can be seen, quite literally, as an upside-down, curled-up foetus. Points on the body correspond with the represented foetal position of the body part on the ear.

The Chinese combined Nogier's embryo theory with the theories of organs and channels in traditional Chinese medicine . The result of this was two sets of maps, one Chinese and the other European, and a loose agreement about the location and naming of many points.

(right) Self-ear massage

Having two separate ear maps may seem confusing at first, but many points are at the same or almost the same location. Some points are named differently but in the same place, and other points have the same name but in a different place.

As with other areas of Oriental medicine, it is not a question of who is right and who is wrong but a question of what works. If we are presented with two points that have both proved to be effective for a particular problem, then we have double the chance of treating effectively.

For the purposes of this book, the points indicated are those that best help the problem regardless of whether they originate from the European or Chinese auricular maps.

Techniques

- It is important not to massage the ear for too long, as it can move too much qi, leaving the body weaker.
- It is important to do acupressure only on a point

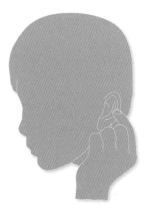

that is sore under a little pressure. Do not just follow an ear chart and blindly massage according to the instructions given. Feel your own ears and look for the point that needs to be massaged. This may be exactly on the point suggested, somewhere nearby, or at a completely different location.

- Use the nail of your index finger to press on the relevant sore points several times. It is important not to keep your nail static pressing on the point; you should knead the point but stop when there is pain. At the same time, use your thumb to support the back of the ear.
- Apply gentle pressure at first to find the sore points, then increase pressure with a circular movement until the soreness improves.
- A matchstick or other blunt, thin object can be used to apply pressure. Many Oriental medicine suppliers sell metallic ear probes for just such a purpose.

Precautions

Avoid ear manipulation altogether if you are pregnant and have a history of miscarriages. In general, avoid the uterus point, ovary point, and endocrine point, if you are pregnant. (See the ear point location section for their exact location).

Healthy ear massage

The following is a general daily ear massage sequence to maintain health and balance in the body. Use the pad of your index finger to apply circular pressure and move up and down the ear in a continual spiral.

The thumb moves down with your finger and provides support at the back. Once at the bottom, go back and repeat several times.

Start by gently stretching the ear with the following two sequences:

STRETCH 1: Pinch the ear and pull the cartilage outwards away from the body. Pull the bottom half of the ear diagonally downwards and the top of the ear diagonally upwards.

STRETCH 2: Twist the ear with your thumb and finger. The thumb slides up the back of the ear, while simultaneously the finger pushes down. You should feel a slight strain at the bottom of the ear. Repeat several times.

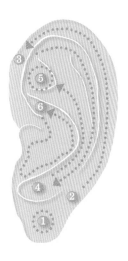

Healthy Ear massage

Now, do the following sequence in one continuous movement:

MASSAGE 1: Massage the ear lobe between your thumb and index finger, the index finger at the front of the ear and the thumb supporting the back.

MASSAGE 2: Knead upwards along the outside of the ear to the top, then follow the bend round to where the ear meets the head. While massaging, gently pull the ear outwards and upwards.

MASSAGE 3: Move slightly inwards towards the centre of the ear, and knead downwards following the contour of the ear.

MASSAGE 4: At the bottom of the ear, again move inwards slightly and massage upwards along the ridge. Follow the contour of the ear and drop into the dip at the end.

MASSAGE 5: Massage this dip in a circular fashion.

MASSAGE 6: Drop down into the central cavity and again knead in a circular fashion.

MASSAGE 7: Knead down the back of the ear with your thumb.

MASSAGE 8: Search around for any sore points with the nail of your index finger. You may have noticed some in the previous exercise. Knead any sore points several times.

Chapter 12
氣 Scraping

(left) Scraping
down the back

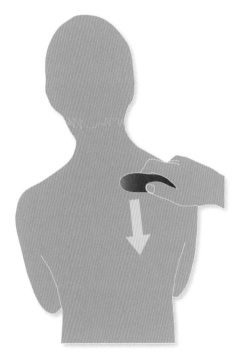

staff to try it themselves, but curiously, I never had any takers.

Scraping has a long history of use in a variety of Far Eastern countries, where it is known as *gua sha* or *cao gio*, and has traditionally been used as folk medicine to treat colds, flu, and muscle aches and pains.

The idea behind Scraping is to bring a red discoloration to the surface of the skin. Of course, if you scrape the skin with this technique it is going to temporarily turn pinky-red; however, the discoloration that sometimes comes out in Scraping therapy has additional characteristics. The skin goes pinky-red as normal, but some parts begin to resemble tiny red dots of varying intensity and are clearly distinguishable from the rest of the skin. This is known as petechiae and occurs when capillary blood vessels are broken.

(right) Strong
petechiae on the
skin after scraping

Scraping therapy can appear rather strange at first glance. Using a splash of oil for lubrication, someone repeatedly drags a blunt object along the skin until it appears reddish or sometimes purple. The end result, if you are not familiar with how the technique works, can cause more than a little jaw-dropping, gasps, and sometimes looks like the recipient has just had some kind of major trauma.

In reality, of course, this is far from the case, but I recall sending my children to school with preemptive explanatory letters every time I did Scraping on them to relieve a cough or a cold. "When changing for PE class today, you may notice that my son has red marks on this upper back, this is not because . . . " I always ended my letter by inviting anyone on the teaching

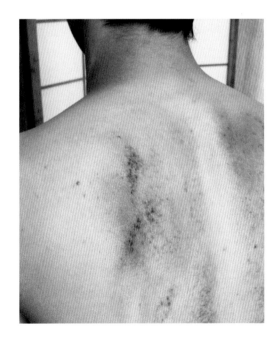

These red or purple dots will remain on the skin after the rest of the redness has died down, and they do not usually fade for days. They appear on the skin because they are reflecting what is just under the skin. This is usually the qi or blood stagnation that lies below the surface within the muscles and tissues but, in actual fact, the colour of the spots themselves can be very informative as to what has caused them.

PALE SPOTS usually mean that there is a weakness of blood in the body.
RED SPOTS suggest that wind, cold, damp, or heat have recently become stuck in the body.
DARK RED SPOTS are caused by the presence of heat.
PURPLE OR VERY DARK SPOTS normally indicate long-standing stagnation of blood.

Scraping is used to treat a variety of health conditions and illnesses, but if used correctly it is very useful in reducing pain. Indeed, research done in the USA found that there is a definite pain-relieving mechanism associated with Scraping.[9]

As a simple but profound home treatment to maintain family health, Scraping has few equals.

Equipment

The tool used in Scraping has to have a rounded edge, so that the Scraping action will not damage the skin and will be relatively painless.

Gua sha scrapers can be bought from specialist

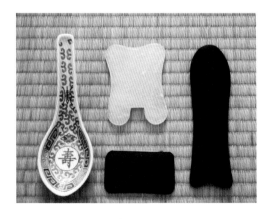

shops. These are often made of animal horn, bone, or jade. A simple Chinese soup spoon made of porcelain, however, is perfectly sufficient as also is the lid of some jam or marmalade jars. The essential thing with whatever you might use is that the edge is firm but rounded.

Techniques

In order to prevent any injury or pain, the area has to be lubricated beforehand with oil. Any massage oil can be used, as can vapour rub.

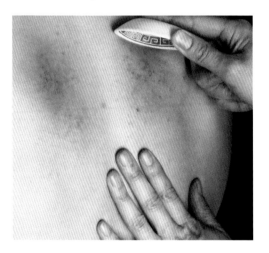

(right) Scraping technique

The general technique is as follows:

1. The oil or vapour rub should be rubbed thoroughly over the area to be treated with both hands.
2. The scraper should be held at a 45-degree angle to the skin in your dominant hand.
3. The area to be treated should be scraped gently at first, with a steady increase in pressure until the strokes are firm, short, and brisk, but still within the comfort zone of the receiver.
4. As a general rule the Scraping should be from top to bottom and from the midline outwards.
5. The Scraping should be continued with varying pressure until red spots appear. If the skin remains pink from the Scraping but shows no tiny spots after several strokes, move on.

(left) Scraping tools

6. Areas where red spots might appear are often tense and resistant under the skin. Once the spots do appear, continue around the area to bring out as much as possible, but pay attention to the comfort of the receiver and check in with them.

7. Any areas with spots can be pressed and kneaded afterwards, but often the Scraping treatment is sufficient.

Areas of treatment

Many conditions have specific areas, but the general areas of treatment are as follows:

Precautions

When Scraping, the scraper will come into contact with body fluids and skin cells, so cross-contamination (especially with hepatitis B or HIV) may potentially occur when using this technique on affected people. Consider wearing medical gloves, to avoid your fingers coming into contact with infected body fluids. Use the scraper only on one person at a time, and clean it thoroughly with disinfectant after use. Other people should ideally have their own dedicated scrapers. Should one scraper be used for different people, it is safest to sterilize it. This can be done simply and cheaply by soaking the scraper in a solution of one part bleach to ten parts water.

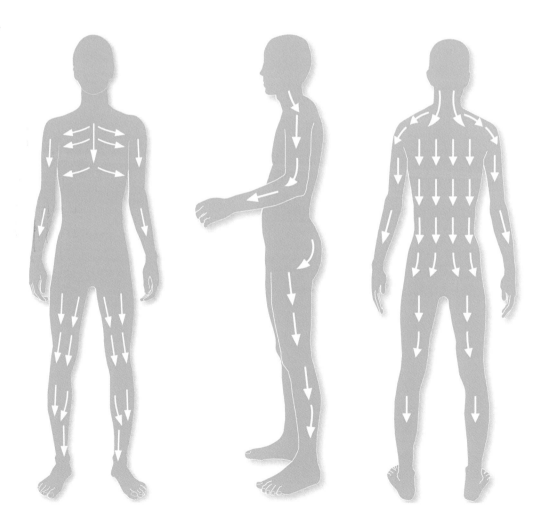

(left) Scraping treatment areas: Front

(middle) Scraping treatment areas: Side

(right) Scraping treatment areas: Back

Do not use Scraping techniques in the following situations:

- With particularly weak, frail people;
- On an area with a fresh injury, including swelling, bruising, cuts and scrapes;
- On an area of skin that is sunburnt;
- On a preexisting skin condition, e.g. a rash or eczema;
- On any moles, blemishes, spots, or raised skin features. These need to be covered with a finger, and care must be taken to scrape the area around them without actually touching them;
- On breast tissue;
- On the abdomen of a pregnant woman;
- Over existing Scraping spots, until they have faded from the skin (this can take a few days).

Chapter 13
氣 **Tapping**

Tapping along the
leg muscles

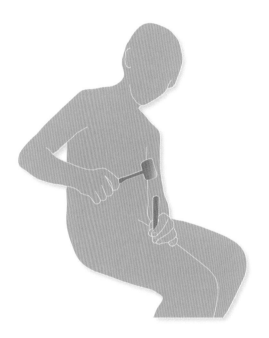

(right) Wooden
hammer and
'needle'

In the imperial court of 16th-century Japan, Tapping was a popular form of treatment. Blunt golden needles known as *uchibari* were tapped on sore points with a small ebony hammer known as *kozuchi,* in a technique known as *dashin.* The emperor's personal doctor, Misono Isai (1557–1616), was credited with popularizing this form of treatment. It was based on what has become known as *mubun style dashin,* whereby all the points of the body were treated on the abdomen.

The Tapping was done rhythmically on the abdominal area in order to treat a wide variety of disorders. The vibration caused changes in qi and was able to scatter what was known as evil qi, or *jaki.*

Jump forward to the 20th century, when a group of doctors reinvigorated the technique with an updated wooden version of the hammer and needle. Among the group was Yoshio Manaka (1911–1989), an innovative doctor who was mindful that, in order for his patients to improve, some form of home therapy was very important. Manaka developed a set of Tapping techniques for his patients to do at home. His rationale was that, if patients could treat the manifestations of daily stress, exhaustion, and tension on themselves, they would have more control over their health and would be less likely to fall ill.

This home therapy entailed the use of the hammer and needle, which according to Manaka's research, produced results not that dissimilar to conventional light acupuncture needling. He also found that the technique can be used not just on the abdomen as practised in *mubun style dashin* but all around the body, wherever the tension lies.

Equipment

In order to do Tapping therapy, you need to have something to tap with – ideally, a wooden hammer and "needle." Dr. Manaka's hammer and needle con-

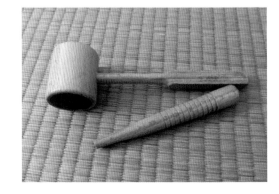

sisted of a blunt wooden peg, 10mm in diameter and 120mm long, and a hammer with a 160mm shaft and a 35mm-diameter head.

Many variations of this wooden hammer and needle can be found, usually at specialist Chinese or Japanese medicine suppliers (see Resources at the back of the book for suppliers). For anyone so inclined, you could make your own wooden hammer. The requirements are that it be small, light, and well balanced, so that it does not strike the wooden needle with undue force.

Technique

The procedure of treating with Manaka's hammer and needle is as follows:

1. Hold the blunt needle between the thumb and forefinger/middle finger of your less dominant hand.
2. Grasp it at the bottom, thinner end of the shaft, much like you would a dart in preparation to throw at a dart board.
3. Place the end of the needle on the point you wish to treat, making sure to keep your hand relaxed. Hold the needle lightly but firmly, and push down slightly into the point, so that the vibration is focused in one place.
4. The other hand can then tap the top of the needle with the hammer with a consistent rhythm. Start lightly and tap each point up to 30 times.
5. The vibration is passed through the needle and into the body. The strength of the Tapping can be adjusted according to sensation, the position of the point, and the strength of qi. Obviously for people with weaker qi and who may bruise easily, the Tapping should be much lighter.

Dr Manaka developed a theory of channel frequencies whereby variations on the rate of the tap will treat different channels. The frequency of the Spleen, for

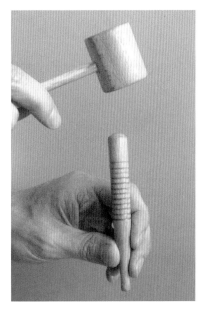

Hammer and needle holding technique

example, is 132 beats per minute so, using a metronome to guide the Tapping rate, the vibration can then resonate to treat the Spleen directly.[10]

This matching of vibration and Tapping can be very effective, but is not necessary to achieve good results at home. Good results come from proper controlled Tapping at the right points on a regular basis.

Precautions

Use caution when performing Tapping therapy in the following situations:

- On frail or weak people;
- On boney areas, and on areas where there is very little muscle;
- On any existing skin condition, such as a rash or eczema.

Do not use Tapping therapy in the following situations:

- On an area with a fresh injury, including swelling, bruising, cuts, and scrapes;
- On the abdomen of a pregnant woman.

Chapter 14
氣 **Exercises**

The importance of performing daily exercises at home cannot be overstressed. Gentle exercise is a major feature of daily life in Oriental cultures, in order to relieve stiffness and tension in the body before they turn into a source of ill health.

In Japan, collective daily exercise is known as taiso and consists of a set routine to simple, repetitive music. This tradition, although gradually dying out in urban areas, was very much alive and kicking in the part of Japan I used to live in (an island of forests, fishermen, and monkeys).

For years, I had to listen to a tortuous recording called Taiso No. 4 every day at precisely 3.00 p.m., played on crackling loudspeakers spaced strategically around our island home so that there was no escape.

In this recording, a man literally barks instructions while pert piano chords keep up the rhythm, until the whole sequence of swinging and swaying comes to a halt minutes later. As far as the music went, it was rather like an annoying pop song that is repeated endlessly on the radio until it becomes so familiar that, despite yourself, you actually start to like it. As for the exercises – simple, repetitive, and invigorating for your health.

The exercises used in this book draw heavily on Japanese stretching exercises (but not that one!) and are variations on what are called sotai and makko ho. I have also included some variations of Chinese qigong (chee gong) exercises, which is a popular meditative practice of combining slow movement and breathing to maintain health.

While there are many levels on which these exercises can be perceived, none requires any special awareness of qi or its movement within the body in order to be effective. For me, this is important. I have designed the sequence of exercises in such a way as to make them accessible to as many people as possible.

Some people prefer to be aware of their qi and use visualization and movement techniques to manipulate it in some way. This is the idea of exercises derived from popular Asian martial arts techniques like tai chi and qigong and from Indian yoga. Other people may find that the very idea of this would put them off, and although they may try out the exercises once or twice, they are ultimately just not comfortable doing activities like this.

So the exercises in this book can be done with or without thinking about qi. Ideally, follow any advice about breathing, but it is the repetitive actions themselves that are of most benefit.

Massaging the five elements

The five-element stretches consist of a set of gentle exercises derived from the tradition of shiatsu in Japan. Each of the exercises is associated with one of the five elements and its corresponding organs.

The exercises were originally developed by Shizuto Masunaga (1925–1981) and consist of yoga-like exercises to maintain good health. When done together, the sequence of exercises reflects the daily cycle of qi and can be very beneficial to ensure that this cycle runs as smoothly as possible.

The following exercises consist of makko ho stretches and variations thereof. They should be done slowly, mindfully (as in relaxed and without distraction), and without any physical strength or effort. They can be completed all in one go as a daily exercise routine, or separately to rebalance an element or organ.

Exercise 1 – Metal
Strengthening the Lungs and Large Intestine

The following exercise stretches the Lung and Large Intestine channels in the fingers, hand, arms, and shoulders.

- Stand with your feet shoulders' width apart, knees slightly bent, and link your thumbs behind your back.

- Breathe in and, keeping the thumbs linked, stretch your fingers out. While breathing out bend your upper body forward, keeping your fingers stretched out but relaxing as much as you can.

- Keep the bent position, breathe in and out slowly and deeply three times and visualize letting go of any tension in the body. As you breathe out the third time, slowly raise the upper body into an upright position. Repeat several times.

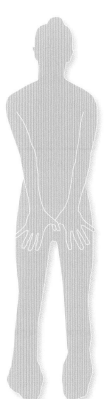

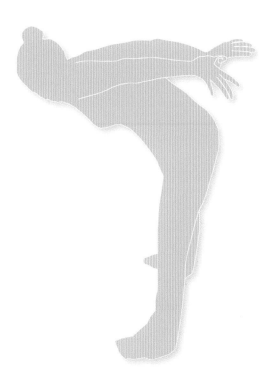

(left) Exercise 1: link your thumbs

(right) Exercise 1: bend forward

Exercise 2 – Earth
Strengthening the Stomach and Spleen

This exercise stretches the Stomach and Spleen channels in the chest, throat, and face, and the lower part of the knees, shins, and feet.

- Kneel on a comfortable flat surface and sit on your heels (a supporting pillow or cushion can be used if necessary).
- Breathe in, and while breathing out, place both hands facing backwards behind you, and lean backwards.
- Allow your head to fall back, so that you can look behind. If possible, lift the hip area upwards and forwards to arch the body backwards.
- Hold the position for a few moments and then return to an upright position.

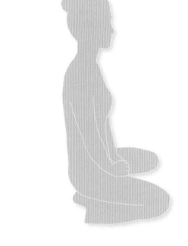

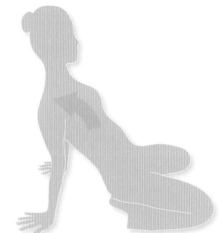

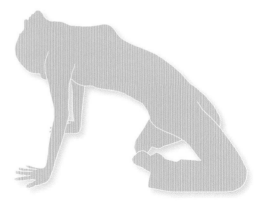

Exercise 3 – Fire
Strengthening the Heart and Small Intestine

This exercise stretches the Small Intestine channel in the shoulders and arms.

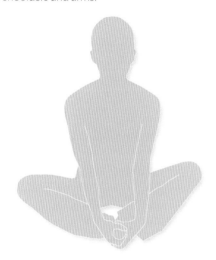

- Sit on the floor with your legs bent and leaning outwards and the soles of the feet touching each other.

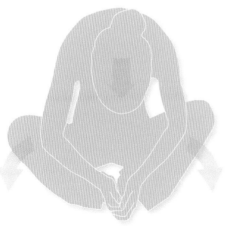

- Keeping your back straight, grab your feet with both hands, and bend forward from your hip as you breathe out. Let your knees fall down to the floor if they can.
- Hold this position while breathing in and out three times, then slowly return to the original position.

Exercise 4 – Water
Strengthening the Kidneys and Bladder

This exercise stretches the Kidney and Bladder channels in the back and legs.

- Sit on the floor, with a straight back and your legs straight out in front of you.

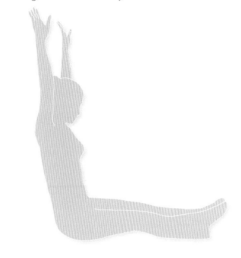

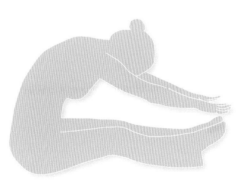

- Raise your arms above your head, and, as you breathe out, bend forward from the hips. Make sure that your knees are kept straight.
- Inhale, then on the exhale, reach as far forward between your legs as you can.
- Hold this position while breathing in and out three times, then slowly return to the original position.

(top left) Exercise 3: soles touching

(bottom left) Exercise 3: bend forwards

(top right) Exercise 4: raise your arms

(bottom right) Exercise 4: reach forward

Exercise 5 – Fire
Strengthening the Pericardium and Triple Burner

This exercise stretches the Pericardium and Triple Burner channels in the arms and shoulders.

Exercise 5: lean forward and stretch

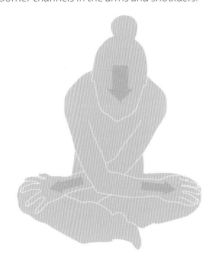

(top right) Exercise 6: stretch your arms

(bottom right) Exercise 6: lean and stretch sideways

- Sit with your legs crossed, right leg over left. Place your left hand on your right knee and your right hand on your left knee so that the right arm is on the outside of the left arm.
- Lean forward and bring your head towards the floor. If you can, stretch your arms farther away from each other to intensify the stretch.
- Hold this position while breathing in and out three times before slowly returning to the original position. Then repeat, swapping arms.

Exercise 6 – Wood
Strengthening the Liver and Gall Bladder

This exercise stretches the Liver and Gall Bladder channels on the sides of the body and legs.

- Sit with a straight back and spread your legs as wide as possible. Link your fingers and stretch your arms above your head, palms up.
- Breathe in deeply and turn to look at your right foot.
- Breathe out and lean your body sideways towards your right, stretching your arms out towards your left foot.

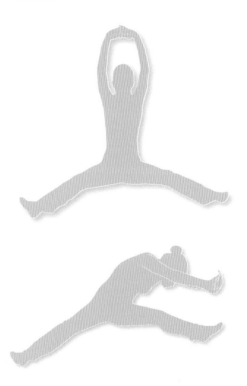

- Facing your right foot, hold the position while breathing in and out three times, then repeat the sequence on the other side.
- End the stretching sequence by leaning forward in the middle, holding, then returning to the original position.

Part Four

How Do You Find the Channels and Points?

In this section, you'll find a selection of points from the main channels, which you will need to use as reference for treating the specific imbalances and medical conditions listed in the treatment chapters of the book that follow.

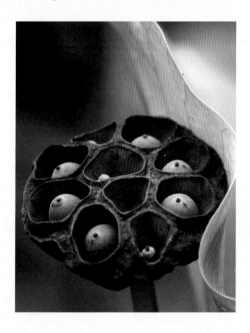

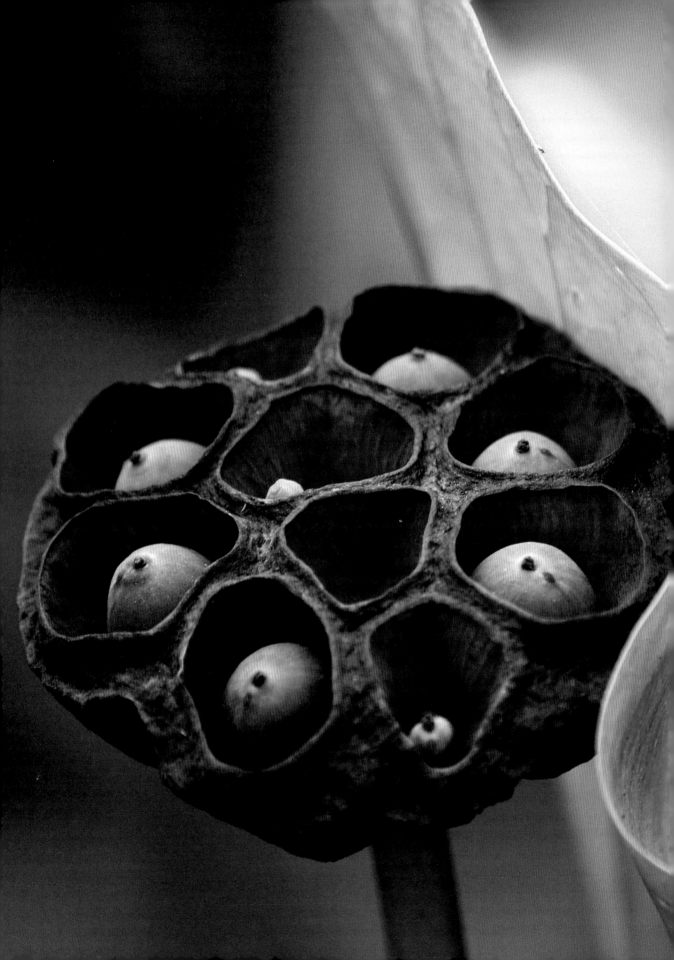

Chapter 15
氣 **Treatment Points on the Body**

I have chosen the following points according to their usefulness, frequency of use, and the ease with which they can be located on the body.

All points have designated Chinese characters and proper names, but to avoid getting distracted by these (they can be rather flowery), I have included the numbering system that is commonly used in the Western world when referring to them. This is made up of an abbreviation of the channel name and then the number of that point along the channel. The abbreviations are as follows:

Lu: Lung; LI: Large Intestine; St: Stomach; Sp: Spleen; He: Heart; SI: Small Intestine; Bl: Bladder; Kid: Kidneys; Pe: Pericardium; TB: Triple Burner; GB: Gall Bladder; Liv: Liver.

The Ren and Du channels are not abbreviated, and you will find that some extra points that do not belong to any channels have been given their proper (usually fairly unpronounceable) names.

The flow of qi along a channel goes in one direction, and this is indicated by the ascending numbers. The Bladder channel, for example, begins at Bl-1 at the eye and ends at Bl-67 in the little toe. So the flow of qi is going downwards towards the toe.

Sometimes the points I give are numbered sequentially as they are on the channel, but you will also find that there are numbers missing in places. This is not an error. It just means that those missing points are not as important for the purposes of home treatment, so there is little sense in including them in this book.

For practical purposes, the treatment points are presented here according to the body area where you will find them, rather than complete channels from beginning to end across the whole body. This is because you will need to use this section as a reference for the self-treatment sections that follow.

NOTE: The distances used in finding some of the points are as follows:

- A finger width: the distance from one side of the middle finger to the other.

A finger width

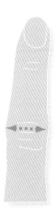

- A thumb width: the distance from one side of the thumb to the other at its widest point.

A thumb width

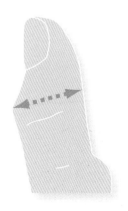

- Two fingers width: the distance across the index and middle fingers.

(top left) Two fingers width

(right) Points on the head: front

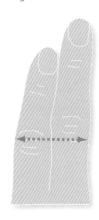

- Three fingers width: the distance across the middle three fingers together.

(middle left) Three fingers width

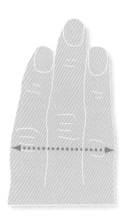

- A hand width: the distance across all four fingers together.

(bottom left) A hand width

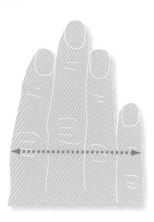

Points on the Head
On the Head 1: Front

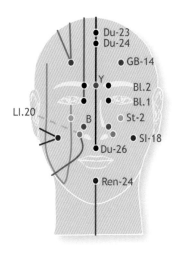

Du-23: On the midline of the head, a thumb width back from the normal hairline. (If your hairline is not where it once was, use your imagination to visualize where it probably would be).

Du-24: On the midline of the head, half a thumb width towards the face from Du-23.

Du-26: On the midline of the face, a third of the distance from the nose to the top lip.

GB-14: On the forehead, a thumb width above the middle of the eyebrow or the pupils, when looking straight ahead.

Bl-1: Just above the inside corner of the eye.

Bl-2: Directly above Bl-1 on the eyebrow.

St-2: Just below the centre point of the lower eye socket.

SI-18: Directly below the cheek bone, on an imaginary line down from the outside of the eye.

LI-20: Next to and level with the midpoint of the flare of the nostrils.

Ren-24: Below the lower lip, on the midline of the chin crease.

Bitong (B): Next to the nose, at the beginning of the flare of the nostrils.

Yintang (Y): Halfway between the eyebrows.

On the Head 2: Back

On the Head 3: Side

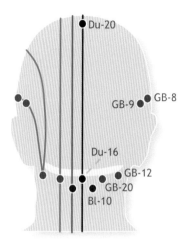

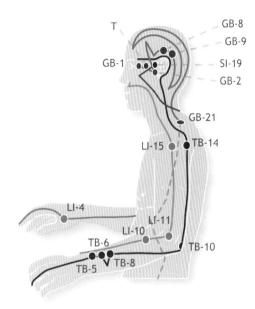

(left) Points on the head: back

(right) Points on the head/arm/shoulder: side

GB-12: Under and just before the end of the base of the skull.

GB-20: Below the base of the skull, halfway between the centre line and GB-12.

Du-16: On the midline of the back of the head, below the base of the skull.

Du-20: On the midline of the head, follow the slanted line of the ear upwards to the top of the head.

Bl-10: Roughly two finger widths outwards from the midline of the neck, one finger width below the base of the skull.

SI-19: In front of the midpoint of where the lower part of the ear attaches to the head. There is normally a curve in the ear here.

GB-1: Follow the corner of the eye outwards towards the temple, just over the ridge of the eye socket.

GB 2: On the side Bl-10: Roughly two finger widths outwards from the midline of the neck, one finger of the face, directly below SI-19, where the ear attaches to the head.

GB-8: On the head, two finger widths above the top point of the ear, when folded over itself.

GB-9: On the head, half a thumb width straight behind GB-8.

Taiyang (T): In the temple, around a finger width and a half behind the end of the eyebrow and the corner of the eye.

Points on the Arm and Shoulders
On the Arms 1: Side

LI-10: Three finger widths towards the wrist from LI-11.

LI-11: At the end of the elbow crease when the elbow is closed.

TB-5: Three finger widths up the forearm from TB-4, in between the radius and the ulnar arm bones.

TB-6: A hand width up the forearm from TB-4, in between the radius and ulnar arm bones.

TB-8: A third of the way from the wrist to the tip of the elbow, in between the radius and ulnar arm bones.

TB-10: Bend the arm at the elbow. The point is a thumb width above the tip of the elbow on the back muscle of the arm.

On the Arms 2: Front

Lu-1: Two finger widths outwards diagonally below Lu-2, in the muscle ridge.

Lu-2: In the hollow at the outside end of the collar bone.

Pc-6: Three finger widths up the forearm from the wrist crease closest to the wrist (some people have a few), in between the two central tendons.

Lu-5: Just to the outside of the biceps tendon at the elbow crease. Flex your biceps and feel the stringy tendons. Make sure you are to the outside of them.

LI-15: Directly under the bone at the shoulder joint on the centre line of the arm.

Jianqian (J): In the shoulder muscle, halfway between the under arm crease and LI-15.

On the Arms 3: Back

SI-8: At the elbow in the gap between the tip of the elbow and the "funny bone."

TB-14: At the shoulder joint, just behind the deltoid arm muscle. At the same level as LI-15 but behind it in the dip.

Points on the Front
On the Front 1: Chest

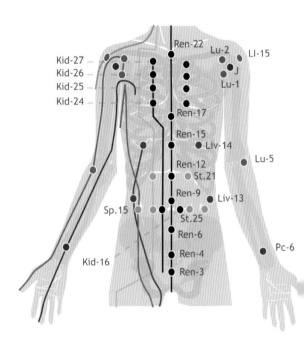

Kid-24: Three finger widths from the centre line of the chest, in between the third and fourth ribs. The nipples are usually in the space between the fourth and fifth ribs in men. So go one above this.

Kid-25: Three finger widths from the centre line of the chest, in between the second and third ribs.

Kid-26: Three finger widths from the centre line of the chest, in between the first and second ribs.

Kid-27: Three finger widths from the centre line of the chest, under the collar bone.

Liv-14: In the sixth rib space, in line with an imaginary line down from the nipple on a man or a little more than a hand's width from the centre line of the chest.

Ren-17: On the midline of the breastbone, level with the fourth rib space (the nipples are usually in the space between the fourth and fifth ribs in men).

Ren-22: On the midline, in the dip just above the top of the breastbone.

On the Front 2: Abdomen

St-21: Three finger widths from the midline of the abdomen level with Ren-12.

St-25: Three finger widths from the midline of the abdomen, or halfway from the farthest line of abdominal muscles (as in those six-pack muscles), level with the belly button.

Sp-15: At the outer line of the abdominal muscles (the six-packs) or a little more than a hand width from and on a line with the belly button.

Kid-16: Half a thumb width outwards from and in line with the belly button.

Liv-13: Just below and forwards of the 11th rib, at the side of the body. The 11th rib is actually below the level of, and not attached to, the rib cage. If you bend your arm and put your elbow at your side, it should be close to this point.

Ren-3: On the midline of the lower abdomen, a thumb width above the top of the pubic bone (the line of bone you hit as you feel down the abdomen).

Ren-4: On the midline of the lower abdomen, a hand width below the belly button or three finger widths above the top of the pubic bone.

Ren-6: On the midline of the lower abdomen, around two finger widths below the belly button.

Ren-9: On the midline of the abdomen, a thumb width above the belly button.

Ren-12: On the midline of the abdomen, halfway between the end of the breastbone and the belly button.

Ren-15: On the midline of the abdomen, a thumb width below the end of the breastbone.

Points on the Back

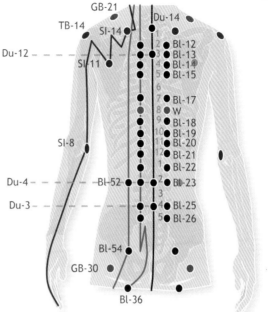

Points on the back

Below you will find lots of references to vertebrae. Should the idea of anatomy fill you with dread, what we are talking about are the boney bits sticking out on the spine. In the illustration, each vertebra in the thoracic (upper back: T1-12) and lumbar (lower back: L1-5) areas of the body are numbered, as they would typically be anatomically, in order to make finding them easier.

On the Back 1: Upper back

SI-11: At the midpoint of the triangular-shaped shoulder blade.

SI-14: A hand width outwards from the first thoracic vertebra (where the neck meets the shoulders), just above the top of the shoulder blade.

GB-21: On the top of the shoulder muscle, halfway between the midline of the neck and the end of the shoulder.

Bl-12: Halfway between the vertical edge of the shoulder blade and the spine (normally about two finger widths), level with the gap between the second and third thoracic vertebrae. (If in any doubt, find Bl-13 first and go up one).

Bl-13: Halfway between the vertical edge of the shoulder blade and the spine, level with the gap between the third and fourth thoracic vertebrae. This is normally found by continuing the diagonal lateral line of the bony spine of the shoulder blade.

Bl-14: Halfway between the vertical edge of the shoulder blade and the spine, level with the gap between the fourth and fifth thoracic vertebrae. (If in any doubt, find Bl-13 first and go down one.)

Bl-15: Halfway between the vertical edge of the shoulder blade and the spine, level with the gap between the fifth and sixth thoracic vertebrae. (If in any doubt, find Bl-13 first and go down two.)

Bl-17: Extend the same vertical line as above in Bl-12 to Bl-15 downwards. It is level with the gap between the seventh and eighth thoracic vertebrae. This is normally found at the same level as the bottom of the shoulder blades.

Bl-18: Extend the same vertical line as above in Bl-12 to Bl-15 downwards. It is level with the gap between the ninth and tenth thoracic vertebrae. (If in any doubt, find Bl-17 first and go down two.)

Bl-19: Extend the same vertical line as above in Bl-12 to Bl-15 downwards. It is level with the gap between the 10th and 11th thoracic vertebrae. (If in any doubt, find Bl-17 first and go down three.)

Bl-20: Extend the same vertical line as above in Bl-12 to Bl-15 downwards. It is level with the gap between the 11th and 12th thoracic vertebrae. (If in any doubt, find Bl-23 first and go up three.)

Bl-21: Extend the same vertical line as above in Bl-12 to Bl-15 downwards. It is level with the gap between the 12th thoracic vertebra and the first lumbar vertebra. (If in any doubt, find Bl-23 first and go up two.)

Bl-22: Extend the same vertical line as above in Bl-12 to Bl-15 downwards. It is level with the gap between the first and second lumbar vertebrae. (If in any doubt, find Bl-23 first and go up one.)

Du-12: On the midline of the spine, in the space between the third and fourth thoracic vertebrae.

Du-14: On the midline of the base of the neck, where the neck meets the shoulders. In the space between the seventh cervical (the last neck vertebra) and the first thoracic vertebra.

Weiguanxiashu (W): Level with the gap between the eighth and ninth thoracic vertebrae, around two finger widths from the centre line of the spine.

On the Back 2: Lower back

Bl-23: Extend the same vertical line as above in Bl-12 to Bl-15 downwards. It is level with the gap between the second and third lumbar vertebrae. This is normally found by finding the bottom of the ribcage at the sides and bringing your hands together at the spine at the same level.

Bl-25: Extend the same vertical line as above in Bl-12 to Bl-15 downwards. It is level with the gap between the fourth and fifth lumbar vertebrae. This is normally at the same level as the top of the pelvic bones at your waist.

Bl-26: Extend the same vertical line as above in Bl-12 to Bl-15 downwards. It is level with the bottom of the fifth lumbar vertebra. (If in any doubt, find Bl-25 first and go down one.)

Bl-36: Directly below the buttock on the midline of the back of the leg.

Bl-52: Extend the line at the edge of the shoulder blade straight downwards. It it is level with Bl-23 and about a hand width from L2 vertebra.

Bl-54: Extend the line at edge of the shoulder blade straight downwards. It is in the buttock level with and about a hand width from the last bony protuberance of the spine.

GB-30: On the hip, one-third of the distance between the bony head of the femur bone and the centre line of the spine.

Du-3: On the midline of the spine, in the space between the fourth and fifth lumbar vertebrae. Two spaces down from Du-4.

Du-4: On the midline of the spine, in the space between the second and third lumbar vertebrae. Usually level with the highest points of the pelvic bone at the sides of the body.

Points on the Hands/Wrists
On the Hand 1: Back

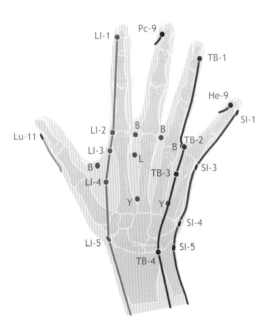

LI-1: Close to the thumb side edge of the nail bed, where the vertical and horizontal lines that mark the edges of the nail meet.

LI-2: Just after the thumb side of the knuckle of the index finger.

LI-3: Just before the thumb side of the knuckle of the index finger.

LI-4: In the web of flesh between the thumb and index finger.

LI-5: Spread open the fingers of your hand, and follow

the gap between the two tendons of the thumb down to the wrist. The point is in the dip at the wrist joint.

He-9: Close to the inside (thumb side) edge of the nail bed of the little finger, where the vertical and horizontal lines that mark the edges of the nail meet.

TB-1: Close to the outside edge of the nail bed of the ring finger, where the vertical and horizontal lines that mark the edges of the nail meet.

TB-2: On the back of the hand, in the web between the ring and little fingers.

TB-3: Make a loose fist. The point lies on the back of the hand, between the third and fourth metacarpal bones and forms an equilateral triangle, with the knuckles of the ring and little finger.

TB-4: Follow the gap between the bones from TB-3, and the point is in the wrist joint before you reach the head of the ulna bone.

Pc-9: In the centre of the tip or close to the outside edge of the thumb-side nail bed of the middle finger, where the vertical and horizontal lines that mark the edges of the nail meet.

SI-1: Close to the outside edge of the nail bed of the little finger. Where the vertical and horizontal lines that mark the edges of the nail meet.

SI-3: Below the little finger joint at the side of the hand. Between the fifth metacarpal bone and palm muscles.

SI-4: On the little finger side of the hand, above the wrist, at the other end of the fifth metacarpal bone to SI-3, between the bone and palm muscle.

SI-5: At the side of the wrist, between the head of the radius bone and hand.

Lu-11: Close to the outside edge of the nail bed, where the vertical and horizontal lines that mark the edges of the nail meet.

Yaotongxue (Y): Two points on the back of the hand, between the metacarpal bones that lead to the second, third, fourth, and fifth fingers. Slide down from between the knuckles, and they are just before the bones meet.

Baxie (B): Make a loose fist, and these points are in the webs between the four knuckles, close to the finger gaps.

Luozhen (L): Below the gap between the second and third knuckles. Put your finger between the knuckles and drop it down on to the back of the hand.

On the Hand 2: Palm

(left) Points on the hands: palm

(right) Points on the legs: back/outside

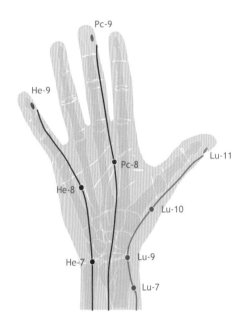

Lu-7: On the thumb side of the lower arm, directly below the head of the radius bone. It should be around two fingers width from the side of the wrist.

Lu-9: In the wrist joint, below the base of the thumb.

Lu-10: In the fleshy part of the hand below the thumb, halfway along and next to the first metacarpal bone that leads to the thumb joint.

He-7: At the little finger end of the wrist crease, next to the small bone (the pisiform bone) at the base of the hand.

He-8: Make a loose fist, and it is where the tip of the little finger touches the palm.

He-9: See back of the hand for its location.

Pc-8: Make a loose fist, and it is where the tip of the middle finger touches the palm.

Pc-9: See back of the hand for its location.

Points on the Legs
On the Legs 1: Back/Outside

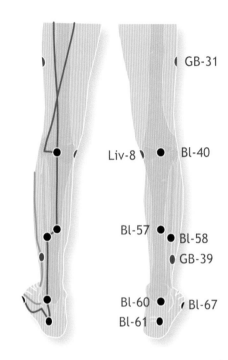

Bl-40: In the middle of the crease at the back of the knee.

Bl-57: On the midline of the back of the lower leg, halfway between the knee crease and the tip of the ankle bone (the lateral malleolus), at the start of the calf muscle.

Bl-58: A thumb width downwards and outwards from Bl-57.

GB-31: On the outside of the thigh, just over halfway between the knee crease and the end of the femor bone. Stand and put your hands relaxed at your sides. Put your middle finger on an imaginary trouser crease running down the sides of the legs. The point should be here.

GB-39: A hand width above the tip of the outside ankle bone (the lateral malleolus), between the fibula bone and the muscle.

On the Legs 2: Front/Inside

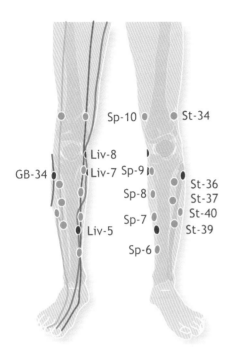

Sp-6: A hand width above the highest point of the inside ankle bone (the medial malleolus), just behind the tibia bone.

Sp-7: A hand width above Sp-6, just behind the tibia bone.

Sp-8: A hand width below Sp-9, just behind the tibia bone.

Sp-9: On the same level as the bottom edge of the bony protuberance below the knee (the tuberosity of the tibia). Feel down from the knee for this lump. The point is at the level of the bottom of this and also GB-34 on the other side of the leg. It is in the muscle just behind the tibia bone on the inside of the leg.

Sp-10: Three finger widths above the top of the knee cap in the thigh muscle, roughly in a straight line from Sp-9.

Kid-7: Three finger widths directly above Kid-3, next to the Achilles tendon.

Liv-5: One-third of the distance from the tip of the inside ankle bone (the medial malleolus) to the knee crease, between the calf muscle and the tibia bone.

Liv-7: In the top of the calf muscle, a thumb width behind Sp-9.

Liv-8: Just after the extreme inside end of the knee crease, when the knee is bent.

St-34: In the thigh muscle, three finger widths above and level with outside edge of the knee cap.

St-36: A hand width below the bottom of the kneecap, one finger-width outwards from the tibia bone.

St-37: A hand width below St-36, one finger width outwards from the tibia bone.

St-39: A hand width below St-37, one finger width outwards from the tibia bone.

St-40: In the lower leg, halfway between the bottom of the knee cap and the midpoint of the ankle bone. Two finger widths outwards from the tibia bone.

GB-34: On the outside of the lower leg, below the knee, a finger width and a half down and towards the centre line of the leg of the knobbly head of the fibula bone.

Points on the Feet/Ankles
On the Feet 1: Sole/Inside

Sp-1: Close to the inside edge of the nail bed, where the vertical and horizontal lines that mark the edges of the nail meet.

Sp-3: Before the ball on the inside of the foot, just below where the first metatarsal bone flares out.

Sp-4: On the inside of the foot, under the first metatarsal bone and three finger widths towards the ankle from Sp-3.

Sp-5: With the foot at a right angle, it lies at the intersection of a line marking the bottom of the inside ankle bone (the medial malleolus) and a line marking the front.

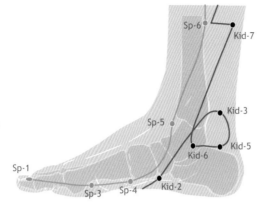

(left) Points on the feet: sole/inside

(right) Points on the feet: top/outside

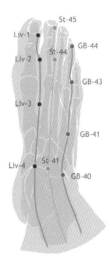

Kid-1: Two-thirds of the way up the sole of the foot, in the dip created when scrunching the foot forwards. For location see Foot massage points: right/left sole. It is in the same place as the Kidney area.

Kid-2: Halfway between the ball of the foot and the heel, under the foot bone on the inside of the foot.

Kid-3: Halfway between the tip of the inside ankle bone (the medial malleolus) and the Achilles tendon.

Kid-5: A thumb width directly below Kid-3.

Kid-6: A thumb width below the tip of the inside ankle bone (the medial malleolus).

On the Feet 2: Top/Outside

Liv-1: Close to the outside nail bed of the big toe, where the vertical and horizontal lines that mark the edges of the nail meet.

Liv-2: In the web between the big and second toes.

Liv-3: In the gap between the bones that lead to the big and second toes. Follow the gap up from Liv-2, and it is before the two metatarsal bones meet.

Liv-4: A thumb width forwards and level with the tip of the inside ankle bone (the medial malleolus).

St-45: Close to the outside edge of the nail bed. Where the vertical and horizontal lines that mark the edges of the nail meet.

St-44: At the web between the second and third toes.

St-41: At the midpoint of the front of the ankle, level with the outside ankle bone (the lateral malleolus).

GB-44: Close to the outside nail bed of the fourth toe, where the vertical and horizontal lines that mark the edges of the nail meet.

GB-43: In the web between the fourth and fifth toes.

GB-41: In the foot, between the metatarsal bones that lead to the fourth and fifth toes. Feel up from the toes to where the two bones meet farther up in the foot.

GB-40: Below the outside ankle bone (the lateral malleolus), where the lines of the forward horizontal and vertical edges meet.

Bl-60: Midway between the tip of the outside ankle bone (the lateral malleolus) and the Achilles tendon. For clearer location see Foot massage points: outside.

Bl-61: Two finger widths below Bl-60. For clearer location see Foot massage points: outside.

Bl-67: Close to the outside edge of the nail bed of the little toe, where the vertical and horizontal lines that mark the edges of the nail meet. For clearer location see Foot massage points: outside.

Chapter 16
氣 **Specific Massage Points on the Hand, Foot and Ear**

The channel points have been covered in the previous chapter. This section goes into more detail on the specific massage points and areas on the hand, foot, and ear.

Points on the Hand

As mentioned earlier, different Asian cultures view the points on the hand slightly differently. For this reason, they have formulated various theories about how the body is reflected on the hand, and where the best treatment areas are located. The following hand map is heavily influenced by older Chinese traditions and includes newer ideas from Chinese medicine, as well as one or two Korean additions.

I have included this map for its ease of use and with self-treatment in mind. Should you come across other maps with slightly different positioning elsewhere, do not be too dismayed. There is more than one path to good health.

A   Chest and respiratory area
B   Stomach, Spleen, and Large Intestine area
C   Head area
D   Essence area
E   Reproductive area
F   Insomnia areas
G   Hypertension areas
H   Dizziness area
I   Heart channel
J   Triple Burner channel
K   Pericardium channel
L   Large Intestine channel
M   Lung channel

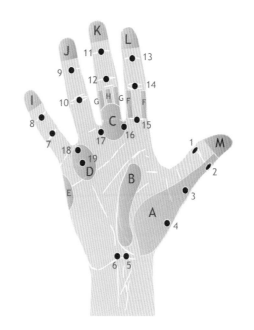

(top) Hand massage points: palm

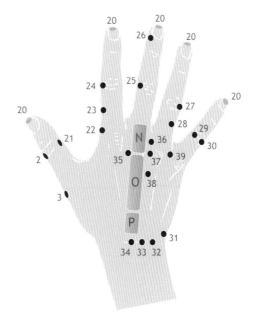

(bottom) Hand massage points: back

N	Cervical area
O	Thoracic area
P	Lumbar area

1	Spleen
2	Chest
3	Ankle
4	Tonsils
5	Reduce blood pressure
6	Heel pain
7	Liver
8	Kidneys
9	Lungs
10	Mingmen
11	Heart
12	Sanjiao
13	Large intestine
14	Small Intestine and Constipation
15	Cough
16	Fatigue
17	Toothache
18	Asthma
19	Palpitations
20	Shixuan
21	Eye
22	Shoulder
23	Knee 1
24	Forehead
25	Top of the head
26	Reduce fever
27	Temples
28	Knee 2
29	Perineum
30	Back of the head
31	Stop itching
32	Thyroid
33	Stop bleeding
34	Raise blood pressure
35	Stiff neck
36	Throat
37	Headache

(left) Foot massage points: right sole

(right) Foot massage points: left sole

38	Diarrhoea
39	Sciatica

Points on the Foot

As with the hand, the areas and points on the foot vary according to country and tradition. Western reflexologists may raise an eyebrow at some of the positioning of points, but Chinese traditional medicine has a slightly different take on how the feet reflect the body.

A	Brain
B	Frontal sinus
C	Eye
D	Ear
E	Nose
F	Neck
G	Thyroid
H	Lungs
I	Liver
J	Adrenal
K	Stomach
L	Pancreas
M	Duodenum

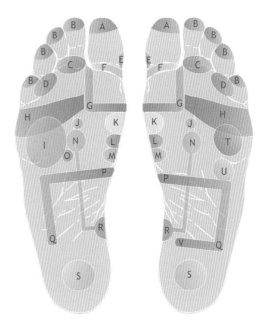

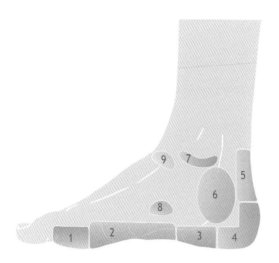

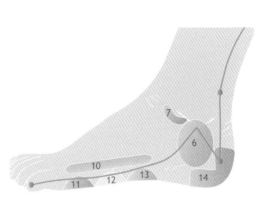

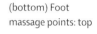

(top left) Foot massage points: inside

(top right) Foot massage points: outside

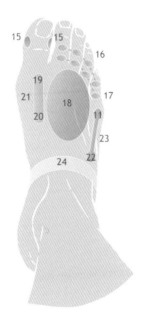

(bottom) Foot massage points: top

N   Kidneys
O   Gall bladder
P   Small intestine
Q   Large intestine
R   Bladder
S   Reproductive organs
T   Heart
U   Spleen
V   Rectum

1   Cervical area
2   Thoracic area
3   Lumbar area
4   Sacrum and coccyx
5   Rectum
6   Uterus or prostate glands
7   Hips
8   Ribs
9   Groin
10 Scapula
11 Elbow
12 Shoulder
13 Abdomen
14 Coccyx
15 Tonsils
16 Upper teeth
17 Lower teeth
18 Chest
19 Larynx
20 Trachea
21 Sternum
22 Shoulder
23 Upper arm
24 Diaphragm

Points on the Ear

As with both the hand and the foot previously, the ear too has no one fixed body map. Different cultures sometimes go in different directions, and so it is with the Chinese and Western ear images. They both share enough similarities, however, that they can be squashed like reluctant bedfellows into the following ear map.

In an attempt to make the map easier to use, the points are colour coded according to the part of the ear they are on.

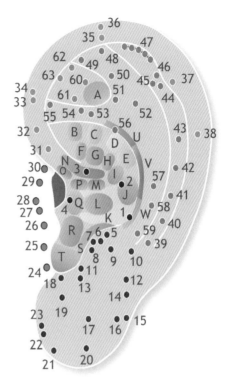

A   Shen Men
B   Bladder
C   Kidneys
D   Pancreas
E   Spleen
F   Large intestine
G   Small intestine
H   Duodenum
I   Stomach
J   Liver
K   Lung
L   Heart
M   Pericardium
N   Ovaries or testes
O   Mouth
P   Esophagus
Q   Trachea
R   Sanjiao
S   Brain
T   Endocrine
U   Lumbosacral area
V   Thoracic area
W   Cervical area
1   Dizziness
2   Muscle relaxation
3   Point zero
4   Throat
5   Occiput
6   Temples

7   Asthma
8   Forehead
9   Vertex
10   Antidepressant
11   Eye disorder 2
12   Upper jaw
13   Frontal sinus
14   Lower jaw
15   Trigeminal nerve
16   Inner ear
17   Eye
18   Blood pressure
19   Tooth
20   Tonsils
21   Nervousness
22   Dental analgesia
23   Master Cerebral
24   Eye disorder 1
25   Tranquilizer
26   Internal nose

27   External nose
28   Appetite control
29   Vitality
30   External ear
31   Rectum
32   Urethra
33   External genitals
34   Sympathetic
35   Allergy
36   Ear apex
37   Liver yang
38   Skin disorder
39   Insomnia 2
40   Master shoulder
41   Shoulder
42   Arm
43   Elbow
44   Wrist
45   Insomnia 1

46   Hand
47   Fingers
48   Toes
49   Ankle
50   Knee
51   Hip
52   Abdomen
53   Buttocks
54   Sciatic nerve
55   Prostate
56   Adrenal gland
57   Chest
58   Thyroid
59   Neck
60   Antihistamine
61   Constipation
62   Hypertension
63   Uterus

Part Five

What are the Main Syndromes and How Do You Treat Them?

Whilst there are intricate relationships and balances within the body on many different levels, they can be grouped together to create a set of generalized patterns common to us all. These patterns of imbalance form the basis of health or ill health and often are at the root of identified health conditions and illnesses. Each pattern comes with a set of symptoms that can identify it. But these are the possible symptoms, and it would be highly unlikely to find someone with all the listed symptoms at the same time. The patterns are not exclusive, and there can be several present at the same time in the same person. If this is so, as regards treatment, you have to decide which of the symptoms seem to be dominant and start there. The chapters that follow deal with symptom patterns that present as Syndromes of Weakness and Syndromes of Fullness, with full descriptions of their symptoms and suggested treatments.

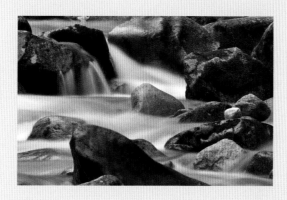

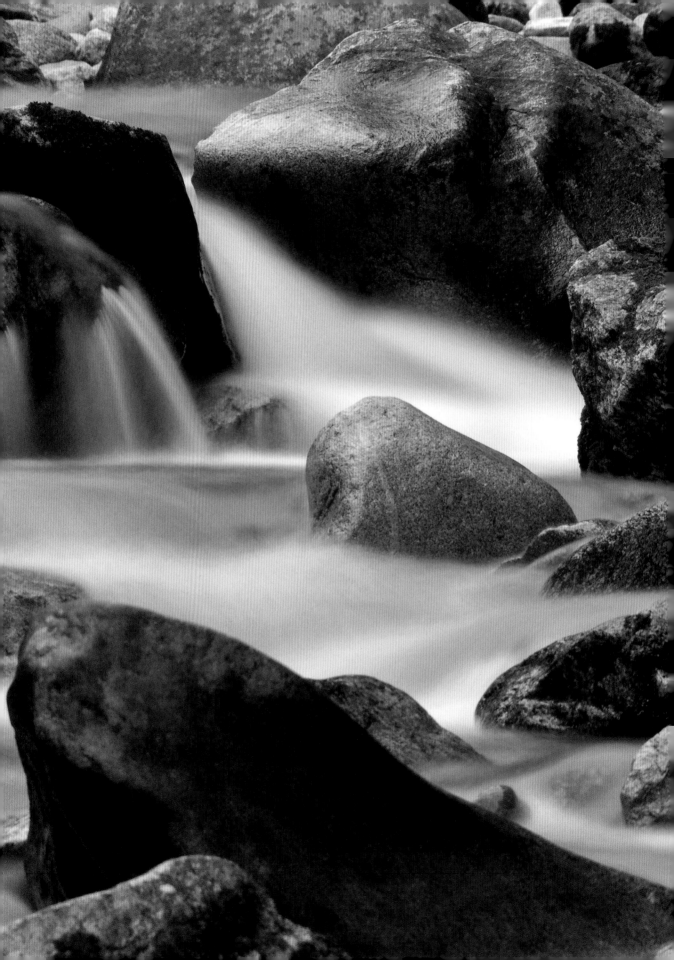

Chapter 17
氣 **Syndromes of Weakness**

Syndromes of Weakness occur when key substances in the body become weak and imbalanced due to:

- Weak qi
- Weak yang
- Weak yin
- Weak blood

Weak QI
Symptoms

Tiredness, low energy, weakness in your arms and legs, pale, loose stools, no appetite, feeling bloated after eating, occasional shortness of breath, easily catch colds.

Signs

A swollen tongue with possible teeth indentations at the sides and trembling when stuck out. Usually pale.

Can include or lead to

Underlying a whole host of medical conditions, both acute and chronic, anything from nasal allergies and chronic fatigue syndrome to depression and persistent back pain.

Common causes

Worrying, overstudying, being inactive, stooping over a desk for long periods, too much cold or raw food, eating in a hurry and at irregular times, emotional stress, chronic diseases, overuse of antibiotics for a cold or flu, smoking, or childbirth.

An explanation

This condition is an extremely common one, as most people exhaust their qi at some point in their lives. Some of us do it all the time!

Qi comes from the food we eat, from the air we breathe, and from the reserves we were born with. If our diet is not appropriate, or the quantity of air we breathe insufficient (through bad posture, for example), or if we lead a stressful lifestyle, sometimes there is not enough qi to keep pace with demand.

This condition often develops gradually over time and is not unlike a car running on empty. It will become slow, sluggish, parts will seize up, and the engine will smoke and rumble, even over short distances.

If there is not enough qi to power the body, it often means that the Spleen, Lungs, or Kidneys have become weak either directly through a poor diet, smoking or doing too much, or indirectly through the effects of emotional stress, which tends to affect the Liver and create blockages of qi.

Whatever the cause, the most effective ways to strengthen qi are those that most people have some degree of control over: diet, exercise, and lifestyle. A few simple changes can make all the difference for maintaining a healthy body.

Dietary factors that can weaken qi

- Irregular eating patterns, especially eating late at night and overeating and drinking too much during meal times, all weaken the digestive process and minimize the creation of qi.

- Microwave cooking tends to deplete the qi in the food being cooked, so while the food comes out cooked, it is no longer so nutritious.
- Cold-natured foods, such as salads, raw fruit, fruit juice, wheat, raw vegetables, tomatoes, tofu, sweet food, beer, brown rice, cold drinks from the refrigerator, and iced water, weaken qi if consumed in excess.
- Too many damp, congesting foods, such as dairy products, ice cream, concentrated orange juice, bread, and peanuts, also weaken qi. In particular, bad fats and refined carbohydrates, such as processed products containing sugar or corn syrup, flaked or puffed grains (breakfast cereals for example), wraps, cookies, chocolate, white flour, and white pasta.
- In small quantities (less than 2 grams a day) Vitamin C reduces heat, but when taken in excess it weakens qi.

Dietary factors that can strengthen qi

- Following a diet similar to the ideal diet, as detailed in the How We Eat section. Complex carbohydrates such as whole grains and legumes are important, as they support qi over a more extended period of time. They should be combined with large quantities of vegetables and with a small amount of good-quality protein and good fats.
- Food should be enjoyed and chewed slowly in a calm atmosphere, and you should follow many of the guidelines in the How We Eat section.
- Soups and stews are preferable, as they often help to strengthen qi and aid digestion.
- Qi can be strengthened with lightly cooked, simple food, such as the following:

FRUIT: cooked or stewed fruits, such as cherries, peaches, figs, grapes, coconut, and dates.

VEGETABLES: cooked vegetables, such as pumpkins, carrots, peas, potatoes, squashes, yams, sweet potatoes, leeks, olives, mushrooms, garlic, onions, and fennel. Preferably fresh and not frozen.

GRAINS: cooked white rice, oats, porridge (oatmeal), millet, corn, barley, and malt (but not cereal bars and most boxed breakfast cereals).

HERBS AND SPICES: warming herbs and spices, such as fresh ginger, sage, thyme, and nutmeg.

LEGUMES, SEEDS, AND NUTS: lentils, chickpeas (garbanzo), black beans, walnuts, and chestnuts.

MEAT AND SEAFOOD: small amounts of beef, lamb, chicken, ham, liver and kidney; also eel, herring, mackerel, salmon, trout, tuna, and anchovies.

DRINKS: Jasmine tea (especially with meals) and drinks at room temperature or above.

OTHERS: Bee pollen and royal jelly.

Acupressure and massage

ON THE LEGS: Thumb-press up the Spleen and Stomach channels to the knee. Knead any sore points, especially Sp-3 and St-36.

ON THE ARMS: Thumb-press up the Lung and Heart channels on the inside of the arm. Knead any sore points, including Lu-9 and He-7 on the palm side of the wrist.

ON THE BACK: Thumb press down the back muscles either side of the spine and hard press Bl-13, Bl-20 and Bl-23.

ON THE FRONT: Hard press Ren-6, Ren-12 and Ren-17 on the centre line of the body.

ON THE HANDS: Do the Healthy Hand massage in the How Can You Treat Yourself? section. Press and knead the following points if sore: Lung, Kidneys, Mingmen, Essence area, Stomach, Spleen, and Large Intestine area.

ON THE FEET: Do the Healthy Foot massage in the How Can you Treat Yourself? section. Also hard-press on the Kidneys, Stomach, Lungs, Pancreas, and Kid-3.

ON THE EARS: Do the Healthy Ear massage in the How Can You Treat Yourself? section. Press and knead the following points if sore: Spleen, Stomach, Heart, Kidneys, Lungs, Vitality, and Shen Men.

Scraping

Scrape down the muscles of the back, either side of the spine. Scrape lightly at first, especially if weak or frail. This can improve the circulation of qi and blood, which are often sluggish when qi is weak.

Tapping

Tap each point up to 30 times. You may need an assistant for the back area.

- Tap at regular intervals along the inner and outer Bladder channels on the back. Begin at the top, and complete both sides before moving downwards.
- Tap at regular intervals down the middle of the body, from the bottom of the breastbone, over the belly button, and down to where the pubic bone begins.
- Tap along the thigh muscles, then the calf muscles.

Exercises

Follow Exercises 1–6 of the five-element stretches, ideally on a daily basis. These stretches can help to strengthen the channels and organs that are weak.

The following Sotai exercises can also be very beneficial in strengthening qi:

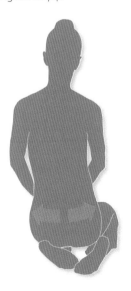

SWING YOUR BOTTOM: Kneel on the floor and rest your bottom on your heels. Move your bottom to one side, then slowly swing it across to the other side. Continue this movement for up to a few minutes.

CROUCH TWIST: Crouch on the floor, with your arms straight and palms and both knees touching the floor. Move your bottom to the right side, and at the same time twist your left shoulder down. Then slowly swing your bottom across to the left, and twist your right shoulder downwards. Repeat this swinging motion for up to a few minutes.

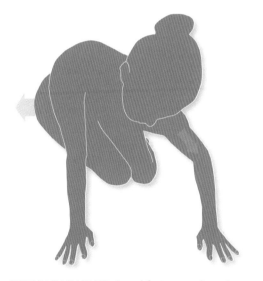

Crouch twist

SWING YOUR WAIST: Stand facing a wall, and press gently into the wall with both palms. Your arms should be slightly bent and the body upright. Swing your bottom slowly from side to side, whilst keeping your hands and feet stationary.

Swing your bottom

BEND YOUR HIP: Stand with your arms at your sides and your feet shoulders' width apart. Put your right hand on your right hip, and bend your body from the hip to the right. Return to the original position, then repeat the same sequence on the other side. Repeat several times on both sides.

ARM SWING: Stand with your arms at your sides and your feet shoulders' width apart. Breathe in and, as you breathe out, put your right hand on your right

(left) Swing
your waist

(centre) Bend
your hip

(right) Arm
swing

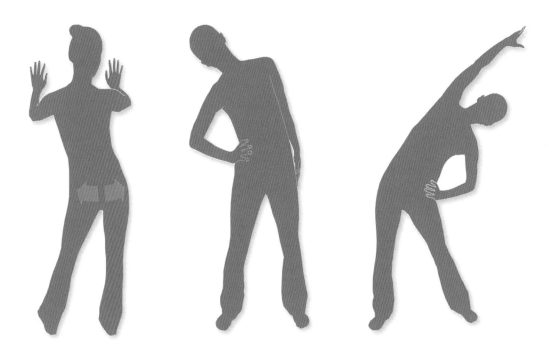

hip and lift up your left arm, as you bend to the right. Swing your arm so that it reaches above your head to the left, and continue to breathe out. Return to the original position, then repeat the same sequence on the other side. Repeat several times on both sides.

Lifestyle advice

- It is essential to take regular moderate exercise in the fresh air rather than indoors. A British review published in 2011 concluded that exercising in the natural environment gives greater feelings of revitalization, increased energy, and less tension, anger, and depression than indoors.[11]
- Breathing deeply, especially when in the fresh air, can strengthen the lungs but is so rarely practised. Most of us, most of the time, take shallow breaths and need to be reminded to fill our lungs.
- If seated for extended periods at work or school, for example, take frequent breaks. More information on this is in the lifestyle section.

Weak Yang
Symptoms

Lower backache, weak and cold knees, feeling cold in your back or abdomen, weak legs, apathy, tiredness, impotence, a desire to lie down, chronic digestive problems, diarrhoea, frequent visits to the toilet, being indecisive, and lacking in motivation.

Signs

A swollen tongue with teeth indentations at the sides and trembling when stuck out. Usually pale.

Can include or lead to

Cystitis, nephritis, prostatitis, urethritis, sexual problems such as frigidity, impotence and premature ejaculation, depression, anxiety, recurrent lumbago, sciatica, rheumatoid arthritis, impaired hearing, and tinnitus.

Common causes

A chronic illness, old age, too much cold or raw food, exposure to a cold or damp environment, overexercise at a young age, worry, overthinking, stress, lack of exercise, or being constitutionally weak.

An explanation

Yin and yang balance each other in the body to maintain good health. There are times of the day when one is more predominant than the other, such as yin at night and yang in the daytime, but there is a constant waxing and waning movement between them throughout the day, as the body reacts to the stresses and strains of our daily life.

Sometimes an imbalance develops that tips the scales too much on one side. This could result from a host of factors, from a poor diet that weakens digestion to a sedentary lifestyle that affects the circulation of qi.

When yang becomes weak, it can no longer exert control over yin, and characteristic yin signs such as a feeling of cold in the lower back or on the abdomen become pronounced. The condition is very much an extension of that detailed in the weak qi section earlier, except with the addition of cold.

In order to help the body rebalance yin and yang, it is essential to strengthen yang by making dietary changes. Diet is often one of the main contributing factors to weak yang.

Dietary factors that can weaken yang

- Eating energetically cold foods such as salad is often considered an essential part of a healthy diet, but if you have weak yang it is not unlike using freezing water to melt ice. For this reason, avoid cool or cold-natured foods, especially raw fruit and raw vegetables, as they can weaken Spleen yang when overconsumed. The following foods should also be avoided or reduced:

FRUIT: citrus fruits, such as grapefruit, lemons, and limes, and all raw fruits, particularly tropical fruit such as mangos, kiwis, and bananas.

VEGETABLES: raw vegetables, salads, tomatoes, summer squash, cucumbers, spinach, and Brussels sprouts.

HERBS AND SPICES: peppermint and excessive amounts of salt.

DRINKS: soy milk, fruit juice, carrot juice, green or black tea, strong alcohol, and iced drinks, including iced water.

OTHER: dairy products, chocolate, ice cream, tofu, vinegar, refined sugars, and excess vitamin C as its strong cooling effect damages yang.

Dietary factors that can strengthen yang

- As with weak qi, in order to strengthen yang, a diet of mostly vegetables and grains and only a small amount of meat or high-quality protein is needed. Warming foods that are pungent help digestion. Salty foods strengthen the Kidneys. Sweet foods strengthen the Spleen and strengthen yang. A combination of these include the following:

FRUIT: stewed fruits, in particular apricots, cherries, peaches, plums, raisins, and dates.

VEGETABLES: lightly cooked onions, leeks, garlic, parsnips, sweet potatoes, onions, pumpkins, squash, carrots, peas, fennel, turnip, and garlic. Preferably fresh and not frozen.

GRAINS: cooked grains, such as rice, oats, roasted barley, and millet (but not cereal bars and most packaged breakfast cereals).

LEGUMES, SEEDS, AND NUTS: black beans, chickpeas (garbanzo), hazelnuts, walnuts, pistachios, and chestnuts.

HERBS AND SPICES: warm spices, such as cloves, black peppercorn, ginger (fresh and dry), cardamom, rosemary, turmeric, nutmeg, black pepper, cloves, and cinnamon.

MEAT AND SEAFOOD: chicken, lamb, beef, mackerel, tuna, anchovies, salmon, prawns, and shellfish.

DRINKS: fennel tea and red grape juice. All drinks should be at room temperature or above.

OTHERS: soups and honey.

Acupressure and massage

ON THE LEGS: Thumb-press up the Spleen and Stomach channels to the knee. Knead any sore points, especially St-36.

ON THE ARMS: Thumb-press up the Lung and Heart channels on the inside of the arm. Knead any sore points, including Lu-9 and He-7 on the palm side of the wrist.

ON THE BACK: Thumb-press down the back muscles either side of the spine, and hard-press Bl-13, Bl-20, Bl-23, and Du-4.

ON THE FRONT: Hard-press Ren-6, Ren-12 and Ren-17 on the centre line of the body.

ON THE HANDS: Press and knead the following points if sore: Lungs, Kidneys, Mingmen, Essence area, and Stomach, Spleen, and Large Intestine area. Do the Healthy Hand massage in the How Can You Treat Yourself? section.

ON THE FEET: Do the Healthy Foot massage in the How Can You Treat Yourself? section. Also hard-press Kidneys, Stomach, Lungs, Pancreas, Sp-3, Kid-3, and Kid-7.

ON THE EARS: Do the Healthy Ear massage in the How Can You Treat Yourself? section. Press and knead the following points if sore: Spleen, Stomach, Kidneys, Lungs, Vitality, and Shen Men.

Scraping

Scrape down the back muscles either side of the spine. Scrape lightly, if frail or weak. As in the case of Weak qi, the Scraping can improve what is normally sluggish circulation.

Tapping

Tap each point up to 30 times. You many need an assistant for the back area.

- Tap at regular intervals along the inner and outer Bladder channels on the back. Begin at the top and complete both sides before moving downwards.
- Tap along the thigh muscles and then the calf muscles.
- Tap at regular intervals down the middle of the body from the bottom of the breastbone over the belly button and up to where the pubic bone begins.

Exercises

Follow Exercises 1–6 of the five element stretches. Ideally, do the sequence daily and without exertion. Do any of the supplementary exercises in the Weak Qi section.

Lifestyle advice

It is very important to dress appropriately for the season and weather, keeping warm, especially around the lower back and abdomen. If it feels comfortable, use a heat source such as a hot water bottle. Take gentle regular exercise but nothing more until you regain your energy reserves. Do not push yourself unless really necessary.

Weak Yin
Symptoms

Lower backache, sweating at night, dizziness, dry mouth at night, dull headache at the back of your head, vertigo, tinnitus, poor memory, deafness, thirsty, sore back, aching in your bones, dark, scanty urine, constipation, strong dreams, dry cough, and feeling worse in the evenings.

Signs

A red tongue with cracks and/or patches where the coating is absent. Also possible red cheeks and dark(ish) urine.

Can include or lead to

Insomnia, migraines, high blood pressure, glaucoma, diabetes, tremors, hypochondriac pain, chronic gastritis, gastric neurosis, recurrent lumbago, anxiety, deafness, and impaired hearing.

Common causes

Emotional stress, overwork, too much sexual activity, long-term worrying, a stressful busy life, a chronic illness, lack of routine, going to bed late, playing computer games, or using a computer for extended periods.

An explanation

The balance between yin and yang is constantly oscillating, and with a busy lifestyle it can be relatively easy for the level of yin to drop below that of yang. The level of yin often drops because of the presence of internal heat drying it up. Any long-standing heat, whether akin to a gentle simmer or a full-blasting furnace, will gradually burn up yin. This heat commonly develops from stagnation resulting from overwork, stress, and unresolved emotional issues.

When the levels of yin are exhausted, yang cannot be contained. The hot, agitated signs of yang appear in the body, especially in the afternoon and at night, when yin is normally dominant. In order to replenish yin and help restore the yin-yang balance, changes in eating habits and lifestyle often have to be made to reduce overstimulation and direct sources of heat.

Dietary factors that can weaken yin

- Hot or warm-natured foods, especially those that are pungent, bitter, and sour, including foods such as citrus fruits, cinnamon, cloves, and ginger, lamb, coffee, red wine, and spirits.
- Avoid roasting and deep-frying as these encourage more heat.

Dietary factors that can strengthen yin

- A wide and varied nourishing diet will help the digestive process and the body's ability to transform food into qi. After being transformed, qi gets sent down to the Kidneys, where it is stored and forms the basis of both the yin and the yang of the body.
- To help yin, it is therefore important to strengthen the Stomach and digestion. The diet for Weak Qi would form a good basis for this, with its stress on complex carbohydrates and vegetables and only a small amount of high-quality protein. The difference here is the addition of more fruit and high-quality, very nutritious fatty foods, such as dairy products (from a cow, goat, or sheep) which strongly benefit yin.
- The predominance of these sweet and sour cooling foods needed to strengthen yin can have negative effects – too many cool-natured foods can damage the Stomach and Spleen. Ideally, foods should involve more stews and steaming. In addition to food to strengthen qi, more of an emphasis on high-quality protein and the following foods will help strengthen yin:

FRUIT: apples, pears, grapes, pineapples, tomatoes, blackberries, strawberries, wolf or goji berries, bananas, and watermelon.

VEGETABLES: peas, spinach, seaweed salad, and asparagus (in moderation: too much asparagus can damage Kidney qi).

GRAINS: corn, rice, and wheat, including pasta and noodles.

LEGUMES, SEEDS, AND NUTS: high-quality protein and omega 3–rich foods, such as flax, pumpkin, sunflower and black sesame seeds, walnuts, chestnuts, and kidney-shaped foods, such as black beans and kidney beans.

MEAT AND SEAFOOD: good-quality pork, duck, fish, and shrimp strengthen yin, but only when eaten in small amounts (about ten percent of your diet).

DRINKS: red fruit juice, citrus juice, milk (goat's or sheep's milk is less damp), and homemade fruit smoothies.

OTHER: olive oil, cheese, eggs, omelettes, and a small amount of salty-flavoured foods, such as miso, sea salt, salted raw sauerkraut, or Korean kimchi.

CAUTION: Many people have weak yin inside but outside have lots of damp (otherwise known as fat). If so, avoid some of the more damp-forming foods and drinks from the above lists. See the section on Damp for more details.

Acupressure and massage

ON THE LEGS: Thumb-press up to the knee along the Liver and Kidney channels on the inside of the leg and the Gall bladder and Stomach channels on the outside. Knead any sore points, and hard-press Liv-8, Sp-6, St-36, and Kid-6 (on the ankles).

ON THE BACK: Thumb- or finger-press down the back muscles either side of the spine. Knead any sore points, and hard-press Bl-15, Bl-18, Bl-21, and Bl-23.

ON THE FRONT: Hard-press Ren-6 and Ren-4 on the midline below the belly button.

ON THE HANDS: Press and knead the following if sore: Kidneys, Stomach, Essence area, Liver, and Mingmen. Do the Healthy Hand massage in the How Can You Treat Yourself? section.

ON THE FEET: Press and knead the following if sore: Kidneys, Liver, and Stomach.

Do the Healthy Foot massage in the How Can You Treat Yourself? section.

ON THE EARS: Do the Healthy Ear massage in the How Can You Treat Yourself? section. Press and knead the following if sore: Kidneys, Spleen, Heart, Vitality, and Shen Men.

Scraping

Scrape down the whole back either side of the spine. Concentrate on the band of muscle that runs parallel to the spine, which can often be tense.

Tapping

Tap each point up to 30 times. You may need an assistant for the back area.

- Press and tap any sore points across the shoulders and down the back muscles on either side of the spine.
- Tap down the muscles on the outside of the upper arm and forearm.
- Tap down the midline of the abdomen from the breastbone to Ren-4.
- Tap Kid-3, Kid-6, and Kid-7 on the foot and leg.

Exercises

Follow Exercises 1–6 of the five-element stretches. Ideally, repeat the stretches on a daily basis, especially Exercise 5, which strengthens the Kidneys and can help rebalance yin.

Lifestyle advice

- Listen to your body. If it is telling you that it has had enough, do not ignore it. It is very easy to push yourself for all sorts of reasons, whether at work, home, or study, but if you are tired, then to preserve your yin, you have to rest.

- When yin is weak, it often helps to reduce all sources of stimulation. This means getting serious (at least temporarily) about shutting down the computer, turning off the television, and avoiding media of any kind. You may gasp with horror at being disconnected from the 21st century, but these activities have a very strong draining effect on yin, especially when they are part of your daily habits.

NOTE: Some medical drugs, such as nonsteroidal anti-inflammatories, can damage Stomach yin when taken regularly.

Weak Blood

Symptoms

Pale lips, dizziness, numb arms or legs, blurred vision, "floaters" in your vision, insomnia and difficulty falling asleep, poor memory, muscular weakness, muscle cramp, headaches, weak nails, painful or light periods, and dry eyes, hair, and skin.

Signs

A pale, dry tongue that may be thin.

Can include or lead to

A whole range of conditions, most notably anaemia, neuroses, dysmenorrhea, amenorrhea, sleepwalking, and mental instability.

Common causes

A diet lacking in nourishment for blood; overexercise; heavy bleeding, especially during childbirth; anxiety; worrying over things you cannot change; going to bed late; too much watching television, looking at a computer screen, or playing video games.

An explanation

For clarity, the term "weak blood" does not refer to an actual physical lack of blood in the blood vessels. The same quantity of blood is present as normal in the body, but the quality is different as it lacks adequately energized cells.

Blood becomes energized through organ interaction in the body. The Spleen transforms food into energy, the Lungs transform energy from the air we breathe, the Kidneys send up energy from the body's stores of qi, the Heart acts as the pumping station, and the Liver acts as a blood storehouse.

Weakness in any one of these can have knock-on effects on the others with regards to how strong the energy within the blood is. The organs most involved are normally the Spleen, Heart, or Liver. If there is insufficient energy or qi in the blood, it can nourish only those areas of the body nearest to where the energy is created and stored. Any parts of the body that are farther away, such as the head, the hands, and the feet, can become prone to undernourishment. Common symptoms include dizziness, numbness, and cramp.

In order to strengthen the blood, you will need to make changes to your dietary habits and include simpler, more nutritious meals, as well as change taxing lifestyle habits so that the body can rest and rejuvenate.

Dietary factors that can weaken the blood

- Warm or hot foods that are also bitter or pungent, such as cinnamon and coffee, have a drying effect on the blood and weaken it.
- Refined carbohydrates, sugary foods, foods with chemical additives, and foods containing high amounts of saturated fats (bad fats) can adversely affect the Liver and Spleen and so also the blood. Spices like dry ginger, pepper, and cinnamon, and also drinks like coffee (decaffeinated included), hot

chocolate, energy drinks, soft fizzy drinks, and strong alcohol can all have a heating effect on the body and weaken the blood.

Dietary factors that can strengthen the blood

- Ideally a lightly cooked diet consisting of neutral foods that are sweet to build up the Spleen and sour for the Liver should be followed.
- Vegetables should form the main part of your diet, especially those high in folic acid such as dark leafy greens and broccoli. This should be supported by complex carbohydrates like rice and lentils or other strengthening grains or legumes. There is a stronger focus here on high-quality protein like meat, seafood, eggs, nuts and seeds.
- The natural colour of foods sometimes plays an important role in how they react in the body. This is particularly true of blood-enriching foods. Dark red and dark green are the key colours of fruit and vegetables for strengthening blood.
- Many of the following foods strengthen blood:

FRUIT: many naturally red fruits such as red apples, grapes, cherries, wolfberries and plums, and also dried apricots, dried figs, prunes, lychees and coconut. Seasonal fruit is preferable.

VEGETABLES: all green leafy vegetables, such as spinach, cabbage, and broccoli, naturally red (ish) vegetables such as carrots and beetroot, and also seaweed and fennel. Preferably fresh and not frozen.

GRAINS: rice, porridge (oatmeal), oats, and millet.

HERBS AND SPICES: parsley and watercress.

LEGUMES, SEEDS, AND NUTS: lentils, mung beans, black sesame seeds, pumpkin seeds, and sunflower seeds.

MEAT AND SEAFOOD: chicken; beef; liver; shellfish, such as mussels, oysters and clams; sardines; crab; eel; and octopus. High-quality (organic or chemical-free) animal protein is rich in Vitamin B12, which is very strengthening for blood.

DRINKS: Small amounts of some alcohol, such as stout and red wine; rosehip tea; hibiscus tea; red grape juice; and water at room temperature or above.

OTHERS: bee pollen, royal jelly, soups, stocks or broths, eggs, and fermented foods such as sauerkraut, kimchi, yogurt, and miso.

Acupressure and massage

ON THE BACK: Thumb-press down the muscles of the back either side of the spine and knead any points if sore. Also hard-press Bl-17, Bl-18, Bl-19, Bl-20, and Bl-23.

ON THE LEGS: Hard-press Sp-6, Sp-10, Liv-8, and St-36.

ON THE HANDS: Do the Healthy Hand massage in the How Can You Treat Yourself? section. Knead any sore points, including Heart, Liver, and Stomach, Spleen, and Large Intestine areas.

ON THE FEET: Do the Healthy Foot massage in the How Can You Treat Yourself? section. Also knead the Liver, Spleen, Heart, and Essence areas, if sore.

ON THE EARS: Do the Healthy Ear massage in the How Can You Treat Yourself? section.

Press and knead the following if sore: Liver, Spleen, Heart, Stomach, and Endocrine.

Scraping

Scrape very softly down the back muscles either side of the spine. Increase pressure only if comfortable for the recipient.

Tapping

Tap each point up to 30 times. You may need an assistant for the back area.

- Tap down the back muscles either side of the spine, especially Bl-18, Bl-20, and Bl-23, if sore.
- Tap Sp-10, St-36, and Liv-8 on the leg.
- Tap Liv-3 on the foot.

Exercises

Follow Exercises 1–6 of the five-element stretches. Do the sequence daily, slowly and methodically. It is also very important not to overdo the exercises, as this can be counterproductive.

Lifestyle advice

- Relaxation and rest are as good as any treatment for this condition and should not be underestimated. Find time to relax and rest, even if your schedule is busy.
- Try to stabilize your day-to-day activities. For example, make sure you eat and sleep at the same time every day.
- Heavy blood loss during periods can be caused by contraceptive devices like the coil. Blood loss may be reduced by changing the form of contraception to one that is less physically invasive.

Chapter 18
氣 Syndromes of Fullness

These patterns occur when key substances in the body become too abundant or forceful due to:

- Qi stagnation
- Yang rising
- Damp
- Phlegm
- Blood stagnation
- Heat
- Cold

Qi Stagnation
Symptoms

Feeling bloated, tight chest, depressed, irritable, easy to upset, burping, wind, nausea, a lump in the throat, tense and stressed, irregular periods, swollen and painful breasts, premenstrual tension, muscle tension in the neck and back, and pain that comes and goes.

Signs

Possible redness or discolouration at the sides of the tongue and a green (ish) colour around the mouth.

Can include or lead to

A whole host of conditions, but especially those of pain, depression, high blood pressure, migraines, menstrual disorders such as premenstrual syndrome, endometriosis, amenorrhea and dysmenorrhea, indigestion, gastritis, hepatitis, neurosis, and chronic fatigue syndrome.

Common causes

Emotional stress, especially when emotions are repressed, frustration that has been building up, resentment, overwork, work stress, lack of regular exercise, and bad posture.

An explanation

Qi should flow around the body smoothly and harmoniously, and it is one of the functions of the Liver to ensure that it does. Sometimes the Liver, which acts like an engine generator, is prevented from maintaining this flow of qi, as it is very susceptible to stress and anger. Both of these cause it to shudder to a halt and create obstructions in vulnerable places in the body.

When an obstruction appears in the flow, qi slows down as it attempts to squeeze past. This often creates a buildup of qi behind it, with associated pressure, agitation, heat, and pain.

The flow of qi is not unlike the road system of a major city. Outside of rush hour the cars move freely, but when commuters leave work and head home the traffic builds up. A traffic accident can then create major holdups: the cars in the midst of the jam have engines running and honk their horns, and drivers become thoroughly frustrated.

Stagnation of qi is very much about getting stuck and agitated. Physically tight muscles can cause pain and discomfort, but mentally, emotions can also get stuck, and it can be difficult to "snap out of it" when irritable, stressed, or depressed.

In order to lessen qi stagnation, it is essential to be aware of the importance of letting out emotions.

Unexpressed emotions tend to fester and deepen stagnation of qi. Dietary habits often need to change and a commitment to regular exercise made.

Dietary factors that can stagnate qi

- Overeating and an irregular diet involving comfort eating or skipping meals will weaken the Stomach and worsen stagnation.
- Some foods are harder to digest than others, and with a condition of stagnation they are best reduced or avoided altogether. The following foods are common examples:

  Oversalted, processed, or sweetened foods and foods high in unhealthy saturated fats and oils (bad fats), such as tinned meat, vegetables, or ready-to-eat meals; cream, cheese, sandwich spreads, eggs, red meat, pizza, French fries, nuts, and margarine; rich, greasy food, such as lamb, beef, and creamy or cheesy sauces.

- Some people with this condition crave spicy, hot food because eating it will temporarily move qi and make them feel better. This is not a good idea, however, as when qi gets stuck, it begins to generate heat. If hot food is then added to this heat, the condition may worsen. For this reason, it is best to avoid hot spices like chilli, cayenne, Tabasco, and pepper.

  Also for this reason, it is preferable to avoid coffee and other sources of caffeine, fizzy soft drinks, fruit-flavoured soft drinks, and alcohol.

Dietary factors that can reduce stagnation

- Eating less is one of the most important strategies. Ideally, the stomach should be only two-thirds full after meals.
- Eating calmly, without distractions, and chewing food well will ease its passage through the body and reduce the likelihood of stagnation.
- A very important point for people with a tendency

towards qi stagnation is to avoid being too fixated on diet. Part of the imbalance of this condition is the tendency to stick unwaveringly to a set of instructions. It is important to be relaxed about any change in diet and not to be totally rigid about what you can or cannot eat. The resulting stress of worrying about your diet may mean you end up with more of the very same condition that you are trying to relieve!

- Strong qi in the Stomach and Spleen can help control the Liver, so food that nourishes qi as described in Weak Qi will also help this condition. The focus of your diet should be on vegetables, supported with smaller amounts of complex carbohydrates and an even smaller amount of high-quality protein. Pungent spices and good fats can be added to encourage the movement of qi.
- The following foods can be of great benefit in removing stagnation:

FRUIT: grapefruit, citrus peel, peaches, cherries, and plums.

VEGETABLES: watercress, onions, beetroot, carrots, garlic, radishes, cabbage, turnips, cauliflower, broccoli, Brussels sprouts, and celery.

HERBS AND SPICES: turmeric, basil, cardamom, marjoram, cumin, horseradish, rosemary, cloves, caraway, coriander, and chives.

LEGUMES, SEEDS, AND NUTS: chestnuts, pine nuts, and black sesame seeds.

MEAT AND SEAFOOD: prawns and shrimp.

DRINKS: fennel, jasmine, aniseed, dill, and chamomile tea.

OTHER: apple cider vinegar and extra virgin olive oil.

Acupressure and massage

ON THE HEAD: Press and knead GB-20 and any other sore points at the base of the back of the head (the occiput).

ON THE BACK: Thumb- or finger-press down the muscles on either side of the spine, and knead any sore areas, especially Bl-18.

ON THE FRONT: Press Liv-13, Liv-14, and around Ren-17, and knead if sore.

ON THE LEGS: Thumb-press along the Liver and Gall Bladder channels up to the knee. Knead any sore points, especially GB-34.

ON THE ARMS: Thumb-press along the Triple Burner channel up to the elbow, and knead any sore points, including TB-6.

ON THE HANDS: Do the Healthy Hand massage in the How Can You Treat Yourself? section. Also knead LI-4, Liver, Sanjiao, and any sore points.

ON THE FEET: Do the Healthy Foot massage in the How Can You Treat Yourself? section. Also press and knead the following, if sore: Liv-3, Liver, Chest, Cervical, Thoracic, and Lumbar areas and Shoulder.

ON THE EARS: Do the Healthy Ear massage in the How Can You Treat Yourself? section. Look for any sore, reactive points; in particular, check Liver, Cervical, Thoracic, and Lumbosacral areas, Shen Men, and Point Zero.

Scraping

Scrape down the neck, across the shoulders, and down the upper back. The muscles may feel tight in these areas, so be aware of any sensitivity. Start lightly and gradually increase the pressure. The spots that appear on the skin can often be deep red and purple if the stagnation is strong.

Tapping

Tap each point up to 30 times. An assistant may be needed for the back area.

- Tap GB-20 at the base of the occiput and then any tender points over the top of the shoulder. Feel for them first with your fingers.
- Tap carefully along the bottom of the ribcage from the breastbone, then down the midline from the bottom of the breastbone to the start of the pubic bone. This involves Tapping down the stomach and abdominal areas, so tap gently.
- Tap down the back muscles on either side of the spine. Tap both sides before moving downwards towards the hips. You can feel for any sore spots with your finger as you go.
- Tap down the Liver channel on the legs, from the knees (Liv-8) to the toes (Liv-1).

Exercises

Do Exercises 1–6 on a daily basis, preferably after waking. Especially useful are Exercises 3, 5, and 6.

Lifestyle advice

- Emotions play a major part in this condition, and the ability to release or express repressed emotions or to remove the cause of these emotions can often have a dramatic effect on a person. This could be anything from confiding in someone to formal therapy.
- Lack of exercise is a major contributing factor to stagnation, so it is essential to do regular exercise. This may mean leaving the car at home and walking, going swimming, cycling, dancing, running – whatever is practicable and enjoyable.
- Some very tense people prefer to play equally tense sports, such as squash, and end up no less tense afterwards than before. It is important, therefore, that there is a sense of relaxation in the exercise.
- Stress and overwork can often be unavoidable but, in order to improve this condition, it is necessary to adapt your home life or working life to lessen them. This can often appear impossible in the busy life most of us lead, but there are always things that can be changed if you have the desire and the will to change them.

Yang Rising

Symptoms

Headache at the temples, behind the eyes, on one side of the head, or only at weekends; migraine; dizziness; ringing in the ears; insomnia; irritability; and a tendency to get angry easily.

Signs

The tongue, eyes, and face may appear red and urine may be dark.

Can include or lead to

High blood pressure, vertigo, ear and hearing problems, Ménière's disease, migraines, hyperthyroidism, menopausal problems, chronic hepatitis, and eye problems like conjunctivitis.

Common causes

Emotional stress, including repressed emotions. In particular, anger or frustration over a long period of time, stress, overwork, and unhealthy eating patterns.

Explanation

Yang rising is the consequence of a strong imbalance between yin and yang. Yin and yang are in constant change but are able to control each other as long as both have sufficient energy to do so. If however one becomes weaker, it no longer acts as a counterbalance, and there is a tendency for the other to dominate. In this case, yin has been weakened and yang has become so agitated that it can no longer be held in its place.

The relationship is similar to a car engine and its coolant system. When you drive the engine heats up, but the amount of heat is regulated by the water in the radiator. If the car is not well maintained, however, the water levels might drop, so that the next time you go for a drive there is nothing to stop the engine temperature from rising. The car might then splutter to a halt in a cloud of steam.

Yin is often weakened by heat generated from stagnation or from a poor diet of heating, fatty foods. The out-of-control yang then rises, like hot steam, all the way through the body up to the head, and as a result often causes symptoms in the top part of the body, such as headaches and dizziness.

In order to prevent the rising of yang, the imbalance between yin and yang has to be addressed, or the same process will happen again and again. This usually involves dietary changes and self-massage as detailed here and in the Weak Yin section.

Dietary factors that can worsen rising yang

- Hot or warm-natured foods, such as lamb, spices, and coffee, can fuel the heat and send even more yang upwards.
- Oily, fatty, processed foods high in bad fats will cause qi to slow down and get stuck, which will then add to the heat. The following foods should be avoided:

FRUIT: citrus fruits and melons.
VEGETABLES: chilies, onions, shallots, leeks, and garlic.
SPICES AND HERBS: pungent spices such as cinnamon, ginger, basil, cloves, and black pepper.
MEAT AND SEAFOOD: lamb, veal, shrimp, and prawns.
DRINKS: warm or bitter drinks like coffee and tea, especially green tea; also beer, red wine, and strong alcohol.
OTHER: vinegar, pickles, tofu, dairy products, and fried food.

Dietary factors that can lessen rising yang

- An ideal diet should include roughly equal proportions of carbohydrates, vegetables (especially green leafy vegetables), and fruit (preferably cooked or stewed) and only a small amount of high-quality protein and fats. As this condition is essentially an extension of weak yin, refer to Weak Yin for more details.

• Sour and bitter cooling foods can help strengthen yin and reduce the heat. NOTE: Eating too many of the following foods may cause other complications, so apply a little common sense, and combine foods and eat in moderation:

FRUIT: plums, rhubarb, radishes, pears, mulberries, blueberries, and blackberries.
VEGETABLES: mung beans, celery, carrots, seaweed, lettuce, cucumber, watercress, and mushrooms.
GRAINS: wheat, oats, rice, millet, barley, and millet.
LEGUMES, SEEDS, AND NUTS: black beans, black soya beans, kidney beans, and black sesame seeds.
MEAT AND SEAFOOD: clams, oysters, and duck.
DRINKS: peppermint tea.
OTHER: extra virgin olive oil, tofu, eggs, and soya milk.

Acupressure and massage

ON THE HEAD: Press the areas around GB-9 and GB-20, and knead if sore.
ON THE BACK: Press and knead GB-21, if sore.
ON THE FEET AND LEGS: Thumb-press along the Liver channel up to the knee. Knead any sore points, including Liv-2 and Liv-3 (both on the feet).
ON THE ARMS: Thumb-press along the Triple burner channel up to the elbow. Knead any sore points, including TB-5.
ON THE HANDS: Do the Healthy Hand massage in the How Can You Treat Yourself? section. Press and knead the following, if sore: Liver, Sanjiao, Kidneys, Head area, Top of the Head, Temples, Forehead, and Back of the Head.
ON THE EARS: Squeeze the front of the ear lobe with the nail of your index finger and look for sore, reactive points. Also press and knead Liver yang and Liver area, if sore.

Scraping

Scrape the upper back, neck, and shoulders. Always scrape either downwards or away from the centre of the body. Be aware that muscles in the neck and shoulder area may be very tight and potentially sore at first.

Tapping

Tap each point up to 30 times. You may need an assistant for the neck/shoulder area.

• Tap GB-20 at the base of the occiput, then any tender points over the top of the shoulder, in particular GB-21. Feel for any sore areas with your fingers first.
• Tap along the Liver and Gall Bladder channels on the leg between the knee and the toes.
• Tap Bl-60 and the area around the Achilles tendon when standing and then LI-4 on the hand when sitting.
• Tap the following nail points:

Fingers: Lu-11, Pc-9, He.9, LI-1, TB-1, and SI-1. Toes: Sp-1, Liv-1, Kid-1 (on the sole), St-45, GB-44, and Bl-67. These should be easy to locate as they are at the corner of the nails.

Exercises

Do Exercises 1–6 of the five-element stretches on a daily basis. Exercises 5 and 6 are particularly useful.

Lifestyle advice

• This condition does not just appear one day out of the blue. It builds up gradually, like a pressure cooker, until one day the lid pops off. So quite often, patterns in your life need to change to reduce the likelihood of this. As yang rising is an extension of yin weakness, the same Lifestyle advice for Weak Yin applies here.

- In addition, there is a strong emotional component – especially when that emotion is being in some way repressed. Smoldering resentment and frustration at being passed over for a job promotion, for example, can quite easily be the pressure increase that pops the lid. It is very important not to let strong emotions like this take hold inside. Usually this means sharing how you feel with family, friends, or people you trust.

Damp

Symptoms

Heavy limbs, heavy head, reduced appetite and weak digestion, a congested feeling in the chest, a bloated feeling, an inability to concentrate, dull aches in joints, swellings, and muzzy headaches.

Signs

A swollen-looking tongue that may have teeth marks at the sides, a yellow colour around the mouth and eyes, and urine might be cloudy.

Can include or lead to

Obesity, arthritis, gastroenteritis, chronic gastritis, chronic colitis, irritable bowel syndrome, Crohn's disease, chronic bronchitis, rhinitis, asthma, bronchiectasis, oedema in legs and ankles, urinary tract infection, cystitis, urinary tract stones, or prostate disorders.

Common causes

A diet high in processed, fatty foods, exposure to the weather, living in a damp environment, worrying about things you cannot change, and overstudying.

An explanation

Body fluids are essential to ensure our bodies are properly lubricated. Sometimes however the body overproduces and accumulates excess body fluids, a situation known as excess "damp".

An excess of damp is often caused by a weakness in the Stomach and Spleen during the digestive process. These two digestive organs are unable to process and digest the food efficiently, usually as a result of a rich diet of fried, processed, damp-forming foods. The weaker these two organs are, the harder they will have to work, and the greater chance that they will generate damp and store it in the form of fat.

Damp can also come from outside the body via the mouth and nose, in the form of wind and damp. This could manifest as a cold, flu, a headache, or even a lung infection. It can also come from being in a damp environment, staying in wet clothes, or not drying wet hair.

Damp is a sticky, thick substance, more like glue than water. It can be very difficult to get rid of. It lingers in the body, sometimes slowing down or blocking essential functions, and can collect in the joints, causing pain. It is often responsible for medical conditions like high cholesterol, heart disease, and obesity.

The most effective way to remove damp is to remove the source. For most people, this can best be achieved by changing dietary habits but could also involve simple changes in lifestyle, such as not sleeping with wet hair.

Dietary factors that can worsen damp

- Overeating and eating late at night can weaken the Stomach and lead to stagnation in the digestive process.
- Excess drinking during meal times can often literally flood the stomach and slow down digestion. It is then less likely to process food efficiently and more likely to accumulate damp.
- Most of the foods that help generate damp conditions in the body are nutrient-dense, so much so that the body can become overwhelmed with too much nutrition at once.

- Fruit juice is one example of this. Many fruits combine sweet and sour flavours, and this alone can have a dampening effect on the body, and a glass of fruit juice, which usually contains the juice of several fruits, concentrates this still farther. Normally, the Stomach and Spleen cannot process this much concentrated nutrition efficiently; as a result, it is often stored as damp.
- The following foods are considered highly nutritious and therefore damp-forming when over-consumed:

FRUIT: bananas, oranges, avocados and too many dried fruits like dates and figs.

VEGETABLES: raw vegetables.

GRAINS: wheat, bread, many kinds of cereal bars and oats, especially when served with milk and sugar.

MEAT: naturally fatty meat, such as pork, lamb, duck, and beef.

LEGUMES, SEEDS, AND NUTS: roasted peanuts.

DRINKS: beer; concentrated fruit juice, especially orange and tomato; milkshakes; yogurt drinks; fruit-flavoured soft drinks; milk; and soya milk.

OTHER: foods high in bad fats (saturated and hydrogenated fats), deep-fried food, and any greasy foods; all dairy produce (from a cow), including milk, cream, butter and spreads, cheese, and ice cream; also mayonnaise, tofu, white sugar, yeast, concentrated sweeteners, processed foods with artificial flavours (often packaged food targeted at children and usually claiming to be "vitamin-enriched"); milk chocolate; eggs; and virtually all junk food.

Dietary factors that can reduce damp

- All food should be cooked and served warm.
- The diet essentially needs to strengthen digestion as in Weak Qi, as a strong Stomach and Spleen can help prevent dampness from collecting in the first place. As carbohydrates tend to be sweet-natured, overconsumption can aggravate damp, so be cautious not to eat too many grains. Most of the diet should be composed of vegetables with a reduced amount of carbohydrates and small amounts of animal protein and quality fats and oils.
- In addition to the foods that strengthen qi, some warming and drying foods are beneficial, especially if also sweet, bitter, or pungent. These have the welcome effects of drying up or expelling the damp and consist of many of the following foods:

FRUITS: lemons, pears, cherries, grapes, cranberries, and papayas.

VEGETABLES: cooked vegetables, such as celery, lettuce, pumpkins, artichokes, turnips, button mushrooms, garlic, onions, broad beans, and radishes.

GRAINS: dry grains such as barley, corn, rye, rye crispbread; also rice, which encourages the production of urine and helps rid the body of excess dampness.

HERBS AND SPICES: watercress and drying and warming spices, such as black pepper, parsley, horseradish (wasabi), cloves, nutmeg, and mustard.

LEGUMES, SEEDS, AND NUTS: kidney beans and aduki beans.

MEAT AND SEAFOOD: small amounts of mackerel, anchovies, clams, chicken, turkey, and white fish.

DRINKS: barley water, chamomile, jasmine and green tea.

Acupressure and massage

ON THE FRONT: Finger- or thumb-press down the midline of the abdomen. Knead any sore points, especially Ren-3, Ren-9, and Ren-12.

ON THE LEGS/FEET: Thumb-press along the Stomach and Spleen channels up to the groin area. Press and knead any sore points, including Sp-3 on the feet, and Sp-6, Sp-9, and St-36 on the legs.

ON THE HANDS: Do the Healthy Hand massage in the How Can You Treat Yourself? section. Knead any sore points, especially in the Stomach, Spleen, and Large Intestine area.

ON THE FEET: Do the Healthy Foot massage in the How Can You Treat Yourself? section. Check the following points, and knead if sore: Stomach, Pancreas, Duodenum, Spleen, Chest, Frontal Sinus, and Small and Large Intestine.

ON THE EARS: Do the Healthy Ear massage in the How Can You Treat Yourself? section. Check the following points, and knead if sore: Lungs, Sanjiao, Stomach, and Spleen.

Scraping

Scrape down the whole back. Pay particular attention to tightness in the muscles of the mid-back.

Tapping

Tap each point up to 30 times. You may need an assistant for the back area.

- Tap along the Spleen and Stomach channels on the leg up to the groin area. Look for any sore points at St-36, Sp-6, and Sp-9.
- Tap down the back muscles either side of the spine. Check Bl-22, and tap if sore.
- Carefully tap down the middle of the breastbone and on to the abdomen, especially check Ren-12 and Ren-9 for soreness.

Exercises

Do Exercises 1–6 of the five-element stretches daily. Exercises 1, 2, and 6 strengthen the Lungs, Spleen, and Liver, all of which are strongly implicated with damp.

Lifestyle advice

- Regular gentle exercise improves the circulation of qi and helps rid the body of damp.
- Avoid bad habits like not drying your hair after washing and going to bed with wet or damp hair. The damp can easily enter the body via the head and neck.

- Watch where you sit outside. Grass is a great place to picnic on a sunny day, but it retains moisture and can happily pass that moisture on to your clothes and into your body.
- In general, warmth and dryness are important factors to combat dampness, so stay warm and dry.

Phlegm

Symptoms

Tiredness, heaviness, an inability to concentrate, dizziness, frequent stuffed nose, persistent cough, sinus problems, lack of appetite, lumps under the skin, overweight, tight chest, dull headache, and ringing in the ear(s).

Signs

There is often a sticky coating on the tongue.

Can include or lead to

Kidney stones, gall bladder stones, swollen lymph nodes, thyroid conditions and fibroids, rhinintis, sinusitis, bronchitis, pneumonia, numbness, oedema in legs and ankles, bone deformities and nodules.

Common causes

A diet of too much greasy, heating food; smoking; repeated lung infections; emotional stress; overthinking; worrying too much over things you cannot change or a long chronic illness.

An explanation

Phlegm and damp (covered in the previous section) are very closely related. Phlegm often develops as a result of damp, which has a tendency to thicken and harden with heat.

The causes of phlegm accumulation in the body are, therefore, often the same as for damp. A weakness in the Stomach or Spleen slows digestion, and the resultant congestion can lead to damp, heat, then phlegm.

Lungs with strong qi should siphon off any excess damp and spread it around the body. But weak Lungs get overwhelmed, and damp and phlegm can find their way into the nose and the lungs. The heat that contributes to the formation of phlegm usually comes from stagnated qi and is often due to stress at work, a repressed emotion, or lack of exercise. It can however develop from other conditions, and if the heat becomes stronger, it can cause phlegm to rise towards the head and affect the mind and clarity of thought.

Ps, causing pain and a sense of numbness and heaviness. It can be behind some psychological conditions and manic behaviour.

As with damp, phlegm should be combated at its source. This often means making dietary changes and avoiding foods likely to add to the problem.

Dietary factors that can worsen phlegm

- Deep-fried or roasted foods, especially when high in bad fats, can be very heating and oily and should be avoided.
- Overeating and eating late at night should be avoided, as these can cause stagnation of food.
- Damp- and phlegm-forming foods should be avoided, including the following:

FRUIT: cool or cold-natured fruit, such as bananas, pineapples, and avocados.
VEGETABLES: raw vegetables and salads.
HERBS AND SPICES: salt
LEGUMES, SEEDS, AND NUTS: roasted peanuts
MEAT: all naturally fatty meat, including pork, lamb, and duck.
DRINKS: coffee, alcohol, soya milk, and fruit juice.
OTHER: all dairy products, including ice cream; sugar; eggs; tofu; chocolate; junk food; and tinned or frozen food.

Dietary factors that can reduce phlegm

- All food should be cooked and served warm.
- An ideal diet should consist of foods that remove damp and phlegm and support the digestive process. This includes small amounts of light, easy-to-digest food. See Weak Qi and Damp for more details.
- Add foods with a bitter and pungent flavour to dislodge the phlegm and damp. Many of the following foods counteract phlegm:

FRUIT: pears, persimmons, grapefruit, lemon, orange, apple, and tangerine peel.
VEGETABLES: cooked leafy greens, olives, garlic, onions, radishes, and seaweed.
GRAINS: strengthening grains, such as rice, corn, and millet.
LEGUMES, SEEDS, AND NUTS: almonds, walnuts, soya beans, and mung beans.
HERBS AND SPICES: watercress, marjoram, thyme, black and white pepper, and licorice.
DRINKS: rice milk.

Acupressure and massage

ON THE HEAD: Press around the top corner of the forehead, just behind the normal hairline and knead if sore.
ON THE ARM: Thumb press along the Lung, the Large Intestine, and the Pericardium channels up to the elbow. Knead any sore points, including Pc-6, Lu-5, and LI-11.
ON THE LEGS: Thumb-press along the Stomach channel up to the knee. Knead any sore points, especially St-36 and St-40.
ON THE HANDS: Do the Healthy Hand massage in the How Can You Treat Yourself? section. Press and knead the following, if sore: LI-4, Stomach, Spleen, and Large Intestine areas, Chest and respiration areas, and the top segment of each of the five fingers.

ON THE FEET: Do the Healthy Foot massage in the How Can You Treat Yourself? section. Press and knead the following if sore: Heart, Lungs, Chest, Scapula, Nose, Stomach, and Spleen.

ON THE EARS: Do the Healthy Ear massage in the How Can You Treat Yourself? section. Press and knead the following points, if sore: Spleen, Stomach, Lungs, Sanjiao, Kidneys, and Shen Men.

Scraping

Scrape down the back muscles either side of the spine. If phlegm is connected to the upper organs (Lungs and Heart) concentrate more on the upper back, especially between the spine and the edge of the shoulder blade.

Tapping

Tap each point up to 30 times. You may need an assistant for the back area.

- Tap down the back muscles either side of the spine as far as the buttocks. Check Bl-20 and Bl-21 for soreness.
- Tap down the midline of the breastbone, including Ren-17, then down the abdomen, including Ren-9 and Ren-6.
- Tap St-40 on the leg and any sore points around it.

Exercises

Do Exercises 1–6 of the five-element stretches daily. Exercises 1 and 2 are useful in strengthening the Lungs and Spleen to prevent phlegm.

Lifestyle advice

Smoking is a direct cause of phlegm and heat in the Lungs, and the only way to prevent this from building up is to stop completely. So if you suffer from phlegm-type symptoms and you smoke, there is no other way to help improve it other than to stop.

Blood Stagnation
Symptoms

Fixed, stabbing pain; painful periods; dark and clotted menstrual blood; abdominal pain; masses in the abdomen; and congestion in the chest.

Can include or lead to

Injuries and broken bones, tumours, fibroids, ovarian cysts, dysmenorrhea, endometriosis, gall stones, and heart disease.

Common causes

Emotional stress, especially when emotions are repressed; an accident or injury; or a long-term illness.

An explanation

Blood and qi usually flow freely around the body to nourish and moisten it. Apart from the mild stagnation of blood in women as blood collects for menstruation, blood should maintain a consistent flow without restriction or obstruction.

When they do happen, obstructions to the flow of blood often come in the form of an injury. Any kind of accident, injury, twist, sprain, strain, or muscle-pull can cause blood stagnation because the flow of blood has been blocked and the pressure builds up from behind. This usually manifests as bruising, blood clotting, and pain.

Often injuries "heal" without the stagnation involved being removed. When this happens, even though the area has a normal appearance, pain may continue and the area gradually weaken due to stagnated blood and qi preventing nutrients from reaching the muscles, tendons, and tissues in that part of the body.

This is a very common pattern in continuing chronic pain at the site of an old injury. It is also often complicated by the addition of wind, cold, or damp, which collect in the area because of the subsequent weakness and further block and weaken it.

Blood can also become stuck in the absence of any injury, usually as an extension of internal qi stagnation. Qi and blood are intricately related: blood is simply a more condensed form of qi, so qi stagnation is often accompanied by stagnation of blood.

The most common cause of this pattern is emotional stress, which may build up over time and fester in the body, affecting the Liver and blocking qi and blood. This is often the origin of masses in the abdomen, as repressed emotions find a place to express themselves within the body.

To resolve blood stagnation many of the same things can be done as for qi stagnation.

Dietary factors that can worsen blood stagnation

- Cold-natured and raw foods are involved in constricting the circulation of blood and qi, and therefore should be avoided. See the Cold food list for more details.
- Overeating and poor eating habits, such as eating late at night or too quickly, can add to any stagnation.
- Oversalted, processed, or sweetened foods, and foods high in bad fats and oils, such as cream, cheese, eggs, red meat, pizza, chips, nuts, and spreads, are hard to digest and should be avoided.

Dietary factors that can improve blood stagnation

- An ideal diet to combat blood stagnation is very similar to that of qi stagnation. See Qi Stagnation for more details both of the general diet and specific foods as they equally apply here.
- Foods that move blood are considered warm, pungent foods, but if there are clear signs of heat in the body, warm foods can worsen the situation;

therefore, a combination of warming foods and more cooling foods should be considered. The following foods help to move blood:

FRUIT: peaches and hawthorn berries.
VEGETABLES: leeks, onions, garlic, aubergines (eggplants), and scallions.
HERBS AND SPICES: turmeric, chives, ginger, basil, nutmeg, oregano, rosemary, and white pepper.
LEGUMES, SEEDS, AND NUTS: chestnuts and aduki beans.
MEAT AND SEAFOOD: venison, crab, and seaweed.
DRINKS: red wine.
OTHER: vinegar.

Acupressure and massage

ON THE FRONT: Palm-circle clockwise with both hands on top of each other around the belly button. Press and knead St-21 then St-25, either side of the belly button. Press again on the same line, but about a hand width lower. Finger-circle along the breastbone up to the collar bone. Knead any sore points.
ON THE BACK: Thumb-press down the back muscles either side of the spine. Press and knead any sore points, including Bl-17 and Bl-18.
ON THE LEGS: Thumb-press along the Spleen channel up to the groin area and knead any sore points, including Sp-10.
ON THE HANDS: Do the Healthy Hand massage in the How Can You Treat Yourself? section. Press and knead any sore points including LI-4, Liver, and Heart area.
ON THE FEET: Do the Healthy Foot massage in the How Can You Treat Yourself? section. Knead any sore points in between the bones, especially Liv-3.
ON THE EARS: Do the Healthy Ear massage in the How Can You Treat Yourself? section. Press and knead the following points, if sore: Heart, Liver, Sanjiao, and Shen Men.

Scraping

Scrape down the neck, across the shoulders, and down the back, either side of the spine. Pay particular attention to tight, knotted muscles in the mid-back. Any dots that appear on the skin may be dark red or purple and last for several days.

Tapping

Tap each point up to 30 times. You may need an assistant for the back area.

- Tap down the muscles on either side of the spine at regular intervals, and feel for any sore, tight areas.
- Tap along the midline of both calf muscles up to Bl-40 at the knee crease.
- Tap each nail point on the fingers and toes: Fingers: Lu-11, Pc-9, He.9, LI-1, TB-1, and SI-1. Toes: Sp-1, Liv-1, Kid-1 (on the sole), St-45, GB-44, and Bl-67. These are easy to find as they are at the top corners of the toenails.

Exercises

Follow Exercises 1–6 of the five-element stretches. Exercise 6 can help to improve circulation by strengthening the Liver.

Lifestyle advice

In general, movement and warmth help to move blood and qi. So gentle exercise and stretching, and avoiding the cold are usually important in maintaining the natural flow of qi and blood in the body.

Heat
Symptoms

Feeling hot, thirsty, skin conditions with red eruptions, a bitter taste, a sore throat, dark and scanty urine, dizziness, headache, a flushed face, agitation, a tendency to get angry easily, tinnitus, bloating, wind, constant hunger, bleeding gums, and sour regurgitation.

Signs

The tongue and the face are usually red. The skin might be hot to touch.

Can Include or lead to

Gastritis, ventricular and duodenal ulcers, stomatitis, chronic cholecystitis, high blood pressure, hyperthyroidism, halitosis, gingivitis, diabetes, eczema, dermatitis, acne, insomnia, asthma, bronchiectasis, migraine, cystitis, and conjunctivitis.

Common causes

Long-term repressed emotions, a diet with too much greasy, fried food, smoking, drinking too much alcohol, overwork, being overexposed to a hot environment, or catching a cold that never went away.

An explanation

Heat often develops in the body as a result of stagnation. This is often the result of stress, poor eating habits, and overwork, which interrupt the normal workings of the Liver and lead to muscle tightness and discomfort.

The buildup of qi behind a blockage can create agitation and heat. The longer the blockage has been there, the more sustained and widespread the heat that can rise and cause conditions like insomnia, headaches, and a bitter taste in the mouth.

Heat can also be generated from an improper diet. Too many hot-natured, oily, processed foods can damage the Stomach and weaken yin. Weak yin can generate warmth, which over time becomes heat and can cause symptoms like constant hunger, nausea, thirst, and bleeding gums.

Colds, flu, and other lung-related conditions can also generate heat. This heat can be confined to the lungs, as in a barking cough or asthma, or it can spread and go deeper into the layers of the body and cause conditions like dry constipation and abdominal pain.

The obvious solution for too much heat is cold, and dietary changes can be made to add more cold- or cool-natured foods and reduce those foods that are hot- or warm-natured.

Dietary factors that can worsen heat

- Overeating creates stagnation and adds to the heat.
- Frying, roasting, or barbecuing foods will increase their heat-producing properties.
- All hot- or warm-natured foods, no matter what type of taste each has, generate heat. The obvious ones to avoid are:

HERBS AND SPICES: chillies, cinnamon, ginger, salt, black pepper, garlic, mustard, and horseradish.

LEGUMES, SEEDS, AND NUTS: peanuts.

MEAT AND SEAFOOD: red meat, especially lamb, and prawns.

DRINKS: coffee, strong alcohol, and red wine.

OTHER: chocolate, bad-quality heated vegetable oils, cheese, curries, eggs, and creamy foods.

Dietary factors that can reduce heat

- An ideal diet to reduce heat should be high in cooling fruits and vegetables. Be very cautious however about eating too many cold, raw foods as they can weaken the digestive organs and end up causing more heat!
- Cool- or cold-natured foods that are also sweet, bitter, or sour, will help to reduce heat such as the following:

FRUIT: cool-natured fruits, such as grapefruit, lemons, kiwis, watermelons, pears, bananas, and tropical fruits.

VEGETABLES: cool-natured vegetables, such as asparagus, lettuce, aubergines (eggplants), spinach, cabbage, potatoes, peas, watercress, and tomatoes; celery, cucumber, and beetroot are diuretics and encourage urination, which can help reduce heat.

GRAINS: millet, rice, barley, and wheat.

LEGUMES, SEEDS, AND NUTS: mung beans.

SEAFOOD: clams.

OTHER: tofu and yogurt.

DRINKS: water with lemon juice, pear juice, elderflower tea, chamomile tea, and peppermint tea.

Acupressure and massage

ON THE ARMS: Press and knead around LI-11 on the elbow.

ON THE BACK: Thumb- or finger-press down the vertebrae of the spine. Knead any sore points, especially Du-14 at the beginning of the neck.

ON THE HANDS: Do the Healthy Hand massage in the How Can You Treat Yourself? section. Also press and knead the top segments of the five fingers, if sore.

ON THE FEET: Do the Healthy Foot Massage in the How Can you Treat Yourself? section. Press and knead Liv-2, GB-43, and St-44, if sore. These points cool heat.

ON THE EARS: Press and knead the following points, if sore: Ear apex, Vitality, Point Zero, and Endocrine.

Scraping

Scrape across the shoulders and down the back muscles either side of the spine. The Scraping action allows the heat to escape, so the skin may become hot and red quite quickly. Do not overdo the Scraping, if this is the case.

Tapping

Tap each point up to 30 times. You may need an

assistant for the upper back/shoulder area.

- Tap along the Large Intestine channel on the arm, from LI-4 on the hand to LI-11 at the elbow.
- Check for any sore points on the shoulders and upper back and tap if present.
- Tap each nail point on the fingers and toes: Fingers: Lu-11, Pc-9, He.9, LI-1, TB-1, and SI-1. Toes: Sp-1, Liv-1, Kid-1 (on the sole), St-45, GB-44, and Bl-67. These are easy to find as they are all at the corner of the nails.

Exercises

Follow Exercises 1–6 of the five-element stretches daily. Generally strengthening all of the channels can help reduce heat.

Lifestyle advice

If you suffer from a condition of heat, it is time to think about making some changes in your life. Vices such as smoking and drinking alcohol, stress at work, a simpler less rich diet – recognize and then try to remove some of the reasons behind the heat.

Cold
Symptoms

Severe pain or stiffness, better with warmth and worse with pressure, an aversion to the cold, a desire for warm drinks, contraction of tendons, cold arms and legs, thin watery discharges, diarrhoea, and vomiting.

Signs

Usually a thick white coating on the tongue surface.

Can include or lead to

Joint pain, arthritis, back pain, irritable bowel syndrome, uterus disorders, and prostrate problems.

Common causes

Exposure to the cold; sitting on cold, wet surfaces; a diet of excess cold-natured foods; or long-term illness.

An explanation

Cold conditions in the body tend to be associated with pain because of the contracting action of cold on muscles, tendons, and body tissues. They normally affect the stomach, intestine, and uterus and can block channels, linger in joints, and cause tense muscles.

Cold often arises from long-term weakness of yang or through a poor diet, but it can also enter the body from outside, especially when exposed to cold and wet weather.

The most common way to treat cold is through warmth, both on the outside of the body and via food on the inside.

Dietary factors that can worsen cold

- Raw foods, such as salads and fruit, can easily lead to digestive weakness. Fruit should be stewed and all vegetables cooked.
- Cooling foods, such as bananas, grapefruit, persimmons, melons, soya products, tomatoes, watermelons, cucumbers, lettuce, ice cream, and yogurt, will increase cold.

Dietary factors that can improve cold

- Warming cooking styles, such as roasting, grilling, and cooking with alcohol, will help dispel the cold. As weak yang is a cold condition, much of the dietary advice in Weak Yang applies here.
- Add more warm and sweet foods, such as:
FRUIT: cherries and lychees.
VEGETABLES: onions, turnips, sweet potatoes, and leeks.

HERBS AND SPICES: ginger, nutmeg, basil, and black pepper.

MEAT AND SEAFOOD: lamb, chicken, anchovies, shrimp, and mussels.

NUTS: chestnuts and walnuts.

DRINKS: wine (in small quantities).

OTHER: vinegar.

Acupressure and massage

Point selection depends on the location of the cold but the following are good general points to use:

ON THE LEGS: Thumb-press up the Spleen and Stomach channels to the knee. Knead any sore points, especially Sp-6, St-34, Kid-7, and St-36.

ON THE ARMS: Thumb-press up the Large Intestine channel to the elbow. Knead any sore points, including LI-11.

ON THE BACK: Thumb-press down the back muscles either side of the spine, and knead any sore points, including Bl-13, Bl-20, Bl-23, and Du-4.

ON THE FRONT: Thumb- or finger-press down the midline of the breastbone and over the abdomen. Knead any sore points on the abdomen, including Ren-6, Ren-12, Ren-17, St-25, and Sp-15.

ON THE HANDS: Do the Healthy Hand massage in the How Can You Treat Yourself? section. Press and knead the following points, if sore: LI-4, Lungs, Kidneys, Reproductive area, Stomach, Spleen, and Large Intestine area.

ON THE FEET: Do the Healthy Foot massage in the How Can You Treat Yourself? section. Also hard-press the Kidneys, Stomach, Lungs, and Pancreas areas and Kid-3.

ON THE EARS: Do the Healthy Ear massage in the How Can You Treat Yourself? section. Press and knead the following points, if sore: Spleen, Stomach, Kidneys, Lungs, Vitality, and Shen Men.

Scraping

Scrape across the shoulders and down the back muscles either side of the spine. Be sure to scrape over the lower back and into the buttock area.

Tapping

Tap each point up to 30 times. You may need an assistant for the back area.

- Tap across the shoulders and down the muscles on either side of the spine. Check the Bladder channels, and tap any sore points.
- Tap down the back of the upper and lower leg muscles.
- Tap down the midline of the breastbone and then down the abdomen to Ren-4.
- Tap down the front thigh muscles and either side of the lower leg. Tap Kid-7, if sore.
- At the feet, tap Liv-3 and Kid-3.

Exercises

Do Exercises 1–6 of the five-element stretches on a regular basis, as these can bring warmth to the organs and channels.

Lifestyle advice

- Wear appropriate clothing, especially at the change of seasons, when wind and cold can easily enter the body.
- It is important to note that some medical drugs have a very cooling effect on the body. Antibiotics, tranquilizers, diuretics, and anaesthetics can often be a source of internal cold.

Part Six

How Do You Treat Common Medical Conditions?

The essence of Oriental medicine is to prevent illness through the balancing of qi, blood, yin, yang, heat, cold, wind, damp and phlegm, as covered in the previous section. However, it is equally valid in treating imbalances that have already taken hold and which often have been given a familiar Western medical name. In this section, I have included the most common of these, from my experience, to show how the same principles can be applied in treating them.

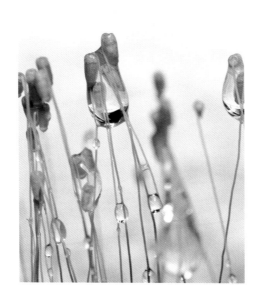

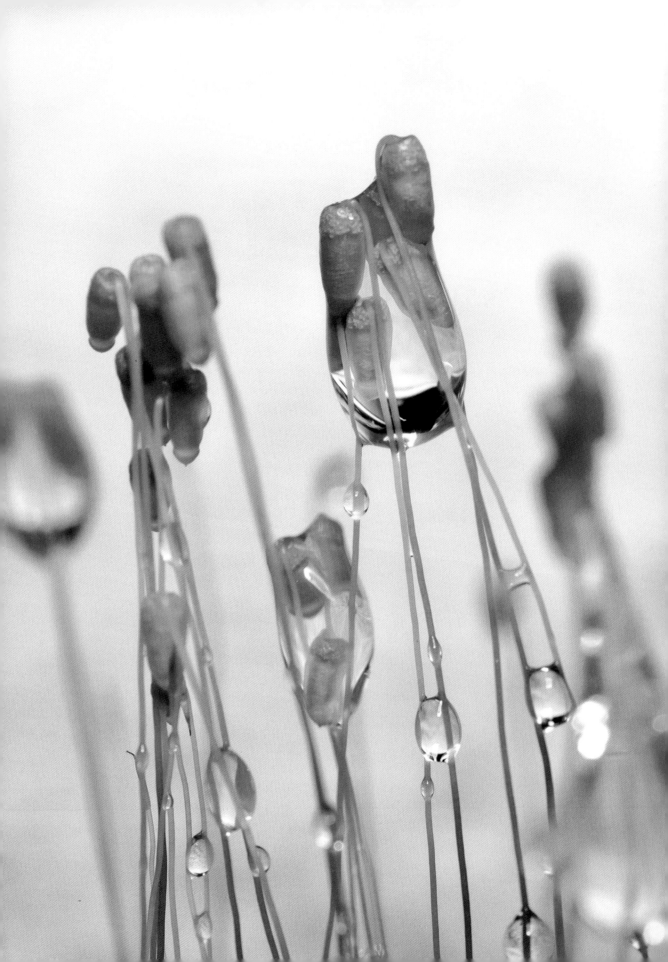

Chapter 19
氣 Head, Neck and Shoulder Area

Headaches
Symptoms

Pain, ache, or discomfort in the head; dizziness; eye pain; earache; tender face or head; sensitivity to light.

Can include or lead to

Migraine, otitis, trigeminal neuralgia, sinusitis, tumour, and spondylitis.

When to see your doctor

If the pains are severe, get worse, and are accompanied by vomiting, a stiff neck, light sensitivity, limb weakness, or tingling.

Common causes

Stress, dehydration, lack of exercise, anxiety, medication, allergies, tight muscles, or emotional stress, especially anger.

An explanation

Headaches manifest in different ways. There is no catch-all treatment for them. This is because headaches are usually caused by an imbalance within the body, not necessarily the head, and that imbalance will vary from person to person.

The exact symptoms of a headache can usually give us useful information about what has happened in the body and what may be causing it:

WIND IN THE HEAD: If the headache is accompanied by cold-like or flu-like symptoms, it is often the case that wind has entered into the Lungs and lodged itself there. Wind can affect the head by causing pain and dizziness. A clear sign of wind being present is the strong desire to stay away from wind, whether it be a gentle breeze or an air conditioner fan.

YANG OR HEAT RISING INTO THE HEAD: An acute headache, where the pain is intense, piercing, or throbbing, suggests heat or yang rising. This is especially so if the headache is mainly felt at the temples on both or either side and also behind the eyes. Sometimes there is an accompanying sensation of heat in the head. This kind of headache can be triggered by emotional stress or the end of the working week.

STAGNATION OF QI IN THE BODY: This is closely related to the kind of headache associated with stagnation of qi, a condition when qi becomes blocked. (See the Qi Stagnation section for more details on this.) It can be brought on by a whole range of factors, from emotional stress and overwork to bad posture and lack of exercise. This kind of headache can feel tight with a piercing sensation, possibly at the forehead or temples. It can be worse before a menstrual period, in stormy weather, and with emotional stress but is relieved with physical activity and as the day draws on.

DAMP AND PHLEGM IN THE HEAD: Damp and phlegm can also cause headaches. The sticky nature of these substances can arise from a weak Stomach and Spleen caused by an improper diet or from a buildup in the Lungs, creating a distinctive heavy feeling in the head. This is often described as a muzzy sensation, like cotton wool surrounding your head, and can be accompanied by difficulty in concentrating and thinking clearly. This kind of headache is often felt at the forehead and can feel worse lying down or in damp weather.

WEAK BLOOD IN THE BODY: Sometimes a weakness of the blood in the Liver can cause a headache. When this happens, the blood does not have the power to nourish the whole body properly, and often a dull headache at the top of the head results. This may feel worse after menstruation, studying, or physical activity.

WEAK KIDNEY QI: There could also be a weakness in Kidney qi; this often happens in old age, as the Kidneys start to wane. This kind of headache may feel dull or empty, come on later in the day, or be relieved by lying down and resting.

Dietary Factors That Can Affect Headaches

Follow the relevant diets for the general patterns, according to the type of headache. For example, for damp conditions see the Damp section, for hot conditions, see Heat, and so on.

Acupressure and massage

ON THE HEAD: Press and knead the following points, if sore: Bl-1, Bl-2, Yintang, and GB-14 on the front of the head; Du-20, GB-20, and Du-16 on the back; and Taiyang at the temples.

ON THE ARM: Thumb-press along the Pericardium, Triple Burner, and Large Intestine channels, up to the elbow. Knead any sore points, especially TB-5.

ON THE LEG: Press and knead St-36 and GB-34, if sore.

ON THE HANDS: Press and knead the following hand points, if sore: LI-4, Temples, Headache, Head areas (Back of the Head, Top of the Head, Forehead), and Eye.

ON THE FEET: Do the Healthy Foot massage in the How Can You Treat Yourself? section. Knead any sore points, including Liv-3, Brain, Frontal Sinus, and Shoulder, and Cervical, Thoracic, and Lumbar areas.

ON THE EARS: Press and knead the following points, if sore: Temples, Occiput, Frontal Sinus, Forehead, Liver, Spleen, Vertex, and Shen Men.

Scraping

Scrape down the neck, across the shoulders and down to the mid-back. There are often sore points in these areas, where the muscle fibres have tightened and caused knots.

Tapping

Tap each point up to 30 times. You may need an assistant for the neck/shoulder area. For any type of headache do the following:

- Gently tap Du-20, Bl-10, and GB-20 on the head.
- Feel over the neck/shoulder for any points that feel sore. Tap these points to relax muscles and tendons.
- Press Du-23 and Du-20 on the head; Liv-2 on the feet; and LI-4, TB-3, and TB-4 on the hands to see if they are sore, and if so, tap them.
- If it feels sore along the Gall Bladder channel on the head, tap GB-20 as above but also Bl-20 on the back, and the Gall Bladder channel on the legs, from GB-31 downwards. In particular, check GB-34, GB-40, and GB-41 on the legs for tenderness; if there is any, focus on these points.
- Palpate the Liver channel and, if sore, tap Liv-3, Liv-4 (on the feet), Bl-18 (on the back), and Pc-6 (on the inside of the arm).

Exercises

Headaches can often be related to the state of several organs or channels at the same time, so it is useful to do Exercises 1–6 of the five-element stretches daily.

Lifestyle advice

Causes of a headache are numerous, so there is no one cure-all remedy for them. The key is knowing what, if anything, is the trigger for the headache. The following can help prevent headaches:

- Posture should be correct for the activity being done. Long-term hunching over a desk, for example, may cause backache, a sore neck, and headaches.
- Your work environment should be adjusted, if necessary. Migraines can sometimes be caused by some types of computer screens.
- Dehydration is a common cause of headaches. This can often be avoided by drinking enough, so that you never actually feel thirsty. Often, if you feel thirsty, then you are already dehydrated.
- Regular doses of painkillers, such as codeine, paracetamol, ibuprofen, and aspirin, can actually cause headaches. They can be effective at reducing the pain of a headache, but like all strong drugs have their own withdrawal symptoms – one of which is something called a "rebound headache." This means that as the drug works its way out of the body, the body then reacts with a headache. This can then result in the need to take strong painkillers again to relieve this rebound headache sometimes leading to a vicious cycle of taking strong painkillers to relieve the effects of taking strong painkillers.
- Finding time for rest and relaxation is often very helpful. Not normally having the time to relax means that lifestyle adjustments sometimes have to be made.

Dizziness
Symptoms

Feeling lightheaded or giddy; blurred vision, floaters, or spots in your vision; and a loss of balance.

Can include or lead to

Viral ear infections, vertigo, Ménière's disease, hypertension, arteriosclerosis, and neurosis.

When to see your doctor

If the symptoms are severe and persistent.

Common causes

Overwork, stress, exhaustion, emotional stress, a diet with too many damp and phlegm-forming foods, depression, anxiety, severe blood loss, a long chronic illness, or drug side effects.

An explanation

YANG RISING INTO THE HEAD: Dizziness is often due to an imbalance of yin and yang. When yin becomes weak, yang becomes much more active and can rise very quickly to disturb the qi in the head. Strong emotions, such as anger or aggression, can also create a similar pattern by obstructing the smooth flow of qi. Dizziness, which is worse when stressed, is often due to this blocked qi that has forced yang upwards.

WEAK BLOOD IN THE BODY: When the blood and qi are weak, they become sluggish and cannot bring enough fresh qi up to the head in time. This is the reason for the feeling of temporary dizziness some people get when standing up quickly. It also explains the mild dizziness that may come from doing too much or staying up too late and will often improve with rest.

PHLEGM IN THE BODY OR HEAD: When there is a lot of phlegm in the body, it can block most of the qi from reaching the head. This can sometimes be accompanied by a lack of clarity and an inability to concentrate. It can also result in very strong dizziness with nausea.

Dietary factors that can worsen dizziness

- To prevent rising yang, avoid hot, pungent spices such as cinnamon, ginger, and black pepper. See Yang Rising for more details.
- When qi and blood are weak, avoid too many bitter, sour, salty, and hot-natured foods. Avoid salads, raw fruit, or vegetables and dairy produce. See Weak Qi for more details.
- For phlegm conditions, avoid damp- or phlegm-forming foods, such as wheat, dairy, bananas, peanuts, processed foods, orange or tomato juice, and fatty meat like pork. See Phlegm for more details.

Dietary factors that can improve dizziness

- To prevent yang from rising, eat more sour and bitter cooling foods like kidney beans, black sesame seeds, watercress, mushrooms, eggs, and rhubarb. See Yang Rising and the Sour and Bitter Foods lists for more details.
- Qi and blood can be strengthened with neutral and warming foods such as rice, pumpkin, chickpeas (garbanzo), parsnips, and cooked fruit. See Weak Qi for more details.
- To remove phlegm, add more of the following to your diet: barley, rye, pumpkin, broad beans, celery, aduki beans, radishes, and extra virgin olive oil.

Acupressure and massage

ON THE HEAD: Press Yintang and knead upwards to the hairline. Press the midpoint of the forehead, and knead outwards to the temples. Knead Taiyang. Press and knead with four fingers together from the temples, around the back of the ear, to the base of the skull (the occiput). Press at the midpoint of the back of the neck, just under the occiput, and knead in a downwards motion to where the neck meets the shoulders. Press GB-20 and Du-23, if sore.

ON THE LEGS: Thumb-press along the Spleen and Liver channels up to the groin area. Knead any sore points.

ON THE HANDS: Press and knead SI-3, TB-3, LI-1, LI-4, and Dizziness and Head areas.

ON THE FEET: Do the Healthy Foot massage in the How Can You Treat Yourself? section. Knead any sore points including Ear, Brain, Neck, and Cervical, Thoracic, and Lumbar areas.

ON THE EARS: Press and knead the following points if sore: Dizziness, Kidneys, Inner ear, Brain, Occiput, Point Zero, and Shen Men.

Scraping

Scrape the upper back and shoulders in an outwards or downwards direction. Reactive areas can sometimes be found between the ribs, below the shoulder blades.

Tapping

Tap each point up to 30 times. You may need an assistant for the back area.

- Tap across the shoulder muscles from the neck area to the shoulder joint. Be careful not to tap directly onto bone. Tap GB-20 at the base of the skull and GB-21 on the top of the shoulder muscles, if sore.
- Tap down the back muscles either side of the spine. Start at the shoulder and tap both sides, before moving downwards at equal spacing, concentrating on the mid-back area.
- Tap along the channels in the legs, in particular the Stomach and Spleen channels and the Liver and Gall Bladder channels. Tap St-40, GB-34, and any sore points in the feet.

Exercises

Do Exercises 4 and 6 of the five-element stretches. These strengthen the Water and Wood channels and organs.

Lifestyle advice

- Keep in mind that widely used drugs, such as tranquilizers, antidepressants, and diuretics, can cause dizziness. If this is the case, you should discuss with your doctor about changing or reducing their use.
- Reduce you workload and level of stress, if possible. Knowing when to stop or when the body has had enough is a key point with reducing some kinds of dizziness.

Sleeping Difficulties

Symptoms

Inability to sleep, difficulty falling asleep, waking up at night, waking up early, strong dreams or nightmares, not rested after sleeping, fatigue, poor appetite, and dizziness.

Can include or lead to

Insomnia, anxiety, and depression.

When to see your doctor

If accompanied by severe mental or emotional symptoms.

Common causes

Emotional stress, overwork, late nights, overexercise, overthinking, excessive study, or pressure from work.

An explanation

WEAK YIN IN THE BODY: Insomnia is very connected to the balance between yin and yang inside the body. In the daytime, yang qi is sent where needed in order for the body to function in its everyday tasks. In particular, it needs yang qi to think, see, smell, hear, and touch effectively. When night falls and yang gives way to yin, yang qi retreats from these areas and disconnects from the senses enough for the body to fall asleep.

If, however, yang qi cannot take its place beside yin for the night, the senses are still "awake" and the body cannot easily switch off. The problem here is not so much with yang but that yin is not strong enough to hold yang in place. This is a common cause of waking up during the night or early in the morning, as the heat from this agitated yang moves upwards and outwards.

WEAK BLOOD IN THE BODY: There is a similar cyclical movement in blood, which if not working properly causes insomnia. As in the case of yang qi, blood is sent around the body during the day to allow us to do our everyday activities. At night the blood, which by its nature is yin, settles in the Liver and adds to the sense of calm that drifts the body into sleep. If the blood is too weak however it cannot gather in the Liver and will "wander" around the body, keeping it awake.

Dietary factors that can worsen sleeping difficulties

- Stimulants like coffee, black tea, tobacco, fizzy soft drinks, energy drinks, alcohol, and recreational drugs can agitate yang qi and worsen insomnia.

Dietary factors that can improve sleeping difficulties

- Blood-strengthening foods include beetroot, seaweed, black sesame seeds, Guinness, and green leafy vegetables. See Weak Blood for more details.
- Yin-strengthening foods include sardines, chicken, sweet potato, black beans, wolf or goji berries, and apples. See Weak Yin for more details.

Acupressure and massage

ON THE HEAD: Rub your palms together until warm, then cover both eyes. Press Yintang, and knead upwards to the hairline. Press the midpoint of the forehead, and knead outwards towards the sides of the head. Knead Taiyang. Press and knead with four fingers together from the temples, around the back of the ear to the occiput. Press and knead Du-20, Bl-2, and GB-20.

ON THE ARMS: Thumb-press along the Heart and Pericardium channels, from the wrist to the shoulder and back again. Pay particular attention to Pc-6 and He-7 (on the palm side of the wrist).

ON THE FRONT/BACK: While seated, rub your belly button on the front and Du-4 on the lower back with the palm of your hand until it feels warm.

ON THE LEGS: Press and knead St-36 and Sp-6, if sore.

ON THE HANDS: Press and knead the following points: Head area, Insomnia areas, Pc-8, Heart, and Kidneys.

ON THE FEET: Rub the Kidney area on the soles of the feet with the palm of your hand.

ON THE EARS: Press and knead the following points: Insomnia 1, Insomnia 2, Heart, Kidneys, Master Cerebral, Point Zero, and Shen Men.

Scraping

Scrape down the muscles on the back, either side of the spine. Pay particular attention to the area between the shoulder blades and spine.

Tapping

Tap each point up to 30 times. An assistant may be needed for the back area. Ideally tap just before going to bed. Select any of the following points if they are sore when pressed:

- On the head: Du-20.
- On the back: Du-12, Bl-18, Bl-20, and Bl-23.
- On the arm: LI-10.
- On the leg: Bl-40, Bl-58, GB-34 Kid-7 and Sp-6.
- On the foot/ankle: Liv-3, Liv-4, and Kid-1.

Exercises

A useful technique to reduce insomnia is to relax your muscles with the following gentle exercises:

1. RELAX THE ARMS, SHOULDERS AND UPPER BODY:

Stand naturally with your arms hanging down at your sides. Raise your arms forward to shoulder level, clench your hands, and tense the muscles of your upper arms while breathing in at the same time.

Then bend your upper body, hang down your arms, and swing them to and fro, to make the muscles of the upper arms and shoulder joints relax fully, exhaling at the same time. Repeat this several times until you feel relaxed.

(left) Relax the arms, shoulders and upper body: tense your arms

(right) Relax the arms, shoulders and upper body: bend and swing

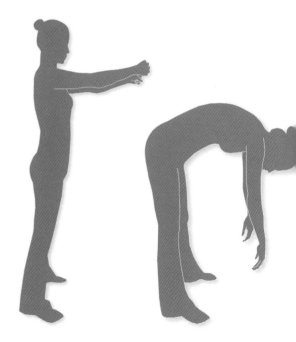

2. RELAX THE HEAD, NECK, AND SHOULDERS: From a seated position, interlock both hands and put them on the back of your head, then push your head backwards while pulling your hands forward in the opposite direction. Tense the muscles of your head and neck while inhaling at the same time. Then relax your head, neck and shoulders, while breathing out. Repeat this several times.

4. RELAX THE FRONT: Lie face up, link your fingers and put both hands on the back of your head. Raise your head slightly and contract your abdomen muscles. Then lower your head and relax, while breathing out. Repeat several times.

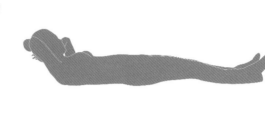

(top left) Relax the head, neck and shoulders

(top right) Relax the front

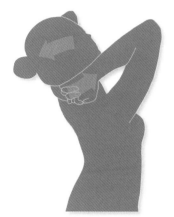

5. RELAX THE LEGS: From a seated position, put your hands on your knees, then push down on each thigh, stamp the floor and tense your leg muscles, while breathing in. Then relax and breathe out. Repeat several times.

(bottom left) Relax the back and sides

(bottom right) Relax the legs

3. RELAX THE BACK AND SIDES: Lie face up and lay your arms down at the sides, palms down. Tense the back and the side muscles, while breathing in. Then relax and breathe out. Repeat several times.

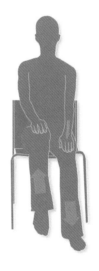

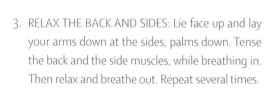
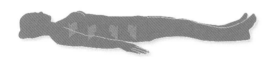

6. RELAX THE HANDS, FINGERS, AND TOES: Lie on your side, with your legs and arms bent slightly and your head resting on the arm closest to the ground. Then contract your fingers and toes and breathe in. Relax and breathe out.

7. RELAX THE WHOLE BODY: Stand with your feet close together and your arms hanging down in front of your body, with the fingers of both hands interlocked. Then lift your heels, raise your arms upward, and contract the muscles all over the body, breathing in at the same time.

Then lower your arms, move your hands apart,

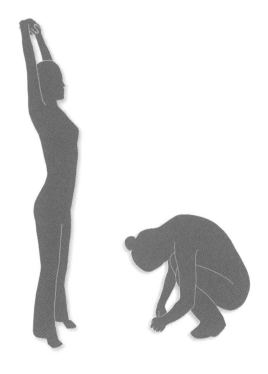

(top left) Relax the hands, fingers and toes

(left) Relax the whole body: raise your arms and contract

(right) Relax the whole body: squat and relax

squat down, and bend your head forward naturally to make the muscles all over the body fully relaxed, while breathing out. Repeat several times.

Lifestyle advice

- Playing video games, watching TV, and staring at a computer screen late at night or for long periods during the day burns up yin qi and should be avoided when there are sleep problems. When yin is weak, it can easily disturb sleeping patterns.
- Avoid taking naps during the day to make up for lost sleep, as this may worsen the pattern. Remember that the problem is often one of an imbalance between yin and yang, so doing yin activities not habitually done in yang time, and vice versa, can mess with the body's balance. This is something that nightshift workers and long-haul travellers know only too well.
- Try to stop what you are doing and just rest at least half an hour before you go to bed. No reading, watching television, talking, or fiddling with smartphones. Just sit down and let the body and mind calm down. Of course, this may not be possible all the time, but the intention should be there.

Anxiety
Symptoms

Constant worry and nervousness, an inability to concentrate, an inability to sleep, dizziness, palpitations, restless, phobias, panic attacks, and irritability.

Can include or lead to

Depression, hyperthyroidism, hypoglycaemia, PMS, menopausal problems, and post-traumatic stress disorder.

When to see your doctor

If the symptoms are severe.

Common causes

Strong emotions such as sadness or grief, depression, stress, overwork, pressure to work hard, too much caffeine, eating too much damp and phlegm-producing food, a side effect of medication or withdrawal symptoms, menopause, hyperthyroidism, heavy bleeding, or sudden shock or trauma.

An explanation

In Oriental medicine, there is no one condition for anxiety. The exact nature of the anxiety differs according to which of the bodily organs are causing the symptoms:

WEAK QI IN THE HEART: The most common condition underlying anxiety is a weakness of Heart qi. Typical indicators of this are if the anxiety gets worse when tired and if there are accompanying palpitations. A weak energetic Heart is also often behind panic attacks and phobias.

WEAK YIN IN THE KIDNEYS: Sometimes a weak Heart affects the Fire-Water balance between the Heart and the Kidneys and weakens the yin of the Kidneys. There is usually more of an element of shock, which can bring on palpitations with this pattern.

PHLEGM AND HEAT IN THE HEART: If there is a buildup of heat or phlegm in other parts of the body, both can rise and affect the Heart. This is often referred to as a mist and is like the steam rising out of the spout of a boiling kettle. This mist clouds the Heart and affects the mind, causing a lack of clarity, nervousness, and waking up before dawn.

Dietary Factors That Can Worsen Anxiety

- Food or drink containing caffeine, such as chocolate, caffeinated soft drinks, energy drinks, coffee, and black tea agitate yang qi and can worsen anxiety. Coffee, in particular, has a bitter flavour that can disperse qi and weaken the Heart.
- Dairy products, soya milk, tofu, and alcohol can worsen anxiety, particularly if there is a phlegm or heat condition. It is also important to strictly limit meat consumption for the same reason. See Phlegm and Heat for more details.
- Warm, pungent foods, such as chillies, black pepper, cayenne pepper, basil, cloves, cinnamon, cumin, rosemary, marjoram, and nutmeg, can exacerbate a weak Kidney yin condition. See Weak Yin for more details.
- Salads, raw fruit and vegetables, dairy products, and ice-cold drinks, and foods that weaken yang must be avoided particularly when Heart qi is weak. See Weak Qi and Weak Yang for more details.
- Important note: do not get overly anxious about the food you eat – you want to get rid of anxiety, not add to it. A little of the above foods is fine once in a while.

Dietary Factors That Can Improve Anxiety

- To reduce phlegm and heat, follow a diet of easy-to-digest fresh foods, including leafy greens, radishes, persimmons, watercress, turnip, and seaweed. See Phlegm and Heat for more details.
- Kidney yin–strengthening foods include pork, kidney beans, black beans, and seaweed. See Weak Yin for more details.
- Heart qi–strengthening foods are those that generally strengthen qi, such as rice, cooked fruit, carrots, and chickpeas (garbanzos). See Weak Qi for more details.

Acupressure and massage

ON THE ARMS: Thumb-press along the Heart and Pericardium channels up to the shoulder. Knead any sore points.

ON THE BACK: Thumb-press along the inner Bladder channel on the back. Pay particular attention to Bl-15, Bl-17, Bl-18, Bl-20, and Bl-23, and knead if sore.

ON THE HANDS: Press and knead the top segment of the middle, ring, and little fingers (the Heart, Triple Burner, and Pericardium channels), Palpitations, Heart, Chest, and respiration areas.

ON THE FEET: Do the Healthy Foot massage in the How Can You Treat Yourself? section. Also knead the Heart, Brain, Liver, and Spleen areas, if sore.

ON THE EARS: Press the following points and knead if sore: Nervousness, Master Cerebral, Tranquilizer, Heart, Point Zero, and Shen Men.

Scraping

Scrape down the back muscles of the upper back either side of the spine. Pay particular attention to the gap between the shoulder blades and the spine. Also scrape down the breastbone and along the rib spaces, avoiding the breast tissue.

Tapping

Tap each point up to 30 times. You may need an assistant for the back area.

- Feel along the shoulder muscles and tap any tightness. Check and tap GB-21, if sore.
- Tap down the back muscles either side of the spine. Start at the shoulder and tap both sides, before moving downwards at equal spacing.
- Tap down the midline of the breastbone, then carefully below the bottom of rib cage in each direction to the side.
- Tap down the outside of the upper and lower legs. Also along the Stomach channel, from the knees to the ankle joints. Check and tap St-40, if sore.

Exercises

- Follow the same sequence of relaxation exercises described in the previous section on Insomnia.
- Perform the Bend Backwards exercise from the Chest Pain section, which is good for releasing tension and stagnation in the upper back.
- Perform Exercises 3 and 5 of the five-element stretches.

Lifestyle advice

- It is vital to reduce external stressors and find ways to relax. But relaxation is more than just the absence of stress; it must be proactive.
- Be sure to get regular exercise, such as walking, and introduce enjoyable activities such as painting, which calm the mind and offer a distraction from worrying.

Depression
Symptoms

In general, feeling pessimistic about life, tired, unmotivated, miserable, sad or weepy, unable to think clearly, and lacking in energy. A more useful distinction here may be to list the possible symptoms by their five-element correspondence. This often gives a clearer indication of where the imbalances may lie:

WOOD: changeable moods, frustrated, feeling stuck or trapped, feeling aggressive, unable to relax, sighing, or timid.

EARTH: feeling insecure, worrying, a lack of support, repetitive thinking, or unable to find a solution.

METAL: grief, sadness, a lack of self-worth, an inability to let go, or a sense of pointlessness.

FIRE: a lack of joy, feeling rejected, feeling hurt, an inability to communicate well, feeling agitated, or being on the defensive.

WATER: fear, dread, an inability to cope, a sense of being overwhelmed or feeling helpless.

Can include or lead to

Clinical depression, mood disorders, dysthymia, seasonal depression, and bipolar disorder.

When to see your doctor

If the symptoms are severe, or if there are suicidal thoughts or urges.

Common causes

Exhaustion, emotional strain, stress, overwork, a poor diet, shock, bereavement, a long-standing illness, pain, or sometimes a constitutional tendency.

An explanation

STAGNATION OF QI IN THE BODY: Sometimes, when the body is confronted by strong emotions, rather than allowing them to be released, we keep them inside. When this happens, a physiological reaction can occur, and unexpressed emotions over time fester in the body in the form of stagnant qi. Stagnant qi slows down the body's internal functions, creating blocks and preventing qi from moving freely. Emotions are like qi, and they too begin to stagnate. It gradually becomes more and more difficult to move from one emotion to another. Instead, like a wheel following a rut in the road, you get stuck in one emotion and are unable to move out of it. This condition is likely to result in many of the Wood symptoms above.

DAMP OR PHLEGM IN THE BODY: If there is too much damp or phlegm in the body due to an improper diet, this too can create blockages. Damp and phlegm are heavy and sticky and can slow the body's processes down.

WEAKNESS OF QI, BLOOD, YIN, OR YANG: If the body has run out of any of the essential substances it needs to function, it will begin to feel weaker, both physically and mentally. This is also true on a much deeper level, as our vitality depends on having the correct balance of substances in the body. When the balance is weak, a lack of drive or will on a very profound almost spiritual level can result.

Dietary factors that can worsen depression

Processed, tinned, fatty foods cannot be digested efficiently by a weak Stomach and can easily lead to stagnation or the accumulation of damp and phlegm. Both of these can lead on to depression.

A five-year British study, published in 2009, found a link between the consumption of processed foods, such as desserts, fried foods, processed meats, and high-fat dairy products and the development of depression. According to the study, participants who followed a processed foods diet were 58 percent more likely to be suffering from depression.[12]

It is, therefore, important to avoid damp-forming foods, such as processed bad fats, junk foods, deep-fried foods, wheat, fatty meat such as pork, and beer in your diet. See Damp for more details.

Dietary factors that can improve depression

- Rice, carrots, onions, cooked fruit, lentils, chickpeas (garbanzos), and other foods that strengthen the Stomach and Spleen, and therefore qi and blood, can be beneficial in removing the underlying cause of depression. See Weak Qi for more details.
- The following foods can also help improve the circulation of qi: grapefruit, citrus peel, watercress, onions, beetroot, spices like turmeric, cardamom and coriander, black sesame seeds, and chamomile tea.

Acupressure and massage

ON THE LEGS: Thumb-press along the Liver and Gall Bladder channels, up to the groin. Knead any sore points, including GB-34.

ON THE HANDS: Do the Healthy Hand massage in the How Can You Treat Yourself? section. Press the following points and knead if sore: the Essence area on the palm, Chest and Respiration, and the Heart, Pericardium, and Triple Burner channel areas at the finger tips.

ON THE FEET: Do the Healthy Foot massage in the How Can You Treat Yourself? section. Press and knead Liv-3 and the Heart area, if sore.

ON THE EARS: Press the following points and knead if sore: Antidepressant, Brain, Master Cerebral, Shen Men, and Point Zero.

Scraping

Scrape across the shoulders and down the back muscles either side of the spine. Scrape down the breastbone and across the chest area in between the ribs, avoiding the breast tissue.

Tapping

Tap each point up to 30 times. You may need an assistant for the back area.

- Press along the Liver and Gall Bladder channels on the legs, and tap any sore points, including GB-34 and GB-40.
- Press down the midline of the breastbone, and tap lightly on any sore points.
- Tap down the back muscles either side of the spine. Start at the shoulder, and tap both sides before moving downwards at equal spacing.

Exercises

1. Do the exercise Bend Backwards from the Chest Pain section. This exercise is good for releasing tension and stagnation in the upper back.
2. Do Exercises 1–6 of the five-element stretches on a daily basis. This can help in reducing stagnation and strengthening any weak organs.

Lifestyle advice

- Regular gentle exercise can help increase the circulation of qi and reduce any blockage of damp and phlegm. The more qi that is circulating, the better

the chances of movement in your emotions. The recommended minimum exercise levels for adults is 30 minutes five times a week and for under 18s at least an hour a day. Only 14 percent of people in the UK actually achieve this.[13]

- Overwork can be bad for your mental health. A UK study found that people who work for 11 or more hours a day are twice as likely to suffer from major depression as those working a standard eight-hour day.[14]

Facial Pain

Symptoms

Pain on one side of the temple, jaw, forehead, or face; a burning feeling; a red face; tiredness or burning in the eyes; toothache; muscle spasms; dizziness; and bad breath.

Can include or lead to

Trigeminal neuralgia, orbital neuralgia, mumps, and rhinitis.

When to see your doctor

If the symptoms are severe.

Common causes

Exposure to the weather; an injury or accident; stress; overwork; emotional stress, especially anger; overworrying; a poor diet of fatty, greasy food; too much alcohol; or a long chronic illness.

An explanation

Pain in the face is normally caused by stagnation of qi and blood in the channels of the face. There are a variety of common causes for this stagnation, both internal and external, which are related to the location and intensity of the pain.

WIND AND HEAT OR COLD: The face is a part of the body that is rarely covered up, and therefore exposed to the environment most of the time. Sometimes a weakness in the layer of defensive qi, which acts as a protective coating around the body, allows wind, cold, or heat to penetrate the pores of the skin and create an obstruction in the face.

If cold has entered the face channels, it can cause pain by contracting the muscles and tendons of the face; heat can cause redness and a burning sensation; and wind may move the pain around or cause tics or muscle spasms.

FIRE RISING FROM THE LIVER: If the wind does not quickly move on, there is sometimes a further complication in that wind lodges itself in the channels of the face and combines with phlegm to create heat.

This heat in the face can worsen if there is any preexisting heat rising up within the body. The most common situation in facial pain is that extreme heat can come raging upwards from the Liver after sustained emotional stress.

Unexpressed emotional energy can fester in the Liver and over time build heat to such a point that it rises, causing intense burning pain in the face. This type of facial pain is usually very sharp and gets worse with strong emotions.

HEAT RISING FROM THE STOMACH: Equally strong heat can rise from the Stomach if it is fed with a diet of greasy, hot-natured, damp-forming food. The Stomach is often implicated in facial pain, as the Stomach channel begins just below the eyes and runs across the face and jawline. It can sometimes get worse after eating certain types of hot-natured foods and can be accompanied by bad breath.

Dietary factors that can worsen facial pain

- Grilling, roasting, and deep frying encourage heat in the body.
- Hot-natured, spicy foods, such as ginger, coriander, turmeric, and other spices; lamb; chillies; coffee; chocolate; and spirits. See Heat for more details.
- Dairy products, bananas, peanut butter, processed junk foods, and some fruit juice are damp-forming foods. See Damp for more details.
- Oily food can strongly affect the Liver and provoke heat.

Dietary factors that can lessen facial pain

- Food should be lightly cooked or boiled with water.
- Cold or cool-natured foods can help to soothe the heat. These include foods like cranberries, grapefruit, melons, bean sprouts, celery, cucumbers and lettuce, peppermint, marjoram, green tea, chamomile tea, and oolong tea. See Cold for more details.
- Salty foods, such as barley, miso, and soy sauce, and bitter foods, such as grapefruit rind, asparagus, watercress, rye, and vinegar, can be generally cooling. See Salty and Bitter food lists for more details.

Acupressure and massage

ON THE HEAD: Press the following points and knead if sore: in the masseter muscle just before the angle of the jaw, the area between the temples and the ear, SI-18 and GB-2. Note: Be careful about massaging the face directly. It can sometimes worsen the condition. If in any doubt, use alternative massage areas.

ON THE LEGS: Thumb-press along the Stomach channel, up to the knee. Knead any sore points, including St-34, St-40, and St-44.

ON THE ARMS: Thumb-press the Large Intestine and Triple Burner channels up to the elbow and back. Also press LI-11 and TB-5, if sore.

ON THE HANDS: Press the following points, and knead if sore: Eye, LI-4, LI-3, TB-2, Forehead, Temples, Liver, and Head area.

ON THE FEET: Press and knead each toe on the top of the foot from the joint up to and around the toenail. This is the frontal sinus area. In particular knead up to the nail on the big toe. Also press and knead Facial area and Eye and Ear.

ON THE EARS: Press the following points and knead if sore: Trigeminal nerve, Upper jaw, Lower jaw, Mouth, and Shen Men.

Scraping

Scrape down the back of the neck, across the shoulders, and down the upper back muscles either side of the spine. The muscles in these areas are usually tense when there is facial pain.

Tapping

Tap each point up to 30 times. You may need an assistant for the back area.

- Tap any sore points over the neck and shoulder area, in particular, the large muscles on the top of the shoulder. Tap GB-20 at the base of the skull and GB-21 on the top of the shoulders, if sore.
- Tap down the back muscles either side of the spine. Focus more on the upper and mid-back.
- Tap along the Large Intestine channel on the forearm, between LI-4 on the hands and LI-11 at the elbows.
- Tap the following points on the fingers and toes, as they help to reduce heat: Fingers: Lu-11, Pc-9, He.9, LI-1, TB-1, and SI-1.
  Toes: Sp-1, Liv-1, St-45, GB-44, and Bl-67.

Exercises

Do Exercise 2 of the five-element stretches, as this strengthens the Stomach channel, which runs across the throat and face.

Lifestyle advice

Stress and emotional factors often feature heavily in facial pain. Wherever possible, these should be worked through to try and stop them being the cause of internal heat. Look at ways of managing stress and of unburdening yourself of emotions that you have kept in for a long time. This may mean anything from talking to those close to you to seeking professional psychological help.

Nasal Allergies
Symptoms

Sneezing, a stuffy nose, an itchy nose and throat, eye irritation and weeping, a headache and runny nose, irritability, and insomnia.

Can include or lead to

Allergic or nonallergic rhinitis, hay fever, nasal congestion, rhinorrhea, conjunctivitis, and pharyngitis.

When to see your doctor

If there are severe symptoms.

Common causes

Lack of exercise; smoking; overwork; an inherited condition; too many cold-natured, phlegm-forming foods; repressed emotions, in particular grief; repeated use of antibiotics in childhood; overthinking; or worry.

An explanation

Nasal allergies are widespread. More than one-third of the populations of Europe and Australasia are thought to suffer from nasal allergies,[15] while in the United States, that number is 60 million people,[16] an estimated 40 percent of them children.[17]

While pollen seasons are worsening worldwide due to global warming and early and long springs, how we cope with allergies depends very much on the state of our qi, particularly "defensive qi," which surrounds us like a protective coating to stop the elements getting in. Defensive qi is fuelled by the qi of the Kidneys and is spread out all over the body by the Lungs.

WIND IN THE BODY: When defensive qi is weak, it is easily compromised by wind, which manages to find its way into the nose. A clear indicator of this is tiredness and lethargy and a tendency to catch colds. If the wind enters with coldness, it can cause sneezing and a runny nose; if it enters with heat, an itchy throat and eyes, and thirst.

If an individual has enough energy to reinforce their defensive qi, the wind, cold, or heat will only be temporary visitors, and everything should return to normal. If, however, their defensive qi remains weak, there is no way for the body to expel wind, cold, or heat entering the body, and they can remain there indefinitely, free to cause nasal problems at will. This is the situation for people suffering from rhinitis.

WEAK QI IN THE LUNGS AND KIDNEYS: The most important organs are the Lungs and the Kidneys, both of which have a direct effect on defensive qi. If they remain weak, the condition can be difficult to change.

WEAK QI IN THE SPLEEN: The Spleen is also important as Earth (the Spleen) has a direct effect on Metal (the Lungs) and Water (the Kidneys). This is where a strengthening diet for the Stomach and Spleen becomes essential as it can help bolster qi by strengthening all the organs involved.

Cold-natured, damp-producing foods, accompanied by improper eating habits, will weaken the Spleen and lead to an accumulation of phlegm in the Lungs, and by default, the nose. A key indicator of this is when symptoms are triggered by smoke, perfume, or fumes, as strong smells spread qi in the Lungs and agitate phlegm and damp.

Dietary habits that can worsen nasal allergies

- Overeating cold-natured, damp-forming foods, such as dairy products, bananas, tofu, soya milk, and fatty foods, can damage Spleen qi and pile up more phlegm in the Lungs. See Damp and Phlegm for more details.

Dietary habits that can improve nasal allergies

- Lightly cooked, simple foods strengthen the Spleen, Stomach, and Lungs. See Weak Qi for more details.
- Add foods that remove phlegm and help clear the sinuses, such as radishes, turnips, onions, watercress, garlic, ginger, and horseradish. See Damp and Phlegm for more details.

Acupressure and massage

ON THE HEAD:
- Circle your face with your fingers to relax the facial muscles.
- Press on the point in the midline of the forehead. Then finger-press outwards on both sides to the temples. At the temples, circle Taiyang.
- Repeat at equally spaced points on the midline up to the middle of the eyebrows. Hard-press Yintang, Bitong, and Bl-2.
- From the eyebrows to the midpoint of the nose, gently finger-press outwards along the eye socket to the temples. At the temples, circle.

- From the midpoint of the nose to the bottom of the chin, finger-press outwards to the corner of the jaw bone and circle.
- Press and knead LI-20 at the flare of the nostrils.

ON THE BACK:

- Finger-circle outwards at the base of the skull towards the ear and back again. Press and knead GB-20, if sore.
- Finger-circle down the neck on either side of the spine.
- Finger-circle along the shoulder muscle.
- Press and knead Bl-20 and Bl-23, if sore.

ON THE LEGS: Thumb-press along the Stomach channel up to the knee, and knead St-40 and St-36, if sore.

ON THE HANDS: Press and knead the following points, if sore: LI-4, LI-2, Lungs, Chest, Head area, Lung, and Large Intestine channel areas and Chest and Respiration area.

ON THE FEET: Do the Healthy Foot massage in the How Can You Treat Yourself? section. Press and knead the following points: Frontal Sinus, Nose, Lungs, Ear, and Eye.

ON THE EARS: Press and knead Internal Nose and External Nose to treat a sneezy, runny nose. Press and knead the following points, if sore: Point Zero, Forehead, Kidneys, Shen Men, Endocrine, and Allergy. Press and knead Eye, if the eyes are irritated.

Scraping

Scrape down the neck, across the shoulders, and down the upper back. Pay particular attention to the area between the shoulder blades and the spine.

Tapping

Tap each point up to 30 times. You may need an assistant for the neck/shoulder area.

- Tap Du-20 and Du-23 on the head.
- Tap down the back of the neck and across the shoulders. Check GB-20 and Bl-12 and tap, if sore.
- Tap along the Large Intestine channel on the arms, especially LI-11, LI-10, and LI-4 on the hand.
- Tap down the outside of the lower legs along the Stomach channel, including St-40 and St-36.

Exercises

Do Exercise 1 and 2 of the five-element stretches daily. These strengthen the Lungs and Large Intestine and Stomach and Spleen.

Lifestyle advice

One of the keys to nasal allergy prevention is not to let the qi in your body become weak in the first place. That is easier said than done, of course, as it involves taking regular exercise, eating sensibly (according to the guidelines above), managing stress so that you can remain relatively calm and relaxed, and expressing your emotions in a positive way.

Sinus Problems
Symptoms

Blocked nose, nasal discharge (often yellow or green), no sense of smell, strong headaches, sinuses painful to touch, lack of clarity in thinking.

Can include or lead to

Sinusitis and nasal polyps.

When to see your doctor

There is a nasal discharge after a head injury.

Common causes

Stress; repressed emotions; worry; overthinking; a poor diet with too much greasy, hot-natured food or too much sweet food; or repeated infections.

An explanation

If you have sinus problems, you are not alone. Sinusitis is one of the leading forms of chronic disease, with an estimated 18 million cases and at least 30 million courses of antibiotics per year in the US alone.[18]

WIND AND HEAT: Wind is the main external cause of sinusitis. It enters the Lungs via the mouth or neck, reducing the drainage of fluid from your sinuses and nose. Heat often accompanies the wind and cooks up these fluids into a thick, sticky mucus soup. Unless this mucus is thoroughly cleared, either naturally or with the help of some form of treatment, the condition will keep repeating itself like a bad dream.

The heat can come from a variety of sources. Repressed emotions over time will block the Liver and generate heat, as will continual stress at home and work. Eating too much heating food, such as deep fried food, lamb and alcohol, can also be a cause.

DAMP AND PHLEGM: The mucus that often accompanies this condition is a literal manifestation of damp and phlegm conditions in the body. The degree of additional damp and phlegm produced depends on your diet and the state of the Stomach and Spleen. If your diet consists of too many damp- or phlegm-forming foods, it is highly likely that this excess will be sent up to the Lungs.

Taking certain medications long-term can also be problematic. People suffering from sinusitis, for example, often take antibiotics to address the condition. Antibiotics clear heat and can improve the symptoms for a while by cooling the sinuses, but they do not clear damp. As a result, sinusitis is highly likely to return because the damp state, of which the mucus is a symptom, is still sitting there unaffected by the antibiotics and preparing for more disruption.

WEAK QI IN THE SPLEEN: Repeated use of antibiotics can also weaken the Spleen. And this has a very important implication for sinusitis. When weak, the Spleen is unable to process fluids and gets clogged up with damp.

WEAK QI IN THE LUNGS: This has a direct knock-on effect on the Lungs, which is where all this extra sticky substance has to be stored. It too quickly becomes weak and is unable to send all this excess fluid down to the Kidneys, as it would normally do. Instead, much of it finds its way up into the sinuses.

Dietary factors that can worsen sinus problems

- Hot-natured and damp-forming foods, such as saturated fats, pizzas, deep-fried foods, and beer. See Damp and Heat for more details.

Dietary factors that can improve sinus problems

- Follow a qi-strengthening diet to improve qi in the Lungs and Spleen. See Weak Qi for more details.
- Eat foods that expel phlegm, such as citrus peel, persimmons, radishes, grapefruit, and pears. See Phlegm for more details.

Acupressure and massage

ON THE HEAD:
- Circle your face with the fingers to relax the facial muscles.
- Press Yintang, then finger-press outwards on both

sides to the temples. At the temples, circle Taiyang.

- Repeat at equally spaced points on the midline up to the middle of the eyebrows. Hard-press Yintang, Bitong, and Bl-2.
- From the eyebrows to the midpoint of the nose, gently finger-press outwards along the eye socket to the temples. At the temples circle.
- From the midpoint of the nose to the bottom of the chin finger press outwards to the corner of the jaw bone and circle.
- Press and knead LI-20 at the flare of the nostrils.

ON THE BACK:

- Finger-circle outwards at the base of the skull towards the ear and back again. Press GB-20.
- Finger-circle down the neck on either side of the spine.
- Finger-circle along the shoulder muscle.

ON THE ARMS: Thumb-press along the Large Intestine channel up to LI-11, and knead any sore points.

ON THE HANDS: Press the following points, if sore: LI-4, LI-2, Lungs, Chest, Lung, and Large Intestine channel areas, Nose area and Chest and Respiration area.

ON THE FEET: Press and knead Frontal Sinus on the toes, Lungs, Chest, Eye, and Ear.

ON THE EARS: Press the following points, if sore: Internal Nose, External Nose, Frontal Sinus, Forehead, Occiput, Point Zero, and Shen Men.

Scraping

Scrape down the neck, across the shoulders, and down the upper back muscles either side of the spine. Concentrate on the area between the shoulder blades and the spine.

Tapping

Tap the following points up to 30 times if they are sore when pressed:

- On the head: Du-20 and Du-23.
- On the back: GB-20 and Bl-12.
- On the arm and hand: LI-10 and LI-4.
- On the leg: St-36.

Exercises

Do Exercises 1 and 2 of the five-element stretches daily to strengthen the Metal and Earth organs.

Lifestyle advice

Some people benefit from regularly washing out their sinuses with warm, salty water – the idea being that water should go in and come out the other nostril or the mouth and clean out lingering mucous.

Add 1–2 level teaspoons of pure sea salt to one-half litre of lukewarm (previously boiled or sterile) water. Note: Add ¼–½ teaspoon of baking soda to prevent any burning sensation that can occur. Pour the saline solution into a syringe, dropper, or plastic squeeze bottle and use gravity or pressure to wash out the sinuses.

You may also want to invest in a neti pot, a ceramic or plastic travel pot that looks like a genie's lamp. Used as a daily cleansing routine in Indian Ayurvedic medicine, neti pots were once the province of yoga practitioners but are now mainstream, as more health practitioners suggest their use as a preventative technique for nasal allergies. The neti pot has a wide handle and a spout that you insert into the nostril as you tilt the head and the pot, allowing the saline solution to flow through first one nostril, then the other. Saline washes are also available commercially, but it is simpler to just use your own solution.

Eye Problems
Symptoms

Vary according to condition.

Can include or lead to

Orbital neuralgia, glaucoma, uveitis, cataracts, trachoma, conjunctivitis, iritis, keratitis, scleritis, haematopsia, endophthalmitis, and herpes zoster on the eyelid.

When to see a doctor

If the symptoms are severe.

Common causes

Stress, overwork, too long in front of a computer monitor, emotional stress, playing video games, exposure to the weather, late nights, lack of sleep, doing too much, a poor diet of either too much greasy, hot-natured foods or cold-natured raw foods, or a chronic illness.

An explanation

WEAK YIN IN THE LIVER OR KIDNEYS: Underlying most eye conditions is a weakness of yin in the Liver and/or the Kidneys. This imbalance of yin has usually gone on for a long time, often with mild symptoms. These include dry, bloodshot eyes, which can be blurred, sore, and sometimes with spots in your vision like marks on the lens of a camera (known as floaters). Like most yin conditions it may also feel worse in the afternoon or at night.

HEAT IN THE BODY: Over time, the slow burning heat of yin weakness can develop into a raging fire, and symptoms such as red, painful, watering eyes with a sensation of heat and pressure from within the eyes often means that the heat has transformed in the Liver and is burning upwards. This condition frequently gets worse when under emotional stress.

DAMP AND PHLEGM IN THE BODY: An inappropriate diet can also create problems in the eyes. A diet consisting of too many hot-natured, greasy foods or too many cold-natured, raw foods weakens the Spleen and Stomach and leads to an accumulation of damp and phlegm, which can combine with heat or cold to affect the eyes.

Dietary factors that can worsen eye problems

- Deep-fried foods, spices, lamb, coffee, and alcohol increase heat and worsen some eye conditions. See Heat for more details.
- Foods that are highly nutritious and sweet, such as dairy products, orange and tomato juice, and pork, worsen phlegm and mucous. See Damp for more details.

Dietary factors that can improve eye problems

- Cooling foods, such as tomatoes, watermelon, cucumber, lettuce, radishes and mangos, soothe heat. See Heat for more details.
- Barley, celery, pumpkin, turnips, lemons, and onions reduce phlegm and mucous. See Damp and Phlegm for more details.
- Cool-natured, sweet foods, such as apples, pears, tomatoes, peas, and asparagus, strengthen yin. See Weak Yin for more details.
- Foods such as broccoli and carrots can help improve vision by directly benefitting the Liver.

Acupressure and massage

ON THE HEAD:
- Press Yintang (in between the eyebrows) and finger-press outwards along the eyebrow to the temples. Then circle at the temples, and hard-press Bl-2 and Bitong.
- Repeat from the midpoint below the eyebrows and hard-press Bl-1 and GB-1.
- Repeat from the bridge of the nose, and follow the eye socket around to the temples. Circle the temples.

- Repeat a finger width below, and follow below the eye socket to the temples. Hard-press St-2.
- Finger-circle outwards at the base of the skull towards the ear and back again. Press GB-20 and Bl-10.

ON THE LEGS: Thumb-press along the Stomach channel up to the knee. Knead any sore points, including St-36. Thumb-press along the Liver and Gall Bladder channels up to the knee. Knead any sore points, including GB-43.

ON THE HANDS: Press and knead the following points, if sore: LI-4, LI-3, TB-2, Eye, and Liver areas.

ON THE FEET: Thumb-press the middle of the soles of the feet, Eye, and Liver.

ON THE EARS: Press and knead the following points if sore: Eye, Eye disorders 1 and 2, Liver, and Shen Men.

Scraping

Scrape down the neck, across the shoulders, and down the back muscles either side of the spine. Look for any tightness in the mid-back area.

Tapping

Tap each point up to 30 times. You may need help with some of the neck and shoulder points.

- For tired, bloodshot eyes, tap along the Gall Bladder channel on the lower leg, especially the area around GB-34.
- Also gently tap Taiyang, St-2, and Bl-2 on the face.
- For general eye problems, tap around the back of the neck and shoulder area, especially GB-20, Bl-10, and along the base of the skull.

Also carefully tap SI-19 and GB-2 on the face.

Exercises

Do Exercise 6 of the five-element stretches daily. This is to strengthen the Wood organs: the Liver and Gall Bladder. The state of the Liver is closely associated with the state of the eyes.

Lifestyle advice

Many people are putting great demands on their eyes on a daily basis without even realizing it, particularly those who watch a lot of television and those who use computers and play video games for hours at a time. Studies in the United States have shown that regular computer users have a severely diminished blinking frequency. Normally, we tend to blink about 18 times per minute, but when using a computer or playing a video game this reduces to only four times per minute.[19]

As blinking is an action designed to protect the eyes, it is essential to take frequent breaks to rest them and return to blinking properly.

For swollen eyelids, soak thin slices of cucumber in salty water (two tablespoons of sea salt dissolved in a cup of water). Put these over your closed eyes for 10 minutes. Repeat daily. Warmth also soothes your eyes, and a rolled-up hot towel placed over the eyes for several minutes can help.

Earache
Symptoms

Fullness or pain inside or outside the ear, redness, swelling, discharge, a ringing or buzzing sound, deafness, dizziness, and a headache.

Can include or lead to

Otitis media, inflammation, abscess, or infection of the auditory canal or mastoiditis.

When to see a doctor

If the symptoms are severe, the earache continues for more than a few days or is accompanied by a high fever.

Common causes

Exposure to the weather; an improper diet of fatty, greasy food; emotional stress, especially anger or frustration; or an injury or accident.

An explanation

WIND IN THE EAR: Owing to the exposed position of the ears on the sides of the head, wind entering the ear and bringing with it heat, damp, and sometimes cold is often the source of ear problems. Any combination of these factors will cause an obstruction in the movement of qi and blood in or around the ear, often with associated pain or discomfort. The most common pattern is for wind and heat to lodge in the ear, with accompanying sore throat symptoms.

STAGNATION OF QI IN THE BODY: Common internal causes of earache involve the Liver and Gall Bladder, which can become sluggish and blocked when emotionally stressed. The stagnation of qi in these two organs can lead to a buildup in heat, which races upwards via the Gall Bladder channel running around the ears. This then blocks qi and blood around the ears and causes severe pain. It often feels like the problem is deep within the ear. It can be accompanied by swelling, redness, and a fever.

DAMP AND PHLEGM IN THE EAR: A diet that contains too many sweet, fatty, greasy foods can damage the Stomach and Spleen and lead to an accumulation of damp and phlegm. This damp and phlegm can easily find its way upwards into the ear and quite literally block it, causing mild pain. There is often an ear discharge with this condition. It is a very common pattern in children.

WEAK QI IN THE KIDNEYS: For gradual cases of earache that are mild in nature and involve symptoms of deafness, low ringing noise in the ear, and feelings of tiredness, it is quite possible that the pain is coming from a weakness in the Kidneys. Each of the organs is connected to parts of the body, and a weakness in a particular organ (for example, the Kidneys) can adversely affect the corresponding body part (for example, the ear). The state of the Kidneys, therefore, can directly affect the ear and quality of hearing.

Dietary factors that can worsen earache

- Overeating and irregular eating habits lead to stagnation in the digestive process that can develop into more general qi stagnation. See also Qi Stagnation for more details.
- Cow dairy products, concentrated orange juice, and fatty meat such as lamb can create phlegm and mucous buildup in the body. See Damp for more details.

Dietary factors that can improve earache

- A balanced diet that strengthens the digestive system should be followed, including many of the foods in Weak Qi. See also Qi Stagnation for more details.
- Radishes, celery, rye, pumpkin, garlic, and aduki beans reduce damp and phlegm. See Damp and Phlegm for more details.

Acupressure and massage

ON THE HEAD:
- Finger-circle outwards at the base of the skull towards the ear and back again. Press GB-20 and Bl-10.

- Finger-circle from the base of the skull up to a point on the skull above the ear. Press GB-8 and GB-9.
- Finger-circle the skull around the ear, starting at the base of the ear. Press GB-2, GB-12, and SI-19 on the face.
- Hard-press GB-14 on the forehead.

ON THE LEGS: Thumb-press the Gall Bladder channel up to the knee and down again. Knead GB-41, GB-43, and any other sore points on the way. Press St-40, and knead if sore.

ON THE HANDS: Press the following points, and knead if sore: LI-4, TB-2, TB-3, SI-3, Triple burner channel area, and Head area.

ON THE FEET: Thumb-press and knead the balls of the feet. Also knead Ear, Frontal Sinus, and Kidneys, if sore.

ON THE EARS: Press the following points, and knead if sore: Inner Ear, External Ear, Kidneys, Point Zero, and Shen Men.

Scraping

Scrape down the neck (including the sides) and over the shoulder muscles and upper back muscles. Pay particular attention to the top of the shoulder and the area between the spine and the shoulder blades.

Tapping

Tap each point up to 30 times. You may need an assistant for the neck/shoulders area.

- Feel over the neck and shoulder area and tap any sore points.
- Gently tap GB-20 and Bl-10 at the base of the skull and Du-20 on the top of the head.
- Feel along the Gall Bladder channel in the lower leg. Tap GB-34 and any other sore point. Also tap St-40 and St-36 on the legs, if sore.
- Tap LI-4, LI-11, and any other sore points along the Large Intestine channel in the arm.

Exercises

Do Exercise 4 and 6 of the five-element stretches daily. This is to strengthen the Wood and Water organs. The Gall Bladder and Kidneys in particular are associated with the state of the ears and hearing.

Lifestyle advice

- Wherever possible, the ears and neck should be protected from exposure to the elements, especially from the wind.
- Avoid repeated use of antibiotics as they can damage the Spleen and can create damp and phlegm. These sticky substances can easily find their way to the ear and prolong the problem.

Tinnitus

Symptoms

A ringing or buzzing sound in either or both ears, partial hearing loss, earache, and fullness in the ear.

Can include or lead to

Wax buildup or a foreign body in the external ear, otitis media, glue ear, an eardrum injury, and Ménière's disease.

When to see a doctor

If the symptoms are severe.

Common causes

Overwork, stress, lack of sleep, old age, a long chronic illness, strong negative emotions like resentment and envy, an improper diet of lots of damp- or phlegm-forming foods, or exposure to loud noise.

An explanation

WEAK QI IN THE KIDNEYS: The key organ in conditions affecting the ear and hearing is the Kidneys. It is either the cause or a strong underlying factor in any case of tinnitus. Strengthening the Kidneys is, therefore, very important for reducing tinnitus and to ensure it stays that way. The sound of tinnitus – a low-pitch sound in both ears – is caused by weak qi and weak blood. It is usually of gradual onset and may improve with rest.

WIND AND HEAT IN THE EAR: As the ear is normally exposed to the elements, it can be susceptible to wind getting in and lodging there, particularly with heat. This is usually the pattern when there is an infection in the inner ear.

DAMP AND PHLEGM IN THE EAR: The ear can also get blocked by damp and phlegm, which gets into the channels around the ear and actually in the ear itself too. Symptoms of this pattern are more likely to be only in one ear and include a feeling of pressure, possible discharge, and a heavy sensation in the whole head.

STAGNATION OF QI IN THE BODY: Emotional stress, especially anger, resentment, and aggression, can sometimes exacerbate the problem. These emotions stagnate Liver qi, and the heat associated with backed-up qi starts to rise. In this case, though, instead of rising into the head, this heat rises into the ear via the channel of the Liver's paired organ, the Gall Bladder. This pattern is usually accompanied by headaches, pressure in the ears, and symptoms of qi stagnation, or perhaps a high-pitched buzzing sound, pain, and signs of heat.

Dietary factors that can worsen tinnitus

- Excess coffee, alcohol, and hot-natured and spicy foods worsen stagnant qi with heat. See Stagnation of Qi for more details.

- Too many damp-forming foods, such as bananas, dairy products, and wheat, worsen phlegm and damp. See Damp and Phlegm for more details.

Dietary factors that can improve tinnitus

- The qi in the Kidneys can be built up with a qi-strengthening diet. See Weak Qi for more details. In particular the following foods directly strengthen Kidney qi: aduki beans, black sesame seeds, kidney beans, walnuts, parsley, raspberries, and blackberries.
- Radishes, celery, and pumpkin reduce damp and phlegm. See Damp and Phlegm for more details.

Acupressure and massage

ON THE ARMS: Thumb-press the Large Intestine channel up to the elbow, and knead any sore points, in particular LI-11.

ON THE LEGS/FEET: Thumb-press the Spleen channel up to the knee and back. Knead any sore points, in particular Sp-3 in the feet, and Sp-6, and Sp-9 in the lower leg. Thumb-press the Gall Bladder channel up to the knee. Knead any sore points, in particular GB-34.

ON THE HANDS: Press the following points and knead, if sore: LI-1, LI-4, SI-3, TB-2, Triple Burner channel area, Head area, Liver, and Kidneys.

ON THE FEET: Press the following points and knead, if sore: Ear, Kidneys, Liver, Gall Bladder, Brain, and Neck.

ON THE EARS: Press the following points and knead, if sore: Inner Ear, External Ear, Liver, Kidney, Point Zero, and Shen Men.

Scraping

Scrape down the neck, over the shoulders, and down the upper back. Concentrate on the area between the shoulder blades and the spine.

Tapping

Tap each point up to 30 times. You may need help with the neck/shoulder area.

- Palpate the neck and shoulders area, and tap any sore points.
- Gently tap GB-20 and Bl-10 at the base of the skull and Du-20 on the top of the head.
- Feel along the Gall Bladder channel in the lower leg. Tap GB-34 and any other sore point. Also tap St-40 and St-36 in the legs, if sore.
- Tap LI-4 in the hand, LI-11 at the elbow, and any other sore points on the Large Intestine channel in the arm.

Exercises

Do Exercises 4 and 6 of the five-element stretches daily. This is to strengthen the Wood and Water organs. The Gall Bladder and Kidneys, in particular, are associated with the state of the ears and hearing.

Lifestyle advice

- As with Earache, avoid repeated use of antibiotics due to the damage they can do to the Stomach and Spleen's ability to process damp and phlegm. It is very easy for any excess accumulation to make it up to the ear and make things worse.
- If there is a possible stress or emotional component to the problem, try to find ways to limit their extent. Think about where stress might be coming from, as sometimes it is not as obvious as it seems.

Toothache

Symptoms

Pain or increased sensitivity of the teeth, headache, swelling, bleeding gums, insomnia, and agitation.

Can include or lead to

Dental cavities, acute or chronic pulpitis, peridental abscess, and pericoronitis.

When to see a doctor

If the symptoms are prolonged and severe.

Common causes

An improper diet of greasy, fatty foods; too much alcohol; stress; too many dairy products; old age; or a lack of oral hygiene.

An explanation

Often the cause of toothache is obvious, and you only need a simple method of pain reduction before or after a dental visit. Sometimes, however, the pain in the teeth has no clear dental cause and can be a symptom of something else happening in the body. For example, more often than not, treatment to relieve stiff shoulders also relieves toothache.

HEAT IN THE BODY: As the Stomach channel runs from just under the eye, over the jaw, to the temple, then down the front of the body all the way to the second toe, it can have quite an influence on the sensations felt in the teeth. Sometimes, severe toothache is due to heat rising through this channel to the face. The heat is usually from an accumulation of heat in the stomach and intestine area over some time, normally caused by an inappropriate diet. If this is the case there will probably be other signs of digestive heat like constipation.

WEAK YIN IN THE KIDNEYS: The Kidneys ensure that your bones and teeth are properly nourished with qi and blood to make them strong and durable. When the Kidneys become weak in yin, your teeth can also become weak and can become loose, wobbly, or even fall out. This condition can also lead to a dull toothache that comes and goes.

WIND IN THE BODY: Wind can sometimes enter the body and lodge in the channels in the face. This can happen on a windy day, when the body's defences are low, or when blood becomes so weak that it actually generates its own wind. Like all wind-type conditions, there is a tendency for the pain to come and go or move from one place to another.

Dietary factors that can worsen toothache

- Hot-natured, spicy foods, such as black pepper, chilli, ginger, and paprika worsen heat in the body, as do fried or roasted foods. See Heat for more details.

Dietary factors that can improve toothache

- Cold-natured foods, such as bananas, tomatoes, grapefruit, cucumbers, lettuce and radishes, lessen heat in the body. See Heat for more details.
- Foods such as beetroot, dark leafy greens, peas, apricots, dates, pears, and honey strengthen yin and blood. See Weak Blood and Weak Yin for more details.
- Foods such as parsley specifically strengthen the teeth.

Acupressure and massage

ON THE HEAD: Hard-press the masseter muscle just before the angle of the jaw, the area between the temples and the ear, SI-18, and LI-20. Keep the pressure on any sore points, release, and repeat several times.

ON THE ARMS: Thumb-press the Large Intestine channel up to the elbow, and knead any sore points, including LI-11.

ON THE LEGS: Thumb-press the Stomach channel up to the knee. Knead any sore points, in particular St-44.

ON THE HANDS: Press the following points, and knead if sore: Toothache, LI-4, LI-2, Stomach, Spleen, and Large Intestine area and Head area.

ON THE FEET: Press the following points, and knead if sore: Lower Teeth, Upper Teeth, Neck, Brain, and Kidneys.

ON THE EARS: Press the following points, and knead if sore: Tooth, Upper Jaw, Lower Jaw, Dental Analgesia, and Shen Men.

Scraping

Scrape down the neck, over the shoulder muscles, and down the upper back muscles.

Tapping

Tap each point up to 30 times. You may need an assistant for the neck/shoulder area.

- Tap any sore or tight points on the neck and shoulder areas.
- Upper teeth pain: Feel along the Large Intestine channel, and in particular check LI-4, LI-10, and LI-11 for soreness. Also Lu-7 on the arm and St-37 on the leg and, if sore, tap until they become less tender.
- Lower teeth pain: Feel along the Stomach channel, and tap any sore points, in particular St-44 on the foot and St-39 on the leg.

Exercises

Do Exercise 2 of the five-element stretches daily. This can help strengthen the Stomach channel, which is often indicated in toothache.

Lifestyle advice

If the source of the pain is tooth decay, or another obvious dental-related reason, the pain will probably not go away completely until this is treated by your dentist. If not, the advice on stress and emotions in Facial Pain can also sometimes be relevant here.

Sore Throat
Symptoms

Swollen, sore throat and/or tonsils, redness, feeling hoarse, pain when swallowing, dry throat, dry cough, and difficulty in speaking.

Can include or lead to

A cold; flu; acute infections such as laryngitis, pharyngitis, and tonsillitis; vocal chord polyps; fibroma; or cancer of the larynx/throat.

When to see a doctor

If the symptoms of pain and/or soreness last more than a couple of weeks or become severe.

Common causes

Exposure to the weather, smoking, an improper diet of rich spicy food, too much alcohol, doing too much at the same time, living in a dry environment (with central heating for example), regular use of bronchodilating medication (as commonly used for asthma), or prolonged emotional stress.

An explanation

OBSTRUCTION OF QI IN THE THROAT: The immediate pain or discomfort of a sore throat is from a local obstruction of qi and blood, accompanied by heat. As heat rises it is not moving on but accumulates in the throat area, along with the rest of the obstruction.

WIND AND HEAT IN THE NECK: This heat often enters from outside the body and is usually accompanied by wind. It normally enters through the mouth or neck and can easily lodge in the throat. If this is the case, the sore throat would normally be more acute – red, sore, and swollen – and resemble an infection.

HEAT RISING FROM THE BODY: The heat in the throat can also be caused internally from the Lungs (due to smoking), from the Stomach (due to an over-rich diet), or from the Liver (when there is a strong emotional component). Sometimes this heat flares up to the throat and causes acute throat symptoms, as it does with external heat; instead, though, internal heat often smolders like the embers of a bonfire and leads to a slight inflammation that goes on for a long time.

WEAK YIN IN THE BODY: Other internal causes are related more to weakness than to heat. When the condition is chronic, it flares up when the patient is tired and never completely disappears. It can be due to a Lung and Kidney yin weakness, which can come with age, overwork, and regular smoking. As with most yin-deficient conditions, the throat would probably be worse in the evening.

WEAK QI IN THE SPLEEN: The cause may also be a Spleen weakness from over-treatment with too many antibiotics. Antibiotics clear heat but not wind or damp, and their repeated use weakens the Stomach and Spleen, causing the condition to be complicated by even more damp.

In all cases of sore throat, the earlier it can be treated the better. Lingering sore throats can cause damage to the tissues of the upper respiratory tract, and sometimes can develop into more troubling conditions, such as abscesses.

Dietary factors that can worsen a sore throat

• Warming foods, such as coffee, alcohol, lamb, and beef, and warm spices, such as cinnamon, ginger, and fennel, feed heat. See Heat and the lists of Hot and Warm Foods for more details.

Dietary factors that can improve a sore throat

- Moistening foods, such as apricots, lemons, limes, persimmons, strawberries, pears (especially pear juice), watercress, and cucumbers (and their juice) can soothe the throat.
- Cooling foods such as radishes also expel phlegm and are particularly calming for a sore throat.
- Useful homemade recipes to treat sore throats include:
  Dice 3cm of daikon radish (with the peel), and soak it in a little honey. Leave for about an hour, then add a small amount of warm water before drinking the mixture.
  Cook the flesh of a grapefruit with a little water and honey for around five minutes and then eat.

Acupressure and massage

ON THE HEAD: Finger-press and knead any sore points along the base of the skull, especially GB-20.

ON THE ARMS/HANDS: Thumb-press the Large Intestine and Lung channels up to the elbow, and knead any sore points, in particular, LI-4 and LI-11, and Lu-7 and Lu-5. Also knead TB-5, if sore.

ON THE BACK: Press BL-12, Bl-13, and Du-14, and knead if sore.

ON THE FRONT: Finger-circle down the breastbone, and knead Ren-17 and any other sore points.

ON THE LEGS: Press and knead GB-34 and St-40, if tender.

ON THE FEET: Knead the outside of the big toe, from the joint to the tip of the toe. Also press and knead Larynx, Sternum, Trachea, Tonsils, Neck, Chest, and Lungs.

ON THE HANDS: Press the following points, and knead if sore: TB-1, TB-2, TB-4, Lu-10, Lu-11, Throat, Tonsils, Chest and Respiration area, Mouth area, and Head area.

ON THE EARS: Press the following points, and knead if sore: Throat, Mouth, Trachea, and Tonsils.

Scraping

Scrape down the neck (on the sides as well), across the shoulders, and down the upper back either side of the spine.

Tapping

Tap each point up to 30 times. You may need an assistant for the neck/shoulder area.

- Tap GB-20 and Bl-10 and any other sore points at the base of the skull.
- Tap any sore points over the neck and shoulder areas.
- Tap along the Large Intestine channel in the arm, including Lu-11 on the arm, and LI-4 and LI-1 on the hand.
- Tap along the Lung channel on the arm, including Lu-10 on the hand and any sore points on the bulge of muscle below the thumb.
- Tap along the Triple Burner channel on the arm, and tap any tender points, including TB-5.
- Tap gently along the breastbone and then along the bottom of the ribcage.

Exercises

Do Exercises 1, 2, and 6 of the five-element stretches. The state of the Metal, Earth, and Wood organs can easily affect the throat.

Lifestyle advice

- If possible, stay out of the elements and rest. Exposure to wind, cold, or heat can exacerbate the problem.
- Sometimes the sore throat is simply the body telling you to stop. This is particularly the case with someone who leads a very yang lifestyle and is doing too much.

Neck Pain

Symptoms

Pain in one or both sides of the neck – the pain can be acute or chronic; tense muscles and tendons; muscle spasms and stiffness.

Can Include or lead to

Cervical disc hernia, whiplash, torticollis, osteoarthritis, degeneration of the cervical vertebrae, and cervical spondylosis.

When to see a doctor

If the symptoms are severe and steadily getting worse; if there is swelling or bruising; if there is pins and needles in the arms and fingers when touching the neck vertebrae; or if there are any symptoms of shock from a neck injury, such as whiplash.

Common causes

Exposure to the weather, bad posture, overuse, a trauma or injury, overwork, emotional stress, an inappropriate spinal manipulation or massage, a chronic illness; or an inappropriate diet.

An explanation

WIND, DAMP, AND COLD IN THE NECK: Both acute and chronic pain in the neck are often related to wind, damp, and cold, and to the subsequent obstruction of qi in the neck area.

The most common way for wind, damp, and cold to get into the neck is through direct exposure to the elements. It could be something as simple as being outside on a windy day, not covering up after swimming or exercise, or sleeping without a blanket or warm covers.

Precautions to take when using manual therapy to treat the neck

Manipulating the neck when there is neck pain can sometimes produce the opposite result to the one desired. It can sometimes become far worse and take longer to cure. If the neck is very stiff, inflamed, and difficult to move, it is often best to use points away from the neck to treat symptoms. Note, too, that if there is a sensation of pins and needles in the arms and fingers when the neck vertebrae are palpated, it could mean that there is a structural problem with the vertebra, which will need professional medical attention.

Once these elements find their way into the neck, they disrupt the smooth flow of qi in the channels that run over the neck and cause pain.

STAGNATION OF QI IN THE NECK: These channels can also be blocked as a result of some kind of local trauma. This causes blood and yang to drastically weaken and the muscles in the neck to tighten, as they are no longer being nourished, resulting in stiffness and cramping. This is often the case with traumas like whiplash, which are acute, very painful, and difficult to move.

STAGNATION OF QI IN THE BODY: Emotional stress and depression can weigh heavily on the Liver and cause it to slow qi down, which then leads to a general stagnation of qi in the body. This stagnation can sometimes find itself heading up the Gall Bladder channel towards the back of the neck, which will then aggravate any neck pain by causing more local neck stagnation.

WEAK QI AND BLOOD IN THE BODY: Any underlying weakness of qi or blood, as often found in stressed, overworked, or chronically ill people, means that the bones, muscles, and tendons in the neck area are undernourished, causing the whole area to become weaker and more susceptible to stagnation or wind, damp, or cold.

Dietary factors that can worsen neck pain

- If the condition is one of damp or cold in the neck, it is important not to add to it by eating too many damp-forming or cold-natured foods, such as bananas, dairy products, and wheat. See Damp and Cold for more details.

Dietary factors that can improve neck pain

- The weakness underlying neck pain can be helped by following a strengthening diet to build up qi and blood. See Weak Qi and Weak Blood for more details.

Acupressure and massage

ON THE NECK: (See the precaution box)
- Knead the back of neck with four fingers together in a circular motion, from the base of the skull to where the neck meets the shoulders.
- Pinch the neck muscles with thumb and fingers from the base of the skull downwards.
- Press the neck muscle with flat fingers and rub up and down to create heat.
- Press and knead Bl-10, GB-20, and Du-16, and any sore points at the base of the skull.
- Moist heat can sometimes be beneficial and can be applied by soaking a towel in hot water, wringing it out, then placing it on the affected area of the neck. This is then repeated with a new hot towel as the towel cools.

ON THE HANDS AND ARMS:
- Thumb-press along the Small Intestine channel up to the shoulder area. Knead any sore points, in particular SI-1–4 and SI-11. Repeat on both sides of the body.
- Thumb-press along the Triple Burner channel up to the shoulder area. Knead any sore points, in particular TB-8. Repeat this on both sides of the body.

ON THE LEGS: Press and knead Sp-6, GB-34, St-40, and Bl-40, if sore.

ON THE FEET: Press the following points and knead if sore: Neck, Shoulder, Cervical area, Thoracic area, and Liver.

ON THE HANDS: Hard-press Luozhen. Also press the following points, and knead if sore: Stiff neck, Cervical area, and LI-4.

ON THE EARS: Press the following points, and knead if sore: Neck, Cervical area, and Shoulder. Press on the area of the ear corresponding with the location of the pain.

Scraping

Scrape down the neck, across the shoulders, down the upper back, and across the chest area. The tension in the neck often extends into the shoulders and back, and relieving tightness there can often help.

Tapping

Tap each point up to 30 times. You may need an assistant for the neck area. Caution: Do not tap on or near the neck if it is inflamed or very stiff.
- Tap the following points near the neck, if sore: Bl-10, GB-21, and SI-14.
- Tap along the Small Intestine and Triple Burner channels on the arm and hand, including TB-8, TB-5, and SI-3.
- On the legs, tap GB-39 and St-40 and the areas around them, if sore.

Exercises

The following are simple exercises to help strengthen the neck. They should ideally be done sitting down:

1. HEAD TURN SIDEWAYS:
Turn your head slowly to the right, as far as possible. Turn it to the left slightly, then go even farther to the right. Repeat this several times on the left and right.

(top left) Head turn sideways

(top right) Neck resistance

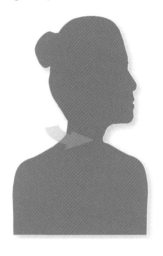

2. HEAD TILT BACKWARDS:
Tilt your head backwards, as far as possible. Bring it forward slightly, then move it farther back. Repeat several times.

(bottom left) Head tilt backwards

(bottom right) Neck circle

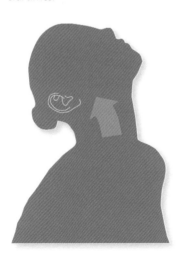

3. NECK RESISTANCE:
Interlink the fingers of both hands, and place them behind your neck. Push your head backwards, and at the same time pull your neck forwards with your hands.

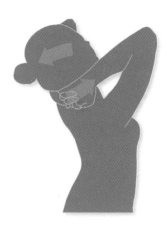

4. NECK CIRCLE:
Relax your head and neck, then slowly turn the head as much as possible and circle it back to center. Do this several times – first, clockwise, then counterclockwise. NOTE: Be careful not to overrotate your neck, to avoid injury.

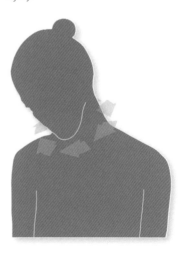

5. BEND FORWARDS:

Stand with a straight back, feet close together and arms at your sides. Breathe in, then gently bend forwards with your upper body. Stop when you reach resistance and hold the position. As you breathe in, lift up your head to see in front. Return slowly to the original position while breathing out.

Also do Exercises 3 and 6 of the five-element stretches.

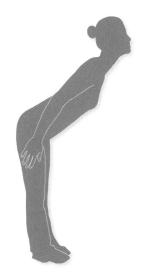

Lifestyle advice

- Protect your neck – not just on windy days but from changes in temperature (usually due to air conditioning and artificial heating systems) – as you engage in simple everyday activities, such as shopping or working at the office.
- Also, do not hesitate to protect your neck from other people's well-meaning massaging fingers. Sometimes a massage can make the pain worse.
- Be cautious when exercising. Any exercise, no matter how healthy it may seem (tai chi or yoga, for example), can cause damage if you go past your limits and overextend you neck.

To ice or not to ice?

For acute injuries, most people automatically reach for the bag of frozen peas sitting in their freezer, but in order for the injury to heal well, you should not overuse ice. As a general guideline, the following may be helpful:

- If pain is from an acute injury, ice can be used to lessen the swelling during the first 24–48 hours.
- After a 24–48-hour period – or when the swelling has gone down, if sooner – the application of ice can sometimes harm healing in the area. This is because cold usually causes more stagnation of qi and blood by contracting the channels, muscles, and tendons.
- Heat in the form of a hot towel, which is replaced as soon as it cools down, does the opposite and is often preferable to aid in healing (provided, of course, the area is not red, hot, and inflamed).

Bend forwards

Shoulder Pain
Symptoms

Pain or stiffness in one or both shoulders, including the shoulder joint, muscles, tendons, and the shoulder blade, and referred pain in the arm and back.

Can include or lead to

Frozen shoulder, periarthritis of the shoulder, synovisitis of the shoulder joint, calcification of the shoulder joint, and tendonitis.

When to see a doctor

If the symptoms are severe and getting worse, and if there is swelling, bruising, or you are unable to move the shoulder joint.

Common causes

Overuse, an injury, exposure to the weather, emotional stress, an improper diet of cold-natured, raw foods or greasy, sweet foods.

An explanation

STAGNATION OF QI IN THE BODY: When Liver qi is weak, it has a weakening effect on the tendons and muscles in the body. They become malnourished and easily affected by disturbances in Liver qi.

Emotional stress is the usual cause of disturbances in the Liver. Irritability, for example, will disrupt the Liver's ability to keep qi moving smoothly around the body. Qi then becomes blocked and causes pain. This pattern is often found in chronic shoulder pain with distending pain down the arm that worsens when stressed.

WEAK BLOOD IN THE BODY: When the body's qi is weak, it is very susceptible to wind either coming in from outside or being generated within the weak blood stored in the Liver. The muscles and tendons can then easily become numb or cramp up, causing pain on movement, especially between the shoulder blades. Sometimes this pain is worse at night, as the weak blood tries to retreat to the Liver.

DAMP OR PHLEGM IN THE SHOULDER: Damp or phlegm also tend to feature prominently in any shoulder pain. The damp or phlegm often comes from weak Spleen qi and often from an inappropriate diet of too much cold-natured, raw or greasy, sweet foods and poor eating habits. The Spleen and Stomach become too weak to prevent the buildup of damp, and the more damp that collects, the greater the chance of blockages. If the condition is one of damp, rainy weather can affect it and, although there is a little movement, it is usually quite stiff.

COLD IN THE BODY: Cold is often due to a weakness of yang qi, or it may be associated with external factors such as being out in cold weather or swimming in the sea. If the pain is due to cold, it will normally be fixed and immovable and can be worse in the morning. This is because cold contracts the muscles and tendons, and it takes time for yang qi to warm them up.

Dietary factors that can worsen shoulder pain

- Inappropriate eating habits, such as overeating or eating late at night, can add to general qi stagnation in the shoulder.
- Processed foods, which often contain chemicals, flavourings, and additives, can weaken blood.
- If cold, damp, or phlegm are present, it is very important to limit the relevant foods that aggravate these conditions in the diet to remove a potential source of problems. See Cold, Damp, and Phlegm for more details.

Dietary factors that can improve shoulder pain

- If cold is present in the shoulder pattern, then a diet with the addition of more warming foods, such as garlic, ginger, black pepper, chestnuts, cherries, and wine, will be of benefit. See Cold for more details.
- If damp or phlegm is present, eat more foods that reduce moisture, such as rye bread or rye crackers, watercress, aduki beans, radish, onions, and pumpkins. See Damp or Phlegm for more details.
- For any underlying weakness of blood, eat more blood-nourishing foods, such as leafy greens, beetroot, chicken soup, and legumes. See Weak Blood for more details.
- Stagnation can be reduced by eating less, at regular times, and in a calm manner. The following foods can also help: spices such as turmeric, ginger, and cumin; turnip; the peel of citrus fruits; and radishes.

Acupressure and massage

If the pain is acute, it is best to use points away from the shoulder so as not to potentially worsen the condition.

ON THE BACK: Press and knead any sore points in the shoulder area, in particular GB-21. Thumb-press down the back muscles either side of the spine. Knead any sore points, including Bl-17 and Bl-18.

ON THE FRONT: Press Lu-1 and Jianqian, and knead if sore.

ON THE ARMS: Thumb-press along the Large Intestine and Triple Burner channels to the shoulder. Knead any sore points, including LI-11, TB-14, and LI-15.

ON THE LEGS: Hard-press Bl-57.

ON THE HANDS: Press the following points, and knead if sore: SI-3, LI-4, LI-3, Lu-9, Lu-10, LI-2, TB-3, Shoulder, Stiff Neck, and Triple Burner and Large Intestine channel areas.

ON THE FEET: Press and knead Shoulder, Cervical area, and Thoracic area.

ON THE EARS: Press the following points, and knead if sore: Shoulder, Master shoulder, Cervical area, Thoracic area, and Shen Men.

Scraping

Scrape down the neck, across the shoulders and tops of the arms, and down the upper back muscles.

Tapping

Tap each point up to 30 times. You may need an assistant for the shoulder area.

- Feel along the Large Intestine, Small Intestine and Triple Burner channels along the arms and over the shoulder. Tap any sore points.
- On the back, press Bl-10, GB-21, SI-14, Du-12, and Jianqian and if tender, tap.

If more acute, tap points further away from the shoulder: LI-10 and LI-11 on the hand, and GB-34 or any sore points along the Gall Bladder channel on the lower leg.

Exercises

The following exercises can relax and strengthen the shoulders:

1. SHOULDER ROTATE:
Bend the waist slightly, stretch both arms out straight, and gently rotate the shoulder joint in a forwards direction.

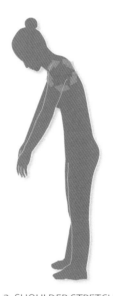

(top right) Shoulder rotate

(below) Shoulder stretch

2. SHOULDER STRETCH:
Stretch each arm upwards while standing in front of a wall, and mark how high they go. Repeat this, and try to increase the height each time.

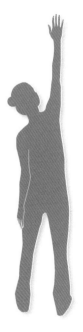

Arm lift

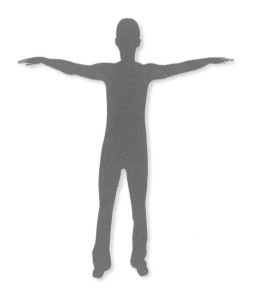

Using your waist as a pivot, twist the top half of your body until you feel resistance, then twist in the opposite direction. Repeat the sequence several times.

5. Do exercise Bend Forwards from Neck Pain, as this gently moves the shoulder.

6. Do exercise Crouch Twist from Weak Qi, as this involves twisting the shoulder joint.

7. Do Exercises 1, 3, and 5 of the five-element stretches daily. These strengthen the channels that run over the shoulder.

Lifestyle advice

If possible, rotate the joint through its full pain-free range of movement daily (in other words, move it until it starts to hurt and do not go any further). If the injury is acute, note the advice about putting ice on it in Neck Pain.

3. ARM LIFT:
Stand with your arms at your sides and your feet shoulders' width apart. Breathe in while gently lifting up both arms to the sides. Stop when the arms reach shoulder height. Breathe out and let the arms fall. Repeat the sequence several times.

4. TWIST THE WAIST:
Stand with your arms at your sides and your feet shoulders' width apart. Lift up both arms to the sides.

Twist the waist

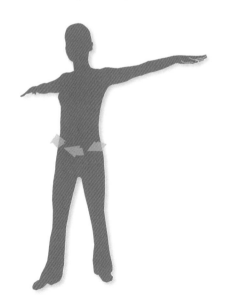

Chapter 20
氣 **Chest Area**

Colds and Flu

Symptoms

Runny nose, sore throat, cough, fever or chills, sneezing, tiredness, stiff and sore neck, muscle aches, and headache.

Can include or lead to

Common cold, influenza, upper respiratory infection, bronchitis, or pneumonia.

When to see a doctor

If severe or symptoms last more than five days.

Common causes

Tiredness; overwork; exposure to the wind, heat, or cold; air-conditioning; going in and out of heated or air-conditioned shops; not wearing appropriate clothing; or sitting in a draught.

An explanation

A layer of qi surrounds our bodies to protect it from the environment, dubbed "defensive qi." Sometimes when it gets weak, it can no longer prevent environmental factors from entering the body and causing disruption.

WIND IN THE LUNGS: When we catch a cold or come down with flu, it usually means that wind has bypassed our defensive qi and found its way into the Lungs via the mouth or nose. It usually is accompanied by either heat or cold, and together they disrupt the Lungs and force them to send qi upwards instead of downwards, causing sneezing and coughing.

If the wind and heat or cold can be expelled effectively within the first 24 hours, the symptoms usually go away fairly quickly. If left to take hold in the Lungs without the right treatment, the condition can often go much deeper within the body and be harder to get rid of.

Dietary factors that can worsen colds and flu

- Overconsumption of damp-producing foods, such as cow dairy products, eggs, fried foods, bananas, and cold drinks from the fridge. See Damp for more details.
- Citrus fruit can also worsen a cold by preventing the body from sweating by closing the pores of the skin.

Dietary factors that can improve colds and flu

- Simple foods that are easy to digest are best. Choose foods such as vegetables or grains in the form of soups or broths, soft rice, and porridge (oatmeal).
- An important distinction to make is whether you feel more chilly (the condition is therefore cold), or more hot and feverish (the condition is therefore hot); different types of foods help each condition:
- If you feel mainly chilly: eat more parsnips, horse-radish, cinnamon, garlic, and onions.

- If you have mainly a fever: eat more parsley, aubergines, carrots, peas, broccoli, turnips, lemon juice, grapefruit, and fruit.
- In both cases, tea can be beneficial, especially when made with sweat-inducing herbs, such as ginger (use fresh ginger root) or chamomile for a cold condition, and peppermint or elderflower for heat. Honey and lemon can be added to the tea to make it taste better.

Acupressure and massage

ON THE HEAD: Press and knead Yintang, Taiyang, and GB-20.

ON THE ARMS/HANDS:

- Thumb-press along the Lung and Large Intestine channels up to the shoulder. Knead any sore points, especially Lu-7 and LI-11 on the arm, and Lu-10 and LI-4 on the hand.
- Thumb-press along the Triple Burner channel on the back of the forearm, and knead any sore points, including TB-5.

ON THE FEET: Press the following points, and knead if sore: Lungs, Chest, Nose, Kidneys, and Diaphragm.

ON THE HANDS: Press the following points, and knead if sore: Head area, Throat, Lungs, Lung, and Triple Burner channel areas, Chest and Respiration area, and Reduce Fever.

ON THE EARS: Press the following points, and knead if sore: Inner Nose, Throat, Lungs, Ear Apex, Occiput, Point Zero, and Shen Men.

Scraping

Scrape down the neck (including the sides), across the shoulders, down the upper back – in particular, the area in between the shoulder blades – and down the back muscles either side of the spine. Also scrape down the middle of the breastbone and along the gaps in the ribs. Be careful not to scrape over breast tissue.

Tapping

Tap each point up to 30 times. You may need an assistant for the neck/shoulder and back area.

- Tap Bl-10, GB-20, and Du-16 and along the base of the skull.
- Feel down the neck and over the shoulder muscles. Tap any sore points.
- Tap down the upper back muscles either side of the spine, including Bl-12 and Bl-17.
- Feel along the Lung and Large Intestine channels in the forearm, and tap any sore points, including Lu-5 and LI-4 on the hand.

Exercises

Do Exercise 1 of the five-element stretches to strengthen the Lungs and prevent yourself from catching colds and flu.

Lifestyle advice

- If you are suffering from a cold or flu, the best place to be is at home resting. If you have to be outside, it is very important to wear clothing that covers and protects your neck.
- The most effective solution to a cold or flu is usually to sweat it out. This literally means getting into bed, covering yourself with a blanket or comforter, wearing extra clothes, and regularly drinking warm, sweat-inducing tea (see earlier in this section). If you are sweating, change any damp clothing or covers promptly.
- If you are in the early stage of a cold or flu and not sweating, a hot bath can help get it started. Afterwards, wrap yourself in a dressing gown or towels for ten minutes, then take a warm shower.
- It is important not to do any physical exercise and, if possible, stop working. The more rundown the body is, the greater the likelihood for the condition to worsen.

- Exercise is very important in cold prevention. A recent British study concluded that the frequency of colds among people who exercised at least five days a week was half that of people exercising once a week or less.[20]

Cough
Symptoms

A cough that may be chronic or acute, dry or wet (brings up mucous), weak, or barking, and with a tight chest.

Can include or lead to

Common cold, upper respiratory tract infection, bronchitis, pneumonia, pulmonary emphysema, and pulmonary tuberculosis.

When to see a doctor

If you are coughing up blood, there is accompanying breathlessness, or the coughing lasts for longer than a week.

Common causes

Overwork, emotional problems such as worry and frustration, too many dairy products and oily, greasy foods, smoking, asthma medication, bad posture, or a long chronic illness.

An explanation

When we breathe in, air rushes into the lungs, where it is converted into qi and sent downwards to mix with the qi extracted from digestion. This enhanced qi is then sent on around the body to energize every last cell and to allow us and all the various parts of us to function. Sometimes, however, this process becomes blocked, and, instead of flowing downwards, qi rises, causing a cough.

WIND AND HEAT OR COLD IN THE LUNGS: Coughs often occur due to wind entering the Lungs, as described in Colds and Flu. They are usually accompanied by heat, with any mucus being thick and yellow or green, or by cold, in which case any mucous would be watery, white, or clear.

DAMP OR PHLEGM IN THE LUNGS: Coughs can also be caused by the accumulation of damp or phlegm in the Lungs, or from an improper diet. A distinctive sign of this is when phlegm is expelled with the cough and a rattling sound can be heard in the lungs. It can often be worse at night or first thing in the morning.

WEAK YIN IN THE BODY: If the yin of the Lungs and Kidneys is weak, there will not be enough moisture for either to function properly, as yang often generates too much heat and dryness. This dry condition is usually worse in the afternoon or evening.

HEAT IN THE BODY: Heat can arise from weak yin, as yang becomes agitated and overactive. It can also come from overactive Liver qi. The Liver can become overactive due to stress and emotional issues, especially if weak and stagnated. This agitation from below can then block the Lung's ability to send qi downwards. With this condition, the cough usually becomes worse with stress and can result in a barking cough that is worse in the afternoon.

Dietary factors that can worsen a cough

- Hot-natured, spicy food and oily or greasy food can worsen any kind of cough. See Heat for more details.
- Dairy products, peanuts, bananas, and other damp-forming foods should be avoided in coughs with lots of mucus. See Damp for more details.

Dietary factors that can improve a cough

- If the cough is dry and due to a weakness of yin in the Lungs, the following foods may help to moisturize the Lungs again: bananas, pears, tangerines, honeydew melons, almonds, sunflower and sesame seeds, milk, and honey.
- If the cough is barking and caused by too much heat, the following foods may be helpful in reducing the heat in the Lungs: apples, pears, asparagus, radish, carrots, tomatoes, mushrooms, mung beans, green tea, and peppermint tea.
- If there is a lot of phlegm with the cough, it is important to add the following foods to your diet: grapefruit, tangerines, citrus peel, watercress, radishes, and lemon juice.

Acupressure and massage

ON THE HEAD: Press Ren-22, and knead if sore.

ON THE FRONT: Finger-press down the middle of the breastbone, and knead any sore points, including Ren-17. Press Lu-1 and Lu-2, and knead if sore.

ON THE BACK: Press Bl-12 and Bl-13, and knead if sore.

ON THE ARMS/HANDS: Thumb-press along the Lung and Large Intestine channels, up to the elbow. Knead any sore points, especially Lu-9, Lu-10, and Lu-11, and LI-4 and LI-11.

ON THE HANDS: Press and knead the following points if sore: Throat, Lung, Asthma, Chest and Respiration area, Lung channel area, Sanjiao, and Large Intestine.

ON THE FEET: Press and knead the top third of the foot, below the toes, on both sides of the feet. This is the Lung and Chest area. Also Sternum, Trachea, Larynx, and Diaphragm.

ON THE EAR: Press and knead the following points, if sore: Asthma, Chest, Antihistamine, Throat, Lungs, Shen Men, and Point Zero.

Scraping

Scrape down the neck (including the sides), across the shoulders, and down the muscles of the upper back. Pay particular attention to the area in between the shoulder blades. Scrape down the breastbone and along the gaps in the ribs. Be careful not to scrape over breast tissue.

Tapping

Tap each point up to 30 times. You may need an assistant for the neck/shoulder area.

- Tap any sore points in the neck and shoulder areas.
- Tap along the Large Intestine channel on the forearm, including LI-11 on the arm, and LI-4 and LI-1 on the hand.
- Tap along the Lung channel on the forearm, including Lu-11 and Lu-10 on the hand.
- Follow the Triple Burner channel on the arm, and tap any sore points. In particular, check TB-5.
- Tap gently along the breastbone and then along the bottom of the ribcage (not on the bone).

Exercises

Do Exercises 1 and 2 of the five-element stretches. These can strengthen the Lungs and reduce phlegm.

Lifestyle advice

- Smoking is a major cause of coughs, and all tobacco product use should be stopped. The action of smoking is the inhaling of a heating substance into the lungs, which can damage the yin of the Lungs. Often simply avoiding tobacco is enough to stop a cough.
- The simplest remedies are often the best. A recent American study of children aged between two and 18 years of age concluded that the effects of buck-

wheat honey on night-time coughs was more soothing than an over-the-counter medication.[21]

Asthma, Breathlessness, and Wheezing

Symptoms

Shortness of breath, wheezing, difficulty in breathing, congestion in the chest, cough, and phlegm.

Can include or lead to

Asthma, Chronic Obstructive Pulmonary disease (COPD), bronchitis, pulmonary tuberculosis, emphysema, pleurisy, and lung cancer.

When to see a doctor

If the symptoms worsen or persist.

Common causes

A constitutional weakness; an improper diet of oily, greasy food; a chronic illness; emotional stress; overwork; or a hectic lifestyle.

An explanation

Asthma is a very common problem – so common, in fact, that it is thought that more than 300 million people worldwide currently suffer from it, and that this number will increase by 50 percent every decade.[22]

Asthma is often caused by wind that has entered the Lungs, usually because of a general weakness in the body's defences, and stayed there, disrupting how qi is sent around the body. This combined with a weak digestive process, often due to a poor diet or overuse of antibiotics, can cause damp and phlegm to accumulate and be sent up to the Lungs.

A combination of this accumulated phlegm at the bottom of the Lungs and the stuck wind can quickly transform into heat and burn up any moisture in the Lungs. This then leaves the Lungs dry and weak and susceptible to further problems.

ACUTE ASTHMA:

- HEAT IN THE LUNGS: If an asthma attack is caused by wind and heat, any mucus is usually yellow or green and is thick and sticky.
- COLD IN THE LUNGS: If an asthma attack is caused by wind and cold, it is often more difficult to exhale. Any mucus is normally watery, white, or clear, and there is usually a feeling of coldness. The condition worsens with cold weather.

CHRONIC ASTHMA:

- WEAK QI IN THE LUNGS AND KIDNEYS: In the young, old, and chronically ill, it is sometimes the case that breathing problems involve a breakdown of the relationship between the Lungs and the Kidneys. There is a close partnership between the Lungs and the Kidneys when we breathe. The Lungs send qi down, and the Kidneys grasp it and pull it down. If the Kidneys do not have enough force to grab the qi, the Lungs can no longer send it, and so the smooth breathing process is interrupted. With this condition, it is usually more difficult to inhale than to exhale. Ironically, prolonged use of the most common asthma medications can make this weakness worse. Salbutamol or Albuterol, commonly known as Ventolin among others, gradually depletes qi in the Lungs, and inhaled corticosteroids such as Pulmicort or Flovent can use up both Lung and Kidney yin.

Dietary factors that can worsen breathing

- Cold-natured, raw foods can solidify the phlegm in the chest and generate more mucus by weakening the digestive process. See Cold for more details.
- Hot-natured, spicy food and seafood can cause heat to build up in the Lungs. See Heat for more details.

Dietary factors that can improve breathing

- Follow a simple, bland strengthening diet to fortify Lung qi. See Weak Qi for more details.
- The following foods can help with asthma:

IN GENERAL: green vegetables, pumpkins, carrots, and apricots can help strengthen and protect the Lungs.

FOR CHEST TIGHTNESS AND SPASMS: anchovies, salmon, mackerel, sardines, and tuna, and pumpkin seeds, dark green vegetables, and blackcurrant can help.

FOR PHLEGM CONDITIONS: the peel of citrus fruits, such as tangerines, lemons, and grapefruit, and horseradish and aduki beans help expel phlegm from the Lungs.

FOR COLD CONDITIONS: garlic, basil, ginger, oats, walnuts, almonds and sunflower seeds.

FOR HOT CONDITIONS: radishes, lemons, and limes may be helpful.

Acupressure and massage

ON THE FRONT:
- Press Ren-22, and knead if sore.
- Finger-circle down the middle of the breastbone, and press and knead any sore points, in particular Ren-17.
- Finger-circle out from the breastbone in the spaces between the ribs. Press and knead any sore points, in particular Kid-24 to Kid-27.
- Hard-press Ren-4 and Ren-6.

ON THE ARMS: Thumb-press the Lung and Large Intestine channels up to the elbow. Press and knead any sore points, in particular the points Lu-5 and Lu-7.

ON THE BACK:
- Thumb-press the Bladder channels, and knead any tender points, in particular Bl-13, BL-17, Bl-20, and Bl-23.

* Finger-circle down the middle of the spine, in the gaps between the vertebrae. Press and knead any sore points in the upper part of the body.

ON THE LEGS: Thumb-press along the Stomach channel up to the knee, and knead any sore points, in particular St-36 and St-40.

ON THE HANDS: Press and knead the following points, if sore: Asthma, Cough, Lu-10, Lu-1, LI-4, Sanjiao, Lung channel area, and Chest and Respiration area.

ON THE FEET: Press and knead Heart and Lung areas in the top one-third of the foot. Also Chest, Ribs, Liver, Kidney, Diaphragm, Larynx, Trachea, and Sternum.

ON THE EARS: Press and knead the following points, if sore: Asthma, Antihistamine, Lungs, Point Zero, Shen Men, Allergy, and Ear Apex.

Scraping

Scrape down the neck, over the top of the shoulders and down the upper back. Also scrape down the breastbone and either side of the breastbone in the gaps between the first four ribs. Scrape sideways, following the rib spaces. Be careful not to scrape over breast tissue.

Tapping

In an acute asthma attack, tap the following points:
- Ren-22 at the top of the breastbone.
- Kid-25, Kid-26, and Kid-27 in between the ribs on the chest.

For chronic asthma:

Tap each point up to 30 times. You may need an assistant for the back area.
- Tap along the Large Intestine and Lung channels of the forearm and hand, especially Lu-5 and LI-11 on the arm and LI-4 and Lu-10 on the hand.
- Tap down the back muscles either side of the spine.

Exercises

Do Exercises 1, 2, 4, and 5 of the five-element stretches to open and strengthen the Lungs and chest.

Lifestyle advice

A variety of preventative measures can be taken to lessen the chances of problems with asthma.

- Weather can affect the Lungs. To prevent problems, it is important to dress appropriately when outside, especially in the wind and cold. The neck especially should be protected.
- Asthma attack triggers include fumes, smoke, or dust. Minimize situations where you are likely to encounter these.
- Posture can affect the Lungs, and habitually bad posture often creates weakness in Lung qi. A 2009 British study concluded that children who spend more than two hours a day sitting down watching TV have double the risk of developing asthma.[23] Extended periods of inactivity, stooping over work, prolonged periods in front of a computer, and working without breaks should therefore be avoided.
- The Lungs can be strengthened by gentle exercise and fresh, clean air. Some form of outdoor activity, such as walking, is essential to support the Lungs.

Chest Pain

Symptoms

Pain, stuffiness, or heaviness in the chest, palpitations, and shortness of breath.

Can include or lead to

Heart problems, pulmonary embolism, pleurisy, angina, depression, hiatus hernia, peptic ulcer, pancreatitis, and hyperventilation.

When to see a doctor

If the symptoms are severe or persistent or include numbness, tingling, or pins and needles in the limbs. Seek immediate medical attention for a crushing chest pain that may extentend to the arms and jaw.

Common causes

An improper diet that weakens the Spleen and Stomach, emotional stress, old age, and repeatedly catching colds or coming down with flu.

An explanation

STAGNATION OF QI IN THE BODY: There is often some form of qi obstruction with chest pain. This often stems from qi stagnation and is caused by stress, repressed emotions, or a sedentary lifestyle. For this reason, the pain can often feel worse when stressed and is more of a discomfort or stuffiness than pain. It often feels better when relaxing and after a big sigh.

PHLEGM IN THE LUNGS: Obstructions can also be caused by phlegm, which can collect in the Lungs as a result of an inappropriate diet. The chest can sound rattly when breathing, owing to the excess phlegm present in the lungs, and coughing can often produce phlegm. If heat is also present with the phlegm, the chest can feel congested, accompanied by a burning sensation.

STAGNATION OF BLOOD IN THE BODY: Should the chest pain be very acute, and there is a stabbing, crushing, or sharp sensation, this suggests the obstruction is caused by a stagnation of blood. This could feel worse at night and would normally signal the need for a rapid hospital visit to check on the condition of your heart.

WEAK QI IN THE HEART: Underlying the above conditions, some form of Heart qi weakness is normally present in cases of chest pain. This normally manifests as palpitations. Unless this weakness is strengthened, the chest pain is likely to either continue or return at a later date.

Dietary factors that can worsen chest pain

- Overeating can cause stagnation in the digestive process, and therefore add to any stagnation in the chest.
- Salads, raw fruit and vegetables, dairy products, ice-cold drinks, and other cold-natured foods can also add to the stagnation. See Cold for more details.

Dietary factors that can improve chest pain

- A diet that strengthens qi and blood can help rebalance the organs within the chest area. See Weak Qi for more details.
- The peel of citrus fruits, such as tangerines, lemons, and grapefruit, horseradish, barley, and aduki beans can help if the condition is one of phlegm in the chest. See Phlegm for more details.
- Herbs and spices such as chives, cloves, marjoram, turmeric, and basil should be emphasized for conditions of stagnation of qi and blood. See Stagnation of Qi and Stagnation of Blood for more details.

Acupressure and massage

ON THE FRONT: Finger-circle along the breastbone, and knead any sore points, including Ren-17. Press Liv-14, and knead if sore.

ON THE BACK: Feel along the neck and back muscles either side of the spine and follow the Bladder channel down to the bottom of the shoulder blades. Press and knead Bl-14, Bl-15, and Bl-17, if sore.

ON THE ARMS: Thumb-press the Pericardium and Triple Burner channels up to the elbow. Knead any sore points including Pc-6 and TB-6.

ON THE LEGS: Thumb-press the Gall Bladder and Liver channels up to the knee. Knead any sore points, including GB-34. Thumb-press along the Stomach and Spleen channels up to the groin. Knead any sore points, including St-40 and Sp-10.

ON THE HANDS: Press the following points, and knead if sore: Chest, Heart, Chest and Respiration area, the top segments of all five fingers, He-9, Pc-8, and LI-4.

ON THE FEET: Do the Healthy Foot massage in the How Can You Treat Yourself? section. Also press the following points, and knead if sore: Chest, Liv-3, Diaphragm, Ribs, Lungs, Sternum, Liver, and Kidneys.

ON THE EARS: Press the following points, and knead if sore: Chest, Heart, Lungs, Liver, Sympathetic, and Shen Men.

Scraping

Scrape down the neck, across the shoulders, and down the back muscles. Pay particular attention to the area around the shoulder blades. Scrape down the breastbone and outwards along the gaps in the ribs. Be careful not to scrape over breast tissue.

Tapping

Tap each point up to 30 times. You may need an assistant for the back area.

- Tap gently outwards from Ren-22 (at the top of the breastbone) at equal spacing above and below the collar bone.
- At the front of shoulder joint, tap Lu-1 and Lu-2.
- Tap gently down the breastbone at equal spacing and along the bottom of the last rib towards the sides.
- Tap GB-20, Bl-10, and Du-16 at the base of the skull, then press over the shoulders. Tap any tender points.
- Follow the Bladder channels down the back muscles, and tap any tender points. Do both sides before moving downwards.

Exercises

1. Do Exercises 1, 2, 3, and 5 of the five-element stretches to open and strengthen the chest area.
2. BEND BACKWARDS:
   Stand with a straight back, feet shoulders' width apart, and put your palms on your lower back. Breathe in, then gently bend backwards from the hip, as you breathe out. Stop when you reach resistance, and hold it for a few seconds. Slowly return to the original position, and repeat the sequence several times.

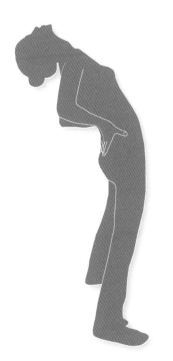

Lifestyle advice

- Stagnation can often be helped with light, regular exercise, especially exercise that involves twisting and stretching the upper back muscles.
- If stress is part of the picture, reduce it with stress management techniques such as managing your time better or just letting things go.

Palpitations and Irregular Heartbeat

Symptoms

A pounding heartbeat, a fluttering feeling in the chest, restlessness, anxiety, insomnia, shortness of breath, and tiredness.

Bend backwards

Can include or lead to

Cardiac arrhythmias, hyperthyroidism, anaemia, menopausal complications, coronary artery disease, neurosis, angina, and depression.

When to see a doctor

If the symptoms are severe and persistent, and if there is breathlessness, chest pain, or dizziness.

Common causes

Emotional stress, depression, prolonged grief, sadness, overwork, medication side effects, or over-exercise.

An explanation

Palpitations and irregularities in the heart beat can be a symptom of a heart condition and should be investigated by a medical professional.

Despite how it may feel, however, for many cases of palpitations, there is little actually wrong with the physical heart itself.

The problem often lies with a weakness of Heart yin or yang qi, and the cause of this imbalance in the Heart in turn can often be found elsewhere in the body.

WEAK YIN IN THE KIDNEYS: As in nature, there is a close relationship between Fire (Heart) and Water (Kidneys) in the body. Both have the ability to directly affect the other by either heating or cooling actions. The balance of yin and yang in the Kidneys is, therefore, directly linked with the balance of Heart yin and yang. If Kidney qi is weak, Heart qi is weak and vice versa.

In practice, what this means is that when Kidney yin becomes weak, it can no longer help contain Heart yang. Heart yang then becomes hot and agitated and affects the Heart, often leading to palpitations, sleeping problems, and a feeling of heat.

WEAK QI IN THE SPLEEN: An improper diet and bad eating habits can often lead to weakness and sluggishness in digestion. This weakness prevents the Spleen from sending enough energized blood to the Heart, which also then weakens Heart yang, causing palpitations, sleeping problems, panic attacks, and dizziness.

PHLEGM IN THE BODY: A weak digestive process can also contribute to the formation of phlegm in the chest, especially when accompanied by a diet of hot-natured, phlegm-forming foods. The phlegm combines with heat to obstruct the Heart and causes restlessness, waking up before dawn, and digestive problems in addition to palpitations.

STAGNATION OF QI OR BLOOD IN THE BODY: Qi stagnation is often caused by the Liver and is related to emotional stress or sedentary lifestyle habits. The stagnation blocks qi in the chest and disrupts correct Heart functioning. Blood stagnation is a much more serious extension of this and can be accompanied by pain or stuffiness in the chest.

Dietary factors that can worsen palpitations

- Coffee, caffeinated soft drinks, alcohol, and other stimulants agitate the Heart.
- Deep-fried foods, fatty meat, junk food, beer, and other hot-natured, phlegm-producing foods will add to the phlegm, heat, and stagnation. See Heat and Phlegm for more details.
- Salads and other cold-natured, raw foods can constrict circulation, also adding to any stagnation of qi and blood. See Cold for more details.

Dietary factors that can improve palpitations

- A general qi-strengthening diet can strengthen the Spleen, Kidneys, and Heart. Wheat, in particular, can be very nourishing for the Heart, while quinoa strengthens the qi of the Pericardium. See Weak Qi for more details.
- For cases of stagnation of qi or blood, add foods that will move qi, such as turmeric, oregano, nutmeg, and ginger. See Qi Stagnation and Blood Stagnation for more details.

Acupressure and massage

ON THE ARMS: Thumb-press along the Heart and Pericardium channels, up to the elbow. Knead any sore points, including Pc-6 on the arm and He-7 on the hand.

ON THE BACK: Thumb-press down the back muscles either side of the spine. Knead any sore points including Bl-15, Bl-17, Bl-18, and Bl-20.

ON THE LEGS: Hard-press Kid-7. This point can reduce palpitations and bring the pulse rate down. Thumb-press along the Stomach channel up to the knee. Knead any sore points, including St-36 and St-40.

ON THE HANDS: Press the following points, and knead if sore: He-8 and He-9; Palpitations, Pericardium, and Heart channel areas; Essence area; Heart; and Chest and Respiration area.

ON THE FEET: Do the Healthy Foot massage in the How Can You Treat Yourself? section. Also press the following points, and knead if sore: Heart, Chest, Diaphragm, Sternum, Lungs, Spleen, and Kidneys.

ON THE EARS: Press the following points, and knead if sore: Heart, Chest, Sympathetic, Pericardium, Shen Men, and Kidneys.

Scraping

Scrape down the neck, across the shoulders, and down the back muscles, either side of the spine. Scrape down the breastbone, then gently scrape along the rib spaces outwards from the breastbone. Be careful not to scrape over breast tissue.

Tapping

Tap each point up to 30 times. You may need an assistant for the back area.

- Follow the Bladder channels down the back muscles, and tap any sore points. Do both sides before moving downwards.
- Tap GB-41, Kid-7, and Bl-58 on the leg and He-7, Pc-6, and LI-11 on the arm/wrist.
- Feel for any sore points on the breastbone, and gently tap if sore.

Exercises

1. Do the exercise Bend Backwards from the Chest Pain section.
2. Do Exercises 3 and 5. When done regularly, both of these can strengthen the chest area and Heart.

Lifestyle advice

- Exercise is essential to prevent stagnation, but it is important to avoid strenuous exercise, such as tennis, squash, and running, as excessive sweating can weaken the yang of the Heart.
- Avoid smoking, as it can cause or add to the accumulation of phlegm and heat in the chest.
- Sometimes there is a strong emotional component to palpitations and heart irregularities, and changes in lifestyle may need to be made. One of the most important is letting your feelings out. This could be talking with someone close or just writing down how you feel on paper.
- If the problem is stress management, think about how this can be resolved. Asking for help is often a major step in the right direction, as is being honest about what works or does not work and letting go of things you cannot change.

Chapter 21
氣 **Stomach and Abdominal Area**

Nausea
Symptoms

Nausea, bloating, acid reflux, loss of appetite, and tiredness.

Can include or lead to

Morning sickness, if pregnant; travel sickness; food intolerance; and gastritis.

When to see a doctor

If the symptoms are severe or persistent.

Common causes

Strong emotions, stress, overeating, an improper diet, overuse of antibiotics, medication side effects, travel, pregnancy, or over-worry.

An explanation

WEAK QI IN THE STOMACH: The Stomach sends qi downwards, so that, when we digest, all the food matter heads down to the intestine. If the Stomach becomes weak, however, it can no longer maintain this downward motion and instead sends the qi upwards causing nausea.

STAGNATION OF QI IN THE BODY: Emotional stress can cause qi to become stuck and stagnate in the Liver. The muscles in the stomach and intestine used to process food downwards then become tense and unable to function properly. Qi then goes sideways, instead of downwards, and disrupts the Stomach. This is how a sudden outburst of anger can cause nausea.

DAMP OR PHLEGM IN THE BODY: The process of digestion can become sluggish from eating an irregular diet or consuming too many damp- or phlegm-forming foods. The Stomach and Spleen cannot process food properly, and as a consequence overproduce damp, which further blocks downwards qi and disrupts digestion.

When nausea is due to morning sickness, it is more a result of a physical imbalance in the abdomen. With pregnancy, blood and qi are concentrated in the lower abdomen. This causes an upward movement of qi from the uterus, which a weak Stomach or Spleen is unable to halt.

Dietary factors that can worsen nausea

- Overeating greasy foods high in saturated fats and also cold-natured, raw foods can weaken the Stomach and Spleen and lead to nausea. See Damp and Cold for more details.

Dietary factors that can lessen nausea

- A diet of easily digestible bland food strengthens the Stomach and Spleen. See Weak Qi for more details.
- Drinks should be sipped frequently rather than drunk in large amounts all at once.
- In cases of morning sickness in pregnancy or drug reactions, where regular nausea is experienced, it

may be necessary to eat many small meals throughout the day.

- Pumpkin or squash seeds, millet, rice, ginger, and spiced teas can help manage nausea. Celery can also help as it directs Stomach qi downwards.
- Several trials have confirmed the efficacy of ginger in significantly reducing nausea in pregnant women.[24] Read the Colds and flu section for more on how to use ginger. One popular method is to drink ginger tea, which can be made by simply pouring boiling water on a small slice of fresh ginger and allowing it to soak. Drink the tea warm, not hot.

Acupressure and massage

ON THE HEAD: Hard-press under the chin and Ren-24 at the same time with thumb and forefinger.

ON THE ARMS: Thumb-press along the Pericardium channel, up to the elbow. Press and knead any sore points. Hard-press Pc-6, and gently knead.

ON THE BACK: Press and kneed any sore points along the inner Bladder channel, especially Bl-20, Bl-21, and Bl-22.

ON THE FRONT: Finger-circle down the middle of the breastbone, and press any sore points. Palm-circle in a clockwise direction around Ren-12.

ON THE LEGS: Thumb-press along the Stomach and Spleen channels, up to the knee, and knead any sore points, including St-36 and St-40.

ON THE HANDS: Press the following points, and knead if sore: Abdomen, Pericardium channel area, and Stomach, Spleen, and Large Intestine areas.

ON THE FEET: Press and knead Stomach, Spleen, Abdomen, Pancreas, Duodenum, St-44, Sp-3, and Sp-4.

ON THE EARS: Press the following points, and knead if sore: Stomach, Pericardium, Inner ear, Esophagus, Spleen, Liver, Shen Men, and Sympathetic.

Scraping

Scrape down the back muscles from the shoulders to the top of the buttocks. Pay particular attention to the mid-back area.

Tapping

Tap each point up to 30 times. You may need an assistant for the back area.

- Feel down the midline of the breastbone, and tap any sore points.
- Follow the back muscles down either side of the spine, and tap any tender points on both sides.
- Tap Pc-6, LI-4, and TB-5 on the arm; Sp-3 and Liv-3 on the foot; and GB-34, St-36, and St-40 on the leg.

Exercises

1. WHOLE BODY STRETCH: This exercise is similar to the Relax the Whole Body exercise in Sleeping Difficulties. In this case, it can help to strengthen the Stomach and prevent nausea.

- Stand with your arms at your sides and feet shoulders' width apart.
- Lift the arms slowly until they are straight above your head, palms upwards.
- Link your fingers and turn the palms. At the same time, lift your heels and look upwards while breathing in.
- Slowly move your body into a squat position, while lower-

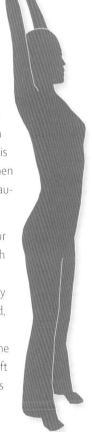

Whole Body Stretch: lift and stretch arms

ing your arms to the sides of the body. Breathe out as you bring your elbows and knees together and the heels flat, exhaling at the same time.

- Repeat several times.

2. BEND BACKWARDS: Do the Bend Backwards exercise from the Chest Pain section, as this stretches the stomach area.
3. Do Exercises 2 and 5 of the five-element stretches to strengthen the digestive organs and reduce nausea.

Whole Body Stretch: squat and relax

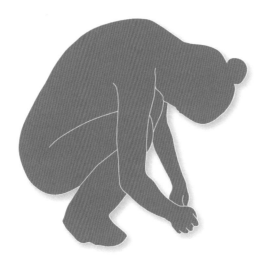

Lifestyle advice

In my short-lived days as a fisherman in Japan, I used to suffer periodic seasickness while out on the ocean, and more than my fair share of stomach contents would regularly empty into the East China Sea. I found that many of the techniques listed above greatly helped counteract the nausea. However, keep in mind the following:

- Activity can worsen nausea, so it is very important to rest but in a position that allows gravity to help you feel better. Rest either in a sitting position or in a supported lying-down position, with pillows.

- Fresh air and being outside often relieves some of the symptoms. Avoid warm, stuffy places, especially if they are not well ventilated.
- Long deep breaths help with relaxation. Adults often get in the habit of breathing shallowly, usually due to stress and bad habits, using only the upper thoracic area and the muscles around the ribs to pull air in. Just using the upper portion of the lungs reduces the availability of cleansing oxygen in the body and prevents the diaphragm from massaging the organs as it expands and pushes down like a bell jar with each breath.
- To see if you are breathing correctly, place one hand on the chest and the other on the abdomen. Inhale slowly and deeply, visualizing the breath moving all the way down into the abdomen. If you are breathing as nature intended, you should feel the belly push out first, then as the diaphragm and chest expand in one full inhalation breath.
- Pause for a moment after inhaling, then slowly exhale, feeling the belly button move toward the spine and the breath move upwards and expand the chest.
- The exhale should be longer than the inhale, allowing the breath to fully expel from the lungs and not remain stagnant in there. Repeat this slowly and methodically several times.

Feeling Bloated
Symptoms

The abdomen feels full, tight, and painful, and can appear uncomfortably swollen and gassy.

Can include or lead to

Gastritis, intestinal obstruction, hiatal hernia, coeliac disease, irritable bowel syndrome, colitis, and peptic/gastric ulcer.

When to see a doctor

If the symptoms are severe or persistent.

Common causes

Emotional stress; overeating; irregular eating habits; a diet of excess cold-natured, raw foods or processed, rich foods; overthinking and worrying; lack of exercise; or constipation.

An explanation

STAGNATION OF FOOD OR DAMP IN THE STOMACH: Bloating often occurs when damp or accumulated food clogs the Stomach and Spleen. This can happen as a result of following an inappropriate diet and overeating at meal times. Digestion then slows down, and Stomach and Spleen qi become weaker.

Like a reservoir behind a dam on a river, fluids collect in the intestine and abdominal walls because the body lacks the digestive power to process them and send them onwards. This leads to discomfort and a sense of fullness. The abdomen often feels soft when pressed, and there is normally little actual pain.

WEAK QI IN THE STOMACH AND SPLEEN: Weak qi in the Stomach contributes to bloating because not enough qi is available to be sent down to the intestine to ensure that stools pass through smoothly during the evacuation process. Peristalsis – the involuntary relaxing and contracting motions in the intestine that allow food to pass through – slows, and the resultant constipated backlog stagnates qi ,which, in turn, furthers the stagnation of qi in the Stomach and Spleen.

With this pattern there are more likely to be weight fluctuations, swollen eyes and fingers, and bloating when tired or at the end of the day.

STAGNATION OF QI IN THE BODY: The relationship between the Stomach/Spleen (the Earth organs) and the Liver/Gall Bladder (the Wood organs) is a close one. Weakness in one brings out weakness or overactivity in the other. When the Stomach and Spleen become weak, the Liver has a tendency to overflow with qi and flood the two Earth organs when the body becomes stressed and agitated.

The Stomach and Spleen effectively act as the lid to a boiling kettle (the kettle being Liver). If the lid stays on the kettle as it boils, then the steam can be released in a controlled way out the spout, and it can cool down quicker. If however the lid does not fit, or is not there at all, the hot water bursts out the top and becomes uncontrollable. This spillage floods the Stomach and Spleen and interrupts the digestive process causing bloating, which can worsen when emotionally affected.

Dietary factors that can worsen bloating

- Overeating and irregular meal times both can add to stagnation and weaken the digestive process.
- Raw, cool, and cold-natured foods will add to the general blockage of qi and food. See Cold and the Cool and Cold Foods lists for more details.
- Dairy products, wheat, bread, bananas, alcohol, and other damp-forming foods can weaken the Stomach and Spleen. See Damp for more details.

Dietary factors that can lessen bloating

- Steam or boil foods to make them easier to digest.
- In general, follow a strengthening diet that will support the Stomach and Spleen. See Weak Qi for more details.
- Carrots, leeks, fennel, garlic, coriander, pepper, and peas can help get the digestive system moving again.

Acupressure and massage

ON THE FRONT:

- Finger-circle down the breastbone. Finger-circle outwards between the ribs. Press and knead Liv-13 and Liv-14, if sore.
- ABDOMEN CIRCLE: Press nine points equally spaced around the belly button with the heel of

Abdomen circle massage

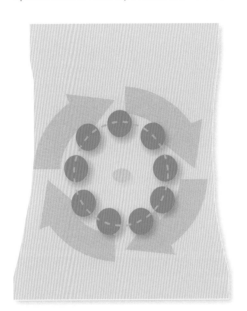

your palm. Work clockwise, and push each point towards the belly button. Press when breathing out and hold for ten seconds.

- Press and knead Ren-12, St-25, and Ren-6 if sore.

ON THE ARMS: Thumb-press along the Large Intestine channel, up to the elbow. Knead any sore points, including LI-10 and LI-11.

ON THE BACK: Press the following points, and knead if sore: Bl-20, Bl-21, and Bl-25.

ON THE LEGS: Thumb-press along the Stomach channel, up to the knee. Knead any sore points, including St-44 and St-37. Press and knead GB-34, if sore.

ON THE FEET: Do the Healthy Foot massage in the How Can You Treat Yourself? section. Press and knead any sore points, including Stomach, Small

Intestine, Liver, and Gall Bladder.

ON THE HANDS: Press the following points, and knead if sore: LI-4, Stomach, Spleen, Large Intestine, Small Intestine, and Abdomen.

ON THE EAR: Press the following points, and knead if sore: Stomach, Small Intestine, Large Intestine, Liver, Spleen, Abdomen, and Shen Men.

Scraping

Scrape down the back muscles, from the shoulders to the buttocks. Pay particular attention to the mid-back area.

Tapping

Tap each point up to 30 times. You may need an assistant for the back area.

- Feel along the Stomach and Spleen channels on the leg, and tap any sore points, including St-36, Sp-7, and Sp-8.
- Tap Bl-18, Bl-20, Bl-25 and any other sore points found in the back muscles either side of the spine.
- Feel along the Large Intestine channel in the arm, and tap any sore points.

Exercises

1. Do the Bend Backwards exercise from the Chest Pain section.
2. Do Exercises 2 and 6 of the five-element stretches, which can help strengthen the Stomach and increase the circulation of qi via the Liver.

Lifestyle advice

- Regular gentle exercise can be very beneficial, as it moves qi and strengthens the main organs involved in bloating.
- Be cautious about the claims of manufacturers of products designed to improve bloating, especially

those whose advertisements use phrases such as "gut flora," "probiotics," and "food intolerance." These broad-based approaches are usually trying to deal with the problem in isolation, without emphasizing the need to look at your eating habits, the type of food you are eating, the strength of your Stomach and Spleen qi, and, of course, the rest of your body. If your diet and eating habits are appropriate, there is normally no need to "help" your digestion with any supplements.

Stomach Pain

Symptoms

Pain or discomfort in the central part of the stomach between the ribcage and the belly button.

Can include or lead to

Gastritis, gastrospasm, gastrointestinal dyspepsia, gastroneurosis, hyperchlorhydria, gastric ulcer, duodenal ulcer, hepatitis, and carcinoma of the stomach.

When to see a doctor

If the symptoms are severe, the pain is worse with movement, or there is abdominal rigidity.

Common causes

A diet containing too many cold-natured, raw foods; stress; overwork; worry; repressed anger; exhaustion; or bad eating habits.

An explanation

The relationship between the strength of the Stomach and Spleen and the nature of the food that it processes is key in understanding many forms of stomach pain.

COLD IN THE STOMACH: A diet containing too many cold-natured, raw foods can lower the internal temperature of the stomach and cause severe, cramping pain as the cold condition contracts the muscles of the stomach lining. This type of stomach pain is often relieved by the application of heat but not with pressure.

HEAT IN THE STOMACH: A diet containing too many processed, hot-natured or spicy foods can increase the temperature of the stomach considerably. The pain is often accompanied by a burning sensation and other signs of heat and agitation.

DAMP HEAT IN THE STOMACH: A diet containing too many damp-forming foods, such as greasy foods, dairy products, and alcohol, can weaken the Stomach and Spleen, causing it to overproduce thick body fluids that, in turn, weaken the Stomach and Spleen further. The subsequent stagnation of fluids generates heat and often causes dull pain, tight chest, and frontal headache.

WEAK QI IN THE STOMACH AND SPLEEN: Poor eating habits and a diet that weakens digestion can lead to weak qi, yin, or yang in the Stomach and Spleen. The accompanying pain is often dull, accompanies eating, and feels better with heat.

STAGNATION OF QI IN THE BODY: The close relationship between the state of the Stomach/Spleen (the Earth organs) and the Liver/Gall Bladder (the Wood organs), as described in the Feeling Bloated section, equally applies here. The same process causes stagnation in the Stomach and Spleen and often results in stomach pain.

Dietary factors that can worsen stomach pain

• Overeating at mealtimes is one of the most common causes of stomach pain, both in the short and long term. Ideally, the stomach should be two-thirds full when you have finished eating.

• Excess damp-forming foods, such as bananas, wheat, processed foods, and foods containing concentrated sweeteners and nuts, can weaken the

Stomach and Spleen. See Damp for more details.

- Deep-fried foods and other hot-natured, oily foods, and black pepper, chilli, ginger, cinnamon, and other pungent spices worsen heat in the body. See Heat for more details.
- Overeating cold-natured foods, such as raw fruit and vegetables, salads, dairy products, and soya products, worsens cold in the body. See Cold for more details.

Dietary factors that can improve stomach pain

- Follow the guidelines for good eating habits in the How We Eat chapter. If eating habits remain poor, the Stomach and Spleen cannot strengthen and the pain will continue.
- A simple diet of broths and thick soups, which reduce the strain on digestion, is beneficial in strengthening the Stomach and Spleen.
- Rice, barley, cucumber, spinach, lettuce, watercress, and yogurt help cool the body. See Heat for more details. NOTE: Too many cooling foods can easily lead to damp and any dietary changes should be in moderation.
- Soups, cooked fruit, ginger, cardamom, and cinnamon help warm up cold conditions in the Stomach. See Cold for more details.
- Rye, radishes, pumpkin, celery, broad beans, and other foods reduce damp conditions in the Stomach. See Damp for more details.

Acupressure and massage

ON THE FRONT:
- Rub in a circular motion around the belly button with your palm.
- Do the ABDOMEN CIRCLE massage in Feeling Bloated.
- Finger-press and knead Ren-12, St-21, and St-25. Press Liv-14, and knead if sore.

ON THE ARMS: Press and knead Pc-6.

> CAUTION: Be cautious when massaging around the stomach and abdomen, as it can worsen the pain. Only use the points mentioned if pressure feels comfortable there.

ON THE LEGS: Thumb-press the Stomach channel up to the knee, and knead any sore points, especially St-36 and St-40.

ON THE BACK: Press and knead any sore points on the Bladder channel, including Bl-18, Bl-20, and Bl-21.

ON THE HANDS: Press the following points, and knead if sore: LI-4, Stomach, Spleen, Large Intestine areas, and Spleen, Liver, and Small Intestine.

ON THE FEET: Press and knead the middle area of the soles of the feet, including the St-44, Stomach, Small Intestine, Duodenum, Spleen, and Liver areas.

ON THE EARS: Press the following points, and knead if sore: Stomach, Liver, Spleen, Duodenum, Abdomen, Sympathetic, and Shen Men.

Scraping

Scrape down the back muscles, from the shoulders down to the top of the buttocks. Pay particular attention to the mid-back, as this is the Stomach area.

Tapping

Tap each point up to 30 times. You may need an assistant for the back area.

- Follow the Ren channel down the middle of the breastbone, and tap any sore points, including Ren-12.
- Follow the Ren channel down the abdomen to the pubic bone, and tap any sore points along the way.
- Press down the muscles on the outside of the leg, and tap any sore points, including St-36.
- Follow the Bladder channels down the back, and tap any tender points, especially Bl-18, Bl-20, Bl-21, and Bl-25.

Exercises

Do Exercise 2 of the five-element stretches to strengthen the Stomach and Spleen.

Lifestyle advice

Taking an overly long siesta in the afternoon can lead to the accumulation of damp in the Stomach and Intestine and should be avoided. A short rest after lunch is, however, very beneficial to the Stomach.

Abdominal Pain

Symptoms

Pain or discomfort around and below the belly button.

Can include or lead to

Enteritis, intestinal neurosis, indigestion, gastrointestinal spasm, duodenal ulcer, ulcerative colitis, irritable bowel syndrome, dysmenorrhoea, fibroids, ovarian cysts, endometriosis, carcinoma, and ascariasis.

When to see a doctor

If there are severe symptoms or abdominal rigidity.

Common causes

Over-worry, emotional stress, a prolonged feeling of frustration or anger, or a improper diet of cold-natured, raw, or hot-natured, spicy food.

An explanation

COLD IN THE ABDOMEN: Cold can enter the body directly and lodge in the intestine or uterus. This could be due to anything, from being inappropriately dressed on a cold day to sitting on a concrete park bench. It can also develop from a diet of cold-natured, raw foods or from an existing weakness of yang. This condition often consists of cramping pain that improves when you apply heat.

DAMP HEAT IN THE ABDOMEN: Heat dries up the moisture in the intestine or uterus and often combines with damp. It can develop from an existing condition of stagnation or weakness of yin or the transformation of a long-standing cold condition. The pain is usually worse with pressure, there is often a burning sensation, and the skin can be hot to the touch. In women, there can be heavy periods, an irregular cycle, and vaginal discharge.

STAGNATION OF QI IN THE ABDOMEN: Stagnation of qi often develops from emotional stress, as the Liver is hindered from regulating the flow of qi. Blockages in qi can find their way into the abdomen, causing pain that initially hurts with pressure then lessens with continued pressure. The pain often worsens with emotional stress and improves with activity or exercise.

STAGNATION OF BLOOD IN THE ABDOMEN: In some long-standing cases of qi obstruction, an actual physical blockage to the free movement of qi and blood develops, in the form of stagnant blood. These masses can sometimes be felt in the abdomen. The resultant pain is often very sharp and fixed, worse with pressure, and often worse at night.

WEAK QI AND BLOOD IN THE BODY: Underlying abdominal pain is often a general lack of strong qi and blood. This can come from an improper diet, an unhealthy lifestyle, a long-term illness, or a variety of depleting factors. Pain deriving from weak qi and blood can be dull and lingering and is usually better with pressure and rest.

Dietary factors that can worsen abdominal pain

- Overeating, eating too fast, and eating late at night add to any stagnation in the abdomen.
- Foods that have been deep fried or roasted aggravate hot conditions.

- Raw foods, especially when served chilled, aggravate cold conditions by forcing the digestive process to work harder at a lower temperature.
- Eating too many sour foods, such as most fruits, leafy greens, olives, pickles, and yogurt, can contract and slow down the digestive system. See the Sour Food list for more details.

Dietary factors that can improve abdominal pain

- Warm-natured foods that are grilled or cooked in the oven can help to reduce a cold condition. See the Warm food list for more details.
- Boiled, steamed, or sometimes raw cooling foods can help reduce a hot condition. See the Cold or Cool foods list for more details.
- In general, a strengthening diet that will help the movement of qi and food solids through the body would be ideal. For more details see chapter Weak Qi.
- Radishes, celery, rye bread, barley, lemons, and horseradish can help reduce damp. See Damp for more details.
- Stagnating qi and blood can often be improved with the addition of vinegar, chives, chilli, garlic, and cloves. See Qi and Blood Stagnation for more details.

Acupressure and massage

ON THE BACK: Finger-press along the Bladder channels, and knead any tender points, especially Bl-20, Bl-21, and Bl-25.

ON THE FRONT:
- Palm-circle with slight pressure around the belly button.
- Do the ABDOMEN CIRCLE massage in Feeling Bloated.
- Press Ren-12 and St-21 in the stomach area, St-25 and Sp-15 in line with the belly button, and Ren-6 below the belly button.

- Finger-press along the sides of the body, from the armpits to the waist. Knead any sore points, especially around Liv-13.

ON THE LEGS:
- Thumb-press along the Stomach channel, up to the knee, and knead any sore points, especially St-36, St-37, and St-39, for their effect on the intestine.
- Thumb-press the Spleen channel, up to the groin, and knead any sore points, in particular Sp-6, Sp-8, and Sp-10. These points are particularly useful in moving blood.

ON THE HANDS: Press the following points, and knead if sore: LI-4, Stomach, Spleen, and Large Intestine areas, Large Intestine, Small Intestine, Perineum, Stomach, and Spleen.

ON THE FEET: Thumb-press and knead Abdomen area on the outside of the foot, Uterus on the inside, and also St-44.

ON THE EARS: Press the following points, and knead if sore: Abdomen, Stomach, Spleen, Large Intestine, Small Intestine, Uterus, Ovaries, Liver, and Shen Men.

Scraping

Scrape down the back muscles, from the shoulders to the top of the buttocks. Pay particular attention to the mid and lower back areas.

Tapping

Tap each point up to 30 times. You may need an assistant for the back area.

- Feel down the muscles of the back either side of the spine, and tap any sore, tense points. Continue until you reach the sacrum (the flat, triangular area at the bottom of the spine that ends at your tail bone). In particular, check Bl-18, Bl-20, Bl-23, and any sore points on the sacrum.

- Check the Spleen, Liver, and Stomach channels in the legs/feet for soreness, and tap if tender. In particular, check Liv-3, Liv-5, Sp-10, Sp-6, St-37, and St-39.

Exercises

1. ABDOMEN IMAGING: This exercise from qigong can be useful in relieving abdominal pain.
- In a relaxed standing or seated position, imagine there is a mass of hot air in the abdomen. Put one hand on top of the other, and place it below your belly button.
- Imagine turning the mass of air, as your hands circle clockwise up to 30 times, then perform the same motion anticlockwise. Be careful not to apply any pressure to the abdomen while doing this.
2. Do Exercises 2, 4, and 6 of the five-element stretches.

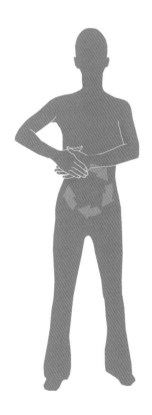

Lifestyle advice

- To prevent any stagnation in the abdomen, it is important to do regular gentle exercise.
- Avoid sitting for long periods, especially cross-legged or kneeling in a meditation position, as this too can add to stagnation.
- As with pain in the stomach, a short rest after lunch is far preferable to a long siesta.

Constipation

Symptoms

Difficulty in passing stools, long gaps between passing stools (once a day or once every two days is considered the norm), or inability to properly evacuate despite a strong desire to do so.

Can include or lead to

Irritable bowel syndrome, diverticulitis, and ulcerative colitis.

Abdomen imaging exercise

When to see a doctor

If the symptoms are severe, are accompanied by bleeding, are getting worse, or are accompanied by vomiting and abdominal bloating.

Common causes

Lack of exercise, an improper diet, emotional stress, frustration, smoking, working in a dry office environment, overeating, excess caffeine, overwork, travel, or changes in routine.

An explanation

The peristaltic movement of the intestine follows the rhythms of yin and yang in controlling body fluids. When yin increases in the intestine, it cools and moistens them and helps the passage of stools. When yang increases, the heat and dryness generated restricts the stools' movement. It is essential, therefore, to have sufficient levels of fluids in the intestine to prevent constipation and ensure the smooth partnership of yin and yang. The following conditions affect this balance:

HEAT IN THE INTESTINE: Heat can usually come from a number of sources.

- It can originate from the Stomach as the result of stagnation of food, bad eating habits, and a poor diet of heating, damp-forming foods.
- It can also derive from the Liver, often related to emotional disturbances or too much rich food and alcohol.
- If not cured properly, sometimes the elements that cause a cold or flu sink deeper into the body and transform into a raging heat with accompanying fever.
- Positioned in the midst of the intestine, if Kidney yin becomes weak, Kidney yang will heat up rapidly and burn up the moisture in the intestine around it.
- In all conditions of heat the stools are normally dry and infrequent.

COLD IN THE INTESTINE: Cold can develop from a weakness of yang or enter directly through exposure to a cold environment and act as an obstruction by constricting the intestine. With this condition, the stools can only be expelled with effort, but are quite often normal in appearance and moisture.

STAGNATION OF QI N THE BODY: Stagnation can come from stress, overwork, and emotional distress, and the subsequent obstruction caused by the Liver can create stools not unlike rabbit droppings. The condition is usually worse when emotionally stressed.

WEAK QI AND BLOOD IN THE BODY: If qi is weak, there is not enough power to push the stools through the intestine. It is often necessary to strain, and the stools are normally soft and long. If the blood is weak, it cannot moisten the intestine, and stools are usually small, round, and dry.

Dietary factors that can worsen constipation

- Drinking during meals floods your stomach and can clog up the digestive process.
- Foods such as barley dry up the moisture in the intestine, and others such as string beans increase yin levels and add to constipation.

Dietary factors that can improve constipation

- It is important to chew food thoroughly before swallowing to trigger the digestive juices needed for digestion and help the passage of food through the intestine.
- Apples, apricots, bananas, pears, peaches, prunes, carrots, cauliflower, spinach, honey, sesame seeds, walnuts, and tofu moisten the intestine and can help the passage of a stool.
- Asparagus, cabbage, black sesame seeds, figs, papayas, sweet potatoes, and castor oil have laxative qualities.

Acupressure and massage

ON THE ARMS: Thumb-press along the Large Intestine channel to the elbow. Press and knead any sore points, especially LI-11. Press TB-6, and knead if sore.

ON THE FRONT:
- Palm-circle with slight pressure in a clockwise direction around the belly button.
- Do the ABDOMEN CIRCLE massage in Feeling Bloated.
- Finger-press St-25, Sp-15, and Ren-12.

ON THE BACK: Press Bl-20, Bl-21, Bl-23, and Bl-25, and knead if sore.

ON THE LEGS: Thumb-press along the Stomach channel, up to the knee. Knead any sore points, including St-36 and St-40. Press GB-34, Sp-9, Sp-6, and Kid-6 (on the ankle), and knead if sore.

ON THE HANDS: Press the following points, and knead if sore: LI-4, Large Intestine, Small Intestine, and Constipation, Stomach, Spleen, and Large Intestine areas.

ON THE FEET: Press the following points, and knead if sore: Large Intestine, Small Intestine, Rectum, Liver, Spleen, Stomach, Abdomen, and Kidneys.

ON THE EARS: Press the following points, and knead if sore: Constipation, Large Intestine, Stomach, Rectum, Abdomen, Sanjiao, and Shen Men.

Scraping

Scrape down the back muscles from the shoulders to the lower sacrum. Pay particular attention to the mid and lower back areas.

Tapping

Tap each point up to 30 times. You may need an assistant for the back area.

- Tap Bl-25 and the muscles in the lower back either side of the spine.
- While sitting or lying down, tap points on the abdomen in a clockwise direction around the belly button. The distance from the belly button should be around three finger widths from all directions.
- Gently tap below St-25 on the abdomen and any tender points nearby.
- Feel along the Large Intestine channel on the forearm, and tap any sore points.

Exercises

The following exercises can help loosen the intestine.

1. ARM CROSS AND STRETCH:
- Stand with the legs shoulders' width apart. Relax and hang your arms loosely at your sides. Clench both fists loosely, and slowly raise them towards your chest while breathing in. Cross over the arms at chest level, so that each fist comes to rest on the opposite shoulder.
- Open the palms, bend your waist, and slowly swing your arms downwards and outwards in a fluid motion while breathing out. The arm movement should end by stretching outwards at right angles to the bent body.
- Repeat this several times.

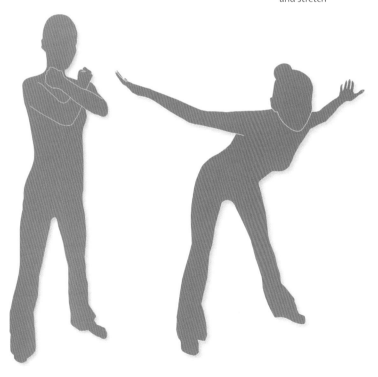

(left) Arm cross and stretch: clench and cross your fists

(right) Arm cross and stretch: swing and stretch

Arm lift

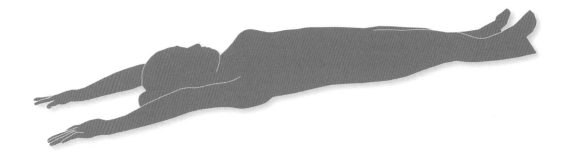

2. ARM LIFT:
- Lie face up on a bed, relax, and place both arms loosely at your sides. Slowly raise both arms while breathing in, and bring them down so that they touch the bed above the head.
- Then on the exhale, bring the arms slowly back to the starting position.
- Repeat several times.

3. Do Twist the Waist from Shoulder Pain, with the focus more on moving your waist than on the shoulders. Repeat the sequence several times.

4. Do exercises Bend Your Hip, Crouch Twist, and Swing Your Waist from Weak Qi to encourage the movement of qi in the abdomen.

5. Do Exercise 1 of the five-element stretches to strengthen the Large Intestine.

Lifestyle advice

1. It is important to exercise regularly to promote the smooth flow of qi, fluids, and blood – both to lubricate the intestine and to ensure the qi does not get blocked or too weak.

2. Avoid taking laxatives regularly, as they can damage yang and actually cause constipation as a side effect. Some people are caught in the vicious spiral of increasing the quantity and dosage of laxatives to combat constipation that the drug itself is causing.

3. Antibiotics are very cooling and can weaken the yang in the Spleen. Strong yang is needed for food to be pumped through the intestine, and weak yang can cause constipation.

4. The body reacts well to routines. Have a toilet routine, and try to keep to it. Energetically, the best time to open your bowels is between 5 and 7 am, as this is when qi is concentrated in the Large Intestine.

Diarrhoea
Symptoms

An increase in daily bowel movements; loose, watery stools; abdominal pain; lack of appetite; tiredness; fever; and gas.

Can include or lead to

Gastroenteritis, food poisoning, food allergies, irritable bowel syndrome, Crohn's disease, and ulcerative colitis.

When to see a doctor

If the symptoms are severe or persistent, with blood or mucus, or if dehydrated.

Common causes

Weak digestion, stress, overwork, repressed emotions, an inappropriate diet, exposure to the weather, or a long chronic illness.

An explanation

WEAK QI IN THE STOMACH AND SPLEEN: The organs with the most influence on diarrhoea are the Stomach and Spleen. Their main function is to transform food into the fuel the body runs on and also to send this fuel up to wherever needed.

    If the Stomach and Spleen become weak, the upwards movement of qi can become more of a downwards motion, and the food rushes through the intestine causing diarrhoea. This condition is usually accompanied by undigested food in the stools, the desire to go to the toilet straight after eating, and sometimes abdominal pain afterwards. If the diarrhoea is early in the morning it may be an extension of this pattern but involve weak Kidney yang.

DAMP WITH HEAT OR COLD IN THE INTESTINE: When weak, the Spleen and Stomach accumulate damp as they slow down the processing of food. They then become more susceptible to dampness from external sources, such as catching a cold or flu.

    The damp sinks and often combines with either heat or cold to stay in the intestine on a long-term basis, causing periodic flare-ups of diarrhoea, sometimes accompanied by blood and mucus.

    This pattern can be acute, with abdominal pain. If the condition is cold, the stools tend to be watery; if the condition is heat, the stools are normally darker or yellowish, and the smell is usually worse.

QI STAGNATION IN THE BODY: When qi stagnates in the Liver, it can also have a destabilizing effect on peristalsis, which moves food through the intestine during the digestive process. This can often result in alternating constipation and diarrhoea, and wind and bloating that may worsen with emotional stress.

Dietary factors that can worsen diarrhoea

- Dairy products, tropical fruits, nuts, junk food, wheat, and other damp-producing foods weaken digestion. See Damp for more details.
- Spices, coffee, alcohol, and other heat-producing foods can add to any heat present. See Heat for more details.
- Cold-natured, raw foods such as salads, soya bean products, and refrigerated drinks aggravate cold conditions. See Cold for more details.
- Apricots, plums, prunes, walnuts, spinach, sesame seeds, and sugary foods, processed foods, and all types of oil aggravate diarrhoea.

Dietary factors that can improve diarrhoea

- Ideally, drink lots of water or diluted juice and eat small meals of easily digestible foods, such as soups and gruels made from rice, oats, and other grains.
- Persimmons, garlic, button mushrooms, carrots, leeks, apples, aubergines (eggplants), olives, string beans, aduki beans, sunflower seeds, blackberry juice, and rice broth can be generally beneficial in combating diarrhoea.
- For cold-type diarrhoea: eat hot-natured foods, such as peppers, ginger, nutmeg, cinnamon, and chestnuts. See Heat for more details.
- For hot-type diarrhoea: eat cold-natured foods such as pineapples, tofu, mung beans, and drink peppermint tea. See Cold for more details.

Acupressure and massage

ON THE FRONT:
- Palm circle with slight pressure in an anticlockwise direction around the belly button.
- Press nine points equally spaced around the belly button with the heel of your palm. Work anticlockwise, and push each point towards the belly button. Press when breathing out, and hold for ten seconds.

Abdomen circle massage (anticlockwise)

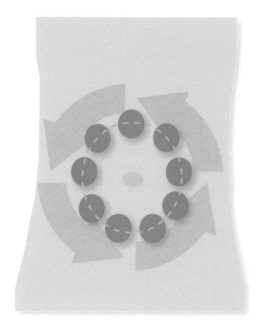

- Press Ren-12, Ren-6, and Ren-4, and knead if tender.
- Hard-press St-25 and Kid-16.

ON THE LEGS:

- Thumb-press along the Stomach channel, up to the knee. Knead any sore points, including St-36 and St-37.
- Thumb-press the Spleen channel, up to the knee. Knead any sore points, including Sp-6 and Sp-9.

ON THE ARMS: Press LI-11, and knead if sore.

ON THE BACK: Thumb- or finger-press down the back muscles either side of the spine. Knead any sore points, including Bl-20, Bl-22, Bl-23, and Bl-25.

ON THE HANDS: Press the following points, and knead if sore: LI-4, Diarrhoea, Large Intestine, Large Intestine channel area, and Stomach, Spleen, and Large Intestine areas.

ON THE FEET: Do the Healthy Foot massage in the How Can You Treat Yourself? section. Press and knead the following areas: Sp-4, St-44, Rectum, Liver, Stomach, Small Intestine, Spleen, and Large Intestine.

ON THE EARS: Press the following points, and knead if sore: Small Intestine, Large Intestine, Spleen, Stomach, Kidneys, Rectum, Shen Men, and Sympathetic.

Scraping

Scrape down the whole back from the shoulders to the lower sacrum. Pay particular attention to the mid and lower back areas.

Tapping

While sitting or lying down, tap points on the abdomen in an anticlockwise direction around the belly button. The distance from the belly button should be around three finger widths from all directions.

Feel down the muscles in the lower back either side of the spine, and tap any sore points.

Exercises

1. Do Exercises 1 and 2 of the five-element stretches to strengthen the Stomach, Spleen, and Large Intestine.
2. Do exercises Bend Your Hip, Crouch Twist and Swing Your Waist from Weak Qi to encourage the movement of qi.

Lifestyle advice

Avoid taking antibiotics for diarrhoea symptoms unless a clear bacterial cause has been identified, or if you have a weakened immune system. Antibiotics can weaken the Stomach and Spleen, which is often the underlying cause of diarrhoea.

Painful Urination

Symptoms

Frequent, painful, or burning urination; pain in the lower back; urine could be clear, dark, or cloudy, or with stones, sand, or blood.

Can Include or lead to

Cystitis, urethritis, vaginitis, herpes, urinary retention, menopausal complications, urinary calculi, prostatitis, and prostatic hypertrophy.

When to see a doctor

If the symptoms are severe or persist.

Common causes

An improper diet of greasy, hot-natured food; emotional stress; repressed frustration or anger; overwork; lack of sleep; dehydration; or extended contact with cold surfaces, such as sitting outside, standing, or lifting excessively.

An explanation

In making a diagnosis, Oriental medicine makes important distinctions between the types of symptoms of painful urination being presented:

DAMP AND HEAT IN THE BLADDER: Symptoms of acute, burning pain when urinating suggest the presence of heat. This is usually the result of a heavy diet of rich, greasy foods and alcohol, but it can also be from heat generated from stagnant qi or from weak yin.

The heat is usually accompanied by damp, which, as it is heavy and clinging by nature, causes the heat to sink into the bladder area. In conditions of heat, the urine is usually darker and more concentrated, and, if cloudy, suggests the presence of damp.

Sometimes there is blood in the urine, as the heat quite literally pushes out the blood from the blood vessels. Antibiotics can help reduce damp and heat (they are cooling by nature), and therefore the symptoms.

QI STAGNATION: If the symptom is either burning pain or more of a dragging discomfort and is relieved by pressure and warmth, it suggests either that there is too little qi or that it has got stuck somewhere. When qi becomes blocked in the Liver, it can directly affect the urinary and reproductive areas because of the location of the Liver channel as it comes up the body (it goes straight through the groin and lower abdominal area). This condition can worsen with emotional stress and cause pain before urination.

WEAK QI IN THE KIDNEYS**:** Chronic pain that recurs and gets worse when tired indicates that there is not enough Kidney qi. It is normally accompanied by other weak qi symptoms, such as lower back pain, pale urine, and pain after urination. For this type of condition, antibiotics may have a temporary relieving effect but can often make the condition worse.

STONES IN THE URINARY SYSTEM: The pain sometimes comes from urinary stones in the kidneys, ureter, or bladder. These are often the end result of long-term damp and heat, whereby the heat solidifies the damp. This could be due to lack of exercise and an inappropriate diet – in particular, a diet that consists of eating a lot of dairy products, spinach, rhubarb, liver, kidney, sardines, and fish roe.

Dietary factors that can worsen painful urination

• Overeating and a diet of hot-natured, damp-forming food, such as hamburgers, pizzas and other fast food, alcohol, and soft fizzy drinks (sodas), can directly lead to damp and heat via the Stomach or Spleen. See Heat and Damp for more details. on this.

- Cheese, milk, rhubarb, spinach, potatoes, liver, kidney, fish roe, sardines, tinned fish, plums, cranberries, chocolate, and alcohol have the effect of hardening phlegm, due to their acidity. This can lead to the formation of calculi, gravel and stones, so it is important to avoid eating them.

Dietary factors that can lessen painful urination

- Melon, watermelon, blueberries, radishes, cucumbers, celery, carrots, asparagus, mushrooms, barley, aduki beans, mung bean sprouts, lemon juice, and cranberry juice can reduce damp and heat in the bladder. See Damp and Heat for more details.
- Smoked fish, lobster, salmon, shrimp, tuna, lentils, black soya beans, and walnuts can strengthen weak Kidney qi. See Weak Qi for more details.

Acupressure and massage

ON THE FRONT: Hard-press Ren-3 and Ren-4.

ON THE LEGS: Press the following points, and knead if sore: Liv-5, Sp-6, Sp-9 and GB-41. Thumb-press along the Bladder channel up to the knee. Knead any sore points, including Bl-40 and Bl-58.

ON THE BACK: Thumb- or finger-press down the back muscles either side of the spine. Knead any sore points, including Du-14, Bl-23, and the sacral area.

ON THE HANDS: Press the following points, and knead if sore: Kidneys, Reproductive area, and the Triple Burner channel area.

ON THE FEET: Press the following points, and knead if sore: Kid-2, Bl-60, Bladder, Hips, Groin, Kidneys, and Liver.

ON THE EARS: Press the following points, and knead if sore: Bladder, Urethra, Kidneys, Shen Men, and Point Zero.

Scraping

Scrape the whole back from the shoulders down to the lower sacrum. Pay particular attention to the mid and lower back areas.

Tapping

Tap each point up to 30 times. You may need an assistant for the back area.

- Tap any sore points on the sacrum and lower back area.
- Tap down the centre-line of the back of the upper and lower legs. Below the calf muscle, look for sore points on the outside of the ankle area and the outside of the foot.

Exercises

1. Do Exercise 4 of the five-element stretches to strengthen the Kidneys and Bladder.
2. Do exercises Bend Your Hip, Crouch Twist and Swing Your Waist from Weak Qi, all of which encourage movement in the lower abdomen.

Lifestyle advice

Regular exercise is very important to prevent the stagnation of qi in the lower body. Avoid extended periods of standing, if possible.

Chapter 22
氣 Back Area

Backache

Symptoms

Pain in the upper, mid, lumbar, sacral, or coccyx areas of the spine.

Can include or lead to

Muscle spasm, herniated disc, spine curvatures, arthritis, fibromyalgia, osteoporosis, and spondylosis.

When to see a doctor

If the symptoms are severe, are getting worse, and are accompanied by bowel or urinary symptoms, numbness, or tingling in the leg.

Common causes

Overwork, stress, a lack of or too much exercise, exposure to the weather, pregnancy, childbirth, or trauma.

An explanation

Backache affects most people at some time in their lives. Often, we presume that back pain must originate from the spine. As a result, it is all too easy to find a slight spinal abnormality and undergo a spiral of sometimes extremely invasive treatments and investigations to "cure" it, only for the pain to continue or even worsen afterwards.

Sometimes back pain is due to spinal disorders or other conditions, such as heart disease, kidney stones, or a bladder infection, but often, back pain sufferers remain in the dark and frustrated as to the real cause of their backache.

WEAK QI IN THE KIDNEYS: Most people with chronic lower backache have Kidney qi weakness. The Kidneys give support and strength to the back, and when weak are unable to ensure there is enough qi and blood to protect the spine.

COLD AND DAMP IN THE BACK: A common cause of backache is cold and damp lodged in the back. This condition often changes with the weather and worsens especially when cold and damp. It can usually be relieved when you apply heat.

STAGNATION OF QI AND BLOOD IN THE BACK: If qi and blood get stuck, the pain is usually sudden and very sharp. This could be from an accident or sudden trauma, but can often appear after an apparently trivial event, such as a sneeze or a stretch. The symptoms of this type of condition are normally much more acute and feel worse with movement.

This stagnation of qi and blood can linger well after the initial incident and be periodically triggered by emotional stress and keeping the same posture for a long time. If there is stagnation of qi lodged in the back, the symptoms are often relieved by doing some form of exercise. If it feels worse after doing exercise, the condition is more likely to be one of weakness of qi and blood.

In practice, most people seem to have a combination of each of the above conditions causing their backache. There is usually stagnation of qi, accompanied by some damp or cold/heat and, underlying it all, weakness in the Kidneys and Spleen.

Dietary factors that can worsen backache

- Eating late at night or overeating can add to stagnation.
- Cold-natured, raw, or damp-forming foods, such as dairy products, bananas, tomatoes, wheat, and tofu, aggravate those conditions. See Cold and Damp for more details.

Dietary factors that can improve backache

- Radishes, aduki beans, turnips, pumpkin, and seaweed help remove damp. See Damp for more details.
- Herbs and spices such as cloves, chives, garlic, turmeric, marjoram, and basil, and citrus peel help warm cold and move any stagnation. See Qi Stagnation for more details.
- Smoked fish, oysters, lobster, salmon, shrimp, tuna, lentils, oats, millet, black soya beans, walnuts, and black sesame seeds strengthen the Kidneys. As the qi in the Kidneys has a strong influence over the back, it is very important to maintain it through diet.

Acupressure and massage

For acute pain press, and knead the following points:
- On the feet: Liv-3.
- On the hand: LI-4 and Yaotongxue.
- On the face: Du-26.
- On the leg: Bl-40.

Other more general points:
ON THE LEGS: Thumb-press along the Bladder channel, from Bl-60 (on the ankle) to Bl-36. Knead any sore points, including Bl-40 and Bl-57. Thumb-press along the Gall Bladder channel, up to GB-30. Knead any sore points, including GB-31 and GB-34. These points are often tender after excessive standing.

> CAUTION: Massaging the back when there is acute pain can often produce the opposite result to the one desired. If in any doubt, avoid manipulating around the area of pain, and use points that are farther away.

ON THE BACK: Thumb-press the Bladder channels on the upper-mid back, depending on where the pain is located.
ON THE ARMS: Press and knead TB-5. This is often sore after excessive sitting.
ON THE HANDS: Press the following points, and knead if sore: Yaotongxue, Cervical, Thoracic, and Lumbar areas and Kidneys.
ON THE FEET: Thumb-press the inside of the foot from the heel to the base of the big toe joint. Knead any sore points, including Cervical, Thoracic, Lumbar, sacrum, and coccyx areas.
ON THE EARS: Press the following points, and knead if sore: Cervical, Thoracic, or Lumbosacral areas, Buttocks, Sciatic nerve, Liver, Kidneys, Spleen, Shen Men, and Muscle Relaxation.

Scraping

Be cautious in scraping the back when back pain is very acute. Be especially cautious if scraping over the area where pain is felt. Be aware that any form of treatment close to an acute condition can often make it worse.

If the pain is more chronic, scrape down the back depending on the location of the pain, include the gaps of the spinal vertebrae, but again be very cautious if there is any spine-related condition. Sometimes the location of the underlying tension that needs to be treated is not where you think it is. For example, scraping the upper back can sometimes relieve lower back pain.

Tapping

Tap each point up to 50 times. You may need an assistant for the back area.

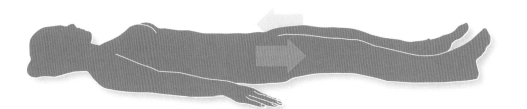

Pelvic stretch

- Feel down the muscles either side of the spine, along the Bladder channels. Tap any tender points and tightness in the muscle, but especially Bl-18, Bl-22, Bl-23, Bl-25, and Bl-52.
- On the leg, tap GB-34, Bl-40, and Bl-58, and any tender points nearby.

Leg stretch

Exercises

The following exercises can strengthen the lower back:

1. PELVIC STRETCH:
- Lie face up on a comfortable flat surface, and relax with your arms at your sides and legs out straight.
- Stretch your left leg away from you as far as is comfortable, and at the same time bend and bring your right leg upwards. The pelvic bone is then stretched, so that it is low on the left and high on the right.
- Repeat this on the other side and alternate up to 20 times.

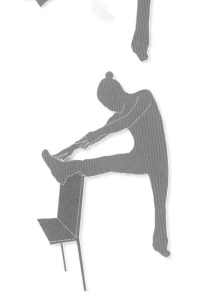

Leg lift

2. LEG STRETCH:
- Stand sideways next to a wall and use the hand closest to the wall to steady the body while you lift the opposite leg.
- Keeping your knee straight, lift your leg sideways as high as possible while breathing in.
- When you reach the highest point, stretch and hold it for a few seconds. At the same time bend your body forward until you can feel strain on the back of your thigh and hip.
- Then slowly lower the leg while breathing out.
- Repeat with the other leg and then continue a total of five times.

3. LEG LIFT:
- Using the support of a wall or a solid object, lift your leg as high as it will comfortably go, and rest it on a chair, table, or other object. Ideally, lift the leg to a 90° angle (but do not over-stretch).
- Stretch both arms forward, and try to touch your toes. Hold for a few seconds.
- Slowly lower the leg and repeat with the other leg. Repeat a total of five times.

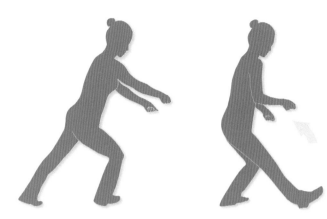

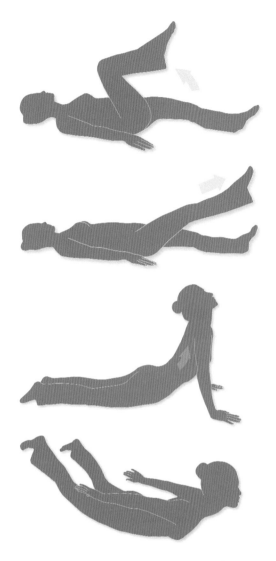

(left) Draw a fishing net: bend forward

(right) Draw a fishing net: draw back the neck

(top right) Leg contraction: bend and raise the knee

(second right) Leg contraction: kick and contract the knee

(third right) Body back twist

(bottom right) Body rocking chair

4. DRAW A FISHING NET:
- Stand with one foot in front of the other, bend the body forwards, and imitate the action of drawing in an imaginary fishing net with both hands.
- As you are bending forward, bring the heel of the back foot off the ground, and breathe in while drawing the net up.
- Then draw the net back and slowly straighten the body. At the same time, breathe out.
- Continue, so that the body is leaning backwards slightly, and bring the heel of the front foot off the ground.
- Repeat up to ten times on either side.

5. LEG CONTRACTION:
- Lie face up, and raise one leg with the knee bent. Kick the leg out straight in the air, then contract the muscles of the leg for a few seconds before bringing it down.
- Repeat with both legs up to 20 times.

6. BODY BACK TWIST:
- Lie face down and, keeping your legs relaxed, lift your body with both arms, as if starting to do a press-up.
- Lift the head and upper body, and stick out the chest. Rest and repeat five times.

7. BODY ROCKING CHAIR:
- Lie face down with arms relaxed at your sides.
- Stretch both arms backwards and both straight legs upwards. This movement raises the upper body and legs simultaneously and resembles the bottom of a rocking chair. Do not over-stretch, and only go as far as is comfortable.
- Hold this position for as long as possible, rest and repeat up to five times.

8. Do the exercise Bend Backwards from the Chest Pain section. This is very strengthening for the back.
9. Do Exercise 4 of the five-element stretches to strengthen the Kidneys and Bladder.

Lifestyle advice

- In most chronic cases of backache, using an ice pack on the pain can do more harm than good (unless there are obvious signs of heat). Heat therapy, such as a hot water bottle or a hot towel, normally has a relieving effect and can help the muscles relax and increase the circulation of qi and blood.
- While it is important to keep the area warm, it is best to avoid hot baths as, although it may relieve the pain, it can appear worse afterwards as the back cools down. Hot showers are preferable.
- Posture is important. Sit in a chair with a back rest that supports your back. Adjust the height so that your knees are level with your hips. Both feet should be flat on the floor or resting on a foot rest. If you are looking at a computer screen, ensure that the top of the screen is about eye level.
- Protect your back from the elements. Dress appropriately, and be very cautious of exposure to wind. After any exercise, change quickly out of sweaty clothing.
- Emotions can sometimes be an underlying issue in back pain. The obvious emotions are fear, which can weaken kidney qi, the main organ of the back, and anger, aggression, and irritability, which can tighten muscles and tendons, causing pain.
- Regular stretching and gentle exercise are usually beneficial. Avoid strenuous exercise or exercise with fast, jerky movements. The most important thing is to keep the back moving and prevent any stagnation.
- If the injury is acute, note the advice about putting ice on it in Neck Pain.

Sciatica
Symptoms

Numbness, pins and needles, stabbing, tingling, or burning pain radiating down the upper or lower leg usually with lower back pain.

Can include or lead to

Muscle sprain, nerve pain, disc hernia of the spine, and osteoporosis.

When to see a doctor

If the symptoms are severe.

Common causes

A diet of too many cold-natured and raw foods, exposure to the weather, long-term back pain, or bad posture.

An explanation

WIND, COLD, OR DAMP IN THE LEG: The pain or uncomfortable sensation felt in sciatica is usually due to a combination of wind, cold, and damp, which block the channels of the leg. They can be the result of an internal disorder, such as weak yang or a weak Stomach or Spleen, which can generate cold and damp in the back. Or they can enter from outside via exposure to cold, damp, or wind in situations such as swimming, cold showers, or inappropriate clothing on a windy day.

Although sciatica can appear independently, it is normally part of a wider area of pain that includes the lower back. Cold is constrictive, and damp is very heavy and obstructive. When these become lodged in the lower back, it is common for them to sink and affect the yang channels of the leg.

The two channels normally affected are the Bladder, when the pain radiates mainly down the back of the leg, and the Gall Bladder, when the pain radiates mainly down the side.

Dietary factors that can worsen sciatica

- Concentrated orange juice, wheat, bananas, dairy

products, peanuts, and other cold-natured or damp-forming foods can add to the stagnation in the yang channels. See Damp for more details.

Dietary factors that can improve sciatica

- Radishes, rye, celery, turnips, and pumpkin improve dampness. See Damp for more details.
- Cold can be warmed by spices such as ginger, black pepper, and nutmeg, also by garlic, onions, and turnips. See Cold for more details.

Acupressure and massage

ON THE BACK: Thumb- or finger-press down the back muscles either side of the spine. Knead any sore points, including BL-23, Bl-25, Bl-52, and any sore points in the sacral area.

ON THE LEGS/FEET:

- Thumb-press along the Gall Bladder channel, down from GB-30. Knead any sore points, especially GB-31, GB-34, and GB-39 on the leg, and GB-41 on the foot.
- Thumb-press the Bladder channel, down from Bl-36. Knead any sore points, especially Bl-40, Bl-57, and Bl-58 on the leg, and Bl-60 on the ankle.
- Press and knead any sore points in the triangle between Bl-54, GB-30, and Bl-36.

ON THE HANDS: Press the following points, and knead if tender: SI-3, LI-4, Sciatica, Thoracic, Lumbar, and Sacral areas.

ON THE FEET: As for Backache, thumb-press the inside of the foot, from the heel to the base of the big toe joint, to cover the spine area. Knead any sore points. Also knead along the Achilles tendon in the ankle, as this is also the Sciatic nerve area.

ON THE EARS: Press the following points, and knead if tender: Sciatic nerve, Buttocks, Lumbosacral area, Hip, Muscle Relaxation, and Shen Men.

Scraping

Scrape down the lower back and sacral area and into the buttock area.

Then scrape either of these two areas:

- For pain radiating down the back of the leg, scrape across the buttocks to GB-30, then down the centre of the back of the thigh to the knee.
- For pain radiating down the side of the leg, scrape across the buttocks to GB-30 at the side. Scrape down the side of the thigh to the knee.

Tapping

Tap each point up to 30 times. You may need an assistant for the back area.

- Press the lower back, sacral, and upper buttock areas, and tap any tender points or tense, contracted muscles.
- Tap down the middle of the back of the leg, from Bl-36 at the buttocks to Bl-57 at the bottom of the calf muscles.
- Feel down the side of the thigh muscle, and follow the Gall Bladder channel down to the foot. Tap any sore points.

Exercises

As there is often a close relationship between sciatica and back pain, many of the same exercises can be practised as detailed in Backache.

Lifestyle advice

Much of the advice given in Backache is also relevant here. It is also very important to avoid staying seated for long periods, to make sure you take regular exercise, and to keep your legs and lower back warm, dry, and protected from the wind.

Chapter 23
氣 Upper Limbs

Elbow pain

Symptoms

Pain in one or both elbow joints, with limited movement.

Can include or lead to

Tennis elbow, a traumatic injury to the elbow joint, rheumatoid arthritis, rheumatism, and muscle strain.

When to see a doctor

If the symptoms are severe, and there is swelling, bruising, or an inability to move the joint.

Common causes

Overuse, overwork, an inappropriate operation, exposure to the elements, or an accident.

An explanation

STAGNATION OF QI AND BLOOD IN THE ELBOW: Pain at the elbow is almost always due to stagnation of qi and blood. This could be due to an accident, a trauma, or an operation, or it could be due to just doing too much – too much work or sport.

One or more of the channels that run over the elbow – the Small Intestine, the Large Intestine, the Lung, and the Triple Burner – and the muscles and tendons around it can become damaged. Blood and qi cannot flow freely over this damaged area and become stuck, causing pain in the elbow.

WIND AND COLD OR HEAT OR DAMP IN THE ELBOW: The elements can often be the cause of qi stagnation, too. If there is even the slightest energetic weakness, wind can invade the elbow and bring with it cold or heat or damp. Cold contracts the muscles and tendons around the elbow and causes sharp pain and stiffness. It will often feel better with the application of heat. Damp lingers and feels fixed in one place, often feeling worse in wet weather. Heat can cause swelling, a burning sensation, and redness. It will often feel better with an ice-pack or a cold towel.

BLOCKAGE OF THE ARM CHANNELS: The location of the pain can often offer a clue as to where the problem lies. Pain at the outside of the elbow suggests a blockage in the Large Intestine channel. Pain at the back could be the Triple Burner channel. Pain on the inside is usually the Small Intestine or the Lung channel.

Dietary factors that can worsen elbow pain

- Overeating and irregular meal times can add to stagnation in the body.
- Milk, cheese, tofu, bananas, and other cold-natured, damp-forming foods can slow digestion and weaken qi and blood. See Damp and Cold for more details.

Dietary factors that can improve elbow pain

- Ideally, follow a diet that is supportive of qi and blood and that will nourish the muscles and tendons. See Weak Qi and Weak Blood.

> CAUTION: If the condition is acute, avoid massaging directly on or around the elbow.

Acupressure and massage

ON THE ARM: Press and knead the following elbow points, if they are sore: LI-11, LI-10, Lu-5, SI-8, and TB-10.

ON THE ARM CHANNELS: Effective treatment depends on locating which of the channels is affected. For this reason, thumb-press up to the elbow on the main channels, and look for sore points, especially the following:

- On the Large Intestine channel: LI-1, LI-3, and LI-4.
- On the Small Intestine channel: SI-3.
- On the Triple Burner channel: TB-1 and TB-3.
- On the Lung channel: Lu-9 and Lu-7.
- On the Heart channel: He-7.

ON THE LEGS: Press the following points, and knead if sore: Sp-6, Sp-9, St-40, and GB-34.

ON THE HANDS: Press the following points, and knead if sore: Shoulder, Large Intestine, and Triple Burner channel areas, and Stiff Neck.

ON THE FEET: Press the following points, and knead if sore: Liv-3, Elbow, Upper Arm, and Liver.

ON THE EAR: Press the following points, and knead if sore: Elbow, Arm, Shen Men, and Muscle Relaxation.

Scraping

Scrape down the neck, across the shoulder muscles, and down the upper back. Scrape down the arm above and below the elbow, preferably in the area of the channel affected. Note: Be very cautious about scraping directly on the elbow area.

Tapping

Tap each point up to 30 times. You may need an assistant for the neck area.

- Tap GB-20 at the base of the skull and down the neck muscles either side of the spine.
- Tap across the shoulder to loosen the muscles.
- Tap any sore points in the shoulder blade area.
- Tap LI-15 and TB-14, at the shoulder joint, if sore.
- Tap down the main muscles of the arm, but stop short of the elbow.
- Tap down the forearm along the main muscles, and stop at LI-4. Tap, if tender.
- Press GB-34, St-36, Sp-9, and Liv-3 on the leg/foot, and tap if sore.

Exercises

The following exercises can help maintain the elbow joint.

1. COVER YOUR EARS:
- Stand with your feet shoulders' width apart and your arms relaxed at your sides.
- Keeping your arms straight, slowly lift them up in front of you as you breathe in.
- When they reach chest level, bend your elbows towards you, and swing your forearms towards your ears.

Cover your ears

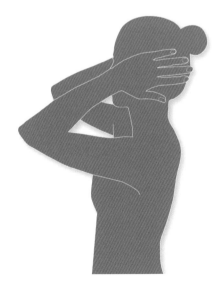

- Both open palms should end up facing your ears, as if you were about to cover them.
- While breathing out, swing the forearm back down, and when it reaches chest level, straighten your arms and bring them slowly down to your sides.
- Repeat for five minutes.

2. Do Exercises 1, 3, and 5 of the five-element stretches, which can strengthen the channels flowing over the elbow.

Lifestyle advice

- Avoid exposing the elbow to the outside elements, especially wind. For chronic pain, if it feels better with warmth, put something warm (like a warm towel) on it every now and again; if it feels better with cold, use a cool towel.
- Immobilizing the elbow is a common treatment, but ideally, moving the elbow joint through its full pain-free range of motion at least once a day helps ensure that the qi does not stagnate and the problem become worse.
- If the injury is acute, note the advice about putting ice on it in Neck Pain.

Wrist Pain
Symptoms

Pain, swelling, numbness, and tingling in the wrist, limitation of movement of the wrist, weakness in the hand, a heavy sensation, and possible soft nodules.

Can include or lead to

Muscle or tendon sprain, carpal tunnel syndrome, rheumatoid arthritis, rheumatic pain, and tenosynovitis.

When to see a doctor

If the symptoms are severe.

Common causes

Overwork, overuse, a traumatic injury, emotional stress, exposure to the weather, or a chronic disease.

An explanation

STAGNATION OF QI AND BLOOD IN THE WRIST: Pain at the wrist is usually because of stagnation of qi or blood. This could be due to a local injury in the wrist area, a weakness in the strength of blood, or wind, cold or damp which have wedged themselves in the joint and are blocking the movement of qi.

STAGNATION OF QI IN THE BODY: Ironically, any stagnation can often worsen with the frustration that comes with not being able to use your wrist as normal. An inability to work or do daily activities without pain or discomfort can in itself be so frustrating that it can disrupt the Liver's function of smoothly pumping qi around the body, causing even more stagnation in the wrist.

WEAK QI AND BLOOD: A numb, tingling sensation in the hand can be due to a weakness in qi and blood, meaning that insufficient strong blood is able to reach the hand to nourish it. This is often more noticeable at night because the yin-yang balance in the body means that energized blood returns to the Liver for storage at night time.

Dietary factors that can worsen wrist pain

- Irregular eating habits and overeating can add to the stagnation of qi.
- Too many damp-forming, oily foods can weaken your digestion and increase the likelihood of damp settling in the wrist. See Damp for more details.
- Too many cold-natured, raw foods can slow digestion and weaken qi and blood. See Cold for more details.

Dietary factors that can improve wrist pain

Ideally, follow a diet that supports qi and blood and nourishes the muscles and tendons. See Weak Qi and Weak Blood for more details.

Acupressure and massage

ON THE WRISTS: Press TB-4, LI-5, and SI-5, and knead if sore.

ON THE HANDS: Do the Healthy Hand massage in the How Can You Treat Yourself? section. Press any sore points, especially LI-3, LI-4, SI-3, and SI-4. Also press the top segments of the five fingers, as all of these channels run through the wrist.

ON THE LEGS/FEET: Thumb-press along the Stomach channel up to the knee, and knead any sore points, especially St-41 on the foot, and St-40 and St-36 on the leg.

Press the main points around the ankles: GB-40, Bl-60, Sp-5, Liv-4, and Kid-3. Knead any sore points. Treating the ankle can often benefit the wrist, and vice versa.

ON THE EARS: Press the following points, and knead if sore: Wrist, Arm, Hand, Shen Men, and Point Zero.

Wrist shake

Scraping

Scrape down the neck, across the shoulders, and down the upper back, particularly around the shoulder blade area. Scrape down the main muscles of the arm to the elbow, then the forearm. Be careful not to scrape over bone and to stop before the wrist.

Tapping

Tap each point up to 30 times. You may need an assistant for the neck/shoulder area.

- Tap down the neck and over the top of the shoulders.
- Tap down the main muscles of the arm, but stop short of the elbow.
- Tap down the forearm along the main muscles, and stop before the wrist.
- Tap LI-4 on the hand, if sore.
- Press the following key points around the ankle, and tap if sore: St-41, GB-40, Bl-60, Sp-5, Liv-4, and Kid-3.

Exercises

The following exercises can help to maintain the wrist joint.

1. WRIST SHAKE:
- Stand with your hands relaxed at your sides.
- Loosen the muscles of your arms, wrists, and hands, and gently shake both wrist joints. Ensure that your wrists and hands are limp. Continue until you feel a slight numbness or pins and needles sensation in the hands.
2. WRIST ROTATION:
- With one hand supporting the wrist of the other hand, rotate your wrist joint in a clockwise direction 10 times.
- Then do the same number anticlockwise.

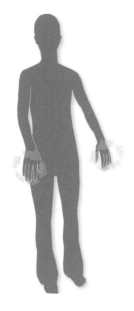

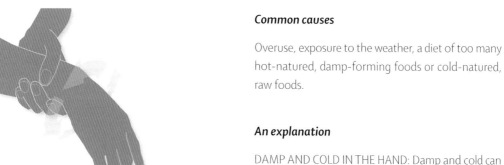

Common causes

Overuse, exposure to the weather, a diet of too many hot-natured, damp-forming foods or cold-natured, raw foods.

An explanation

DAMP AND COLD IN THE HAND: Damp and cold can come via a yang imbalance in the body or direct exposure of the hands to cold or water over a long time. The cold can contract the muscles and tendons in the hand and cause severe pain, swelling, or numbness. It is often worse in damp and cold weather.

DAMP AND HEAT IN THE HAND: Damp and heat also have external and internal causes. Damp can be generated by an inappropriate diet or exposure to water, and heat as a development from damp or stagnation, or from weak yin. The presence of damp and heat can lead to redness and swelling, and it can often be difficult for the hand to grasp.

STAGNATION OF QI AND BLOOD IN THE FINGERS OF HAND: Any local injury can cause stagnation, as well as damp, heat, or cold. The obstruction to qi and blood often causes pain that feels better with movement but is worse at night and can lead to deformities of the bone.

WEAKNESS OF QI AND BLOOD IN THE BODY: If the body does not have enough qi and blood to maintain itself, it often cannot nourish the body parts farthest away. This can result in stiff, weak hands or fingers.

Lifestyle advice

- It is essential to avoid all activities that may aggravate the condition, if possible. The wrist usually cannot heal without time to rest.
- It is also important to adapt any work or home situation so as to lessen any strain in the future. This could mean making major life-changing job decisions, or it could be just a matter of buying a wrist support for clicking on a computer mouse. It depends on the severity of the condition.
- If the injury is acute, note the advice about putting ice on it in Neck Pain.

Pain in the Hands and Fingers
Symptoms

Pain, discomfort, or swelling in the hand or one or more fingers.

Can include or lead to

Osteoarthritis, rheumatoid arthritis, rheumatic fever, chilblains, nerve pain, paralysis or injury of the nerves, and a local injury of the muscles or tendons.

When to see a doctor

If the symptoms are severe.

Dietary factors that can worsen hand or finger pain

Irregular eating habits and overeating, too many damp-forming, oily foods, and too many cold-natured, raw foods can slow digestion, weaken qi and blood, and add to stagnation in the body. See Damp and Cold for more details.

Dietary factors that can help hand or finger pain

As with other joint and bone pain, it is best to follow a diet that is supportive of qi and blood and that will nourish the muscles and tendons. See Weak Qi and Weak Blood for more details.

Acupressure and massage

ON THE HANDS: Do the Healthy Hand massage in the How Can You Treat Yourself? section. Press and knead Baxie. Press the following points, and knead if sore: LI-3, LI-4, TB-3, TB-5, SI-3, and SI-5.

ON THE FEET: Do the Healthy Foot massage in the How Can You Treat Yourself? section.

ON THE EARS: Press the following points, and knead if sore: Fingers, Hand, Muscle Relaxation, and Shen Men.

Scraping

Scrape across the shoulders, then scrape down the upper and lower arms, stopping at the wrist. Be careful not to scrape over bone.

Tapping

Tap each point up to 30 times.

- Feel along the Triple Burner, Large Intestine and Small Intestine channels on the outside of the fore-arm, and tap any sore points. Stop before you reach the wrist.
- Tap LI-4 on the hand and any sore points around it.
- Press Liv-3, St-40, St-44, and Sp-6 on the foot/leg, and tap if sore.
- Tap the nail points on each of the fingers and toes:
  Fingers: Lu-11, Pc-9, He-9, LI-1, TB-1, SI-1
  Toes: Sp-1, Liv-1, Kid-1 (on the sole), St-45, GB-44, Bl-67.

Exercises

1. Do Exercises 1, 3, and 5 of the five-element stretches to increase circulation in the hand channels.
2. Do Relax the Hands, Fingers, and Toes exercise from Sleeping Difficulties.

Lifestyle advice

- When doing daily chores, such as washing dishes, wear protective gloves to minimize external damp, cold, or heat on the hands.
- Avoid certain actions that may make the pain worse, such as making a fist or gripping objects. Instead of a clutch bag, take a shoulder bag. Instead of holding a book while reading, use a book stand. When writing, typing, or using your hands, take a break every 15 minutes, or when your hand feels tired or painful.
- If the injury is acute, note the advice about putting ice on it in Neck Pain.

Chapter 24
氣 **Lower Limbs**

Knee pain
Symptoms

Pain, swelling, or stiffness in either one or both knee joints, or the muscles/tendons around the knee area.

Can include or lead to

Synovitis of the knee, rheumatoid arthritis, fibrositis, local ligament damage, and local nerve damage.

When to see a doctor

If there are severe symptoms or the joint is immovable.

Common causes

Overuse, overexercise, an improper diet with too much greasy food, an injury, an inappropriate knee operation, chronic illness, or old age.

An explanation

STAGNATION OF QI AND BLOOD IN THE KNEE: There is usually some form of stagnation of qi and blood causing pain in the knee, especially if it has been overused through exercise or activity. The stagnation blocks the flow of qi and blood over the knee area and often leads to pain and swelling.

WEAK QI IN THE KIDNEYS: Weak Kidney qi is also often a key factor in knee problems. The Kidneys affect the knees because both the Water channels (the Kidney and Bladder channels) run behind the knee but also because the strength of the Kidneys in turn influences the strength of bones and joints. Weak Kidney qi is implicated if the pain developed gradually and in both knees.

DAMP AND COLD IN THE KNEE: If the knee is swollen, affected by damp and cold weather, and the pain is more on one side, then damp or cold could be lodged in the knee. Cold contracts the muscles and tendons around the knee, causing severe pain, and damp can cause swelling and numbness.

WIND IN THE KNEE: Sometimes the pain can mysteriously jump from place to place, or even from one knee to the other. This is normally caused by wind, which tends to move within the body as it does outside the body. It can develop from long-term conditions of weak blood or from exposure to the weather.

DAMP AND HEAT IN THE KNEE: If wind, cold, or damp remains stuck in the knees for too long, it can transform into damp heat, which can cause swelling, inflammation, and a burning sensation. This condition is often found in people who drink too much alcohol or eat a diet containing too many fatty, greasy foods. In these cases, the damp and the heat in the knee are being fuelled by the damp and the heat coming from the Stomach or Spleen.

Dietary factors that can worsen knee pain

- Processed, junk foods like pizzas and hamburgers, soft fizzy drinks (sodas), and alcohol, can lead to damp and heat in the body, which can then sink to the knees. See Damp for more details.
- Salads, grapefruit, melons, mangos, tomatoes, watermelons, cucumbers, lettuce, ice cream and

other raw, cold-natured foods weaken Stomach and Spleen, and damp can collect in joints. See Cold for more details.

Dietary factors that can improve knee pain

- Radishes, rye bread, celery, and pumpkin improve damp in the knees. See Damp for more details.
- A strengthening diet that allows the Stomach to digest food properly would help ensure that the knee can be nourished with qi and blood. See Weak Qi for more details.

Acupressure and massage

ON THE KNEE: Press St-35 and the equivalent point on the other side of the knee, especially if the pain feels as if it is inside the knee cap. Press and knead any sore points near the knee. Use your palm to gently rub the knee area in a circular motion to create warmth.

ON THE LEG:

- Press and knead St-34 and Sp-10 for pain above the knee.
- Press and knead Sp-9, Liv-7, and Liv-8 for pain on the inside of the knee.
- Press and knead GB-40, St-36, and GB-34 for pain on the outside of the knee.
- Press and knead Bl-40 for pain at the back of the knee. Stretch the leg and repeat several times.
- Thumb-press along the Stomach, Spleen, Liver, Gall Bladder, and the Bladder channels, up to below the knee. Knead any sore points.
- Provided the knee is not hot and swollen, it can be covered with a hot towel to encourage the

CAUTION: If the condition is acute, inflamed, or painful to the touch, avoid massaging the knee directly.

movement of qi and blood. Remove the towel before it cools down.

ON THE FEET: Press and knead Sp-5 for any knee pain location.

Press St-41 with your thumb, and hold. At the same time, push back your foot towards your body. Repeat this several times.

ON THE HAND: Press and knead the following points if sore: LI-4, Knee 1 and 2, and Kidneys.

ON THE EARS: Press and knead the following points, if sore: Knee, Muscle Relaxation, Shen Men, and Point Zero.

Scraping

Scrape down the back muscles, from the bottom of the shoulder blades to the sacrum. Then scrape across the hip and down the sacral area.

Tapping

Tap each point up to 30 times. The same caution for direct massage applies here.

- Press around (but not on) the knee area in a clockwise direction, and tap any sore points. Do this on both knees.
- Feel down both sides of the lower leg muscles until just before the ankle. Tap any sore points.
- Check to see if St-34, Sp-10, Sp-9, and GB-34 on the leg are sore, and if so tap them.

Exercises

The following exercises can strengthen and loosen the knee joint.

1. KNEE ROTATION:
- Stand with both legs together.
- Keeping your legs together, bend from the waist and place one hand on each knee for support.
- Bend your knees slightly, and rotate your legs in a

Knee rotation

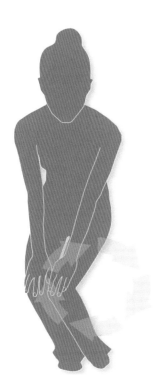

clockwise circular motion for 10 rotations. Then for 10 rotations in an anticlockwise direction.

2. Do Exercises 2 and 6 of the five-element stretches. These strengthen the Earth (Stomach and Spleen) and Wood (Liver and Gall Bladder) channels, all of which flow on or near the knee.

3. Do exercise Swing Your Bottom in Weak Qi, as this involves a gentle movement of the knees.

Lifestyle advice

*   If possible, avoid keeping the knee joint in the same position for any prolonged period of time. While watching television, for example, get up, stretch, and move around every half-hour.
*   At work or at home, adjust the height of your chair to reduce the stress on the knees when getting up. Higher is generally better.
*   If the injury is acute, note the advice about icing it in Neck Pain.

Ankle Pain

Symptoms

Pain or discomfort in one or both ankles with possible restricted movement and swelling.

Can include or lead to

Sprain or dislocation of the ankle, gout, tarsal tunnel syndrome, synovitis, and rheumatoid arthritis.

When to see a doctor

If the symptoms are severe.

Common causes

A traumatic injury; overuse; exposure to the elements; an improper diet of too many greasy, fatty foods; an inappropriate operation; standing for too long; strong emotional problems; or a chronic illness.

An explanation

WEAK QI AND BLOOD IN THE BODY: If the body is weak in blood and qi, the channels that run over the ankle can no longer give enough nourishment to the ankle area. This will lead to an underlying weakness in the ankle and make it much easier to injure.

A weakness in any of the leg channels can adversely affect the ankle, and when there is pain, the obvious clue to help identify which one is affected is its location.

Pain on the outside of the ankle: Stomach, Gall Bladder, or Bladder channels.

Pain on the inside of the ankle: Spleen, Liver, or Kidney channels.

STAGNATION OF QI AND BLOOD IN THE ANKLE: Any injury to the ankle, whether from an accident or overuse, will cause stagnation of qi and blood in the ankle. This can often linger well after the ankle itself mends and can make the ankle more susceptible to environmental conditions, in particular, wind, cold, and damp.

WIND, DAMP, OR COLD IN THE ANKLE: Environmental factors can enter the ankle through exposure. Wind can move the pain from place to place; cold often contracts the tendons and channels around the ankle and leads to severe pain; and damp can numb and swell the ankle with a fixed, heavy pain. Any one of these if left long enough can change into heat and inflame the ankle.

Dietary factors that can worsen ankle pain

Weak qi or blood, and damp, cold, and heat can originate from a poor diet:

- Hot-natured, damp-forming foods, including processed foods high in bad fats can lead to damp and heat in the body. This can then sink to the ankles. See Damp for more details.
- Too many cold-natured, raw foods can cause the Stomach to weaken and cold and damp to collect in the joints. See Cold for more details.

Dietary factors that can improve ankle pain

A strengthening diet that allows the Stomach to digest food properly would be helpful to ensure that the ankle can be nourished with qi and blood. See Weak Qi for more details.

Acupressure and massage

ON THE ANKLE(S):
- For pain on the outside of the ankle, press and knead GB-40, GB-41, and Bl-60.
- For pain on the inside of the ankle, press and knead Sp-4, Sp-5, Kid-3, Kid-5, and Liv-4.

ON THE FEET/LEGS:
- For pain on the outside of the ankle, press St-36, St-41, St-44, and GB-34.
- For pain on the inside of the ankle, press and knead Sp-3, Sp-6 and Sp-9, and Liv-3.

ON THE HANDS: Press the following points, and knead if sore: Ankle and Liver area.

ON THE EARS: Press the following points, and knead if sore: Ankle, Shen Men, and Muscle Relaxation.

Scraping

Scrape down the lower back and sacral areas. Scrape into the buttocks and the hips.

Tapping

Tap each point up to 30 times. The same caution for direct massage applies here.

- Press around the ankle area on both ankles, and tap any sore points.
- Tap the nail points of the toes on both feet: Sp-1, Liv-1, Kid-1, St-45, GB-44, and Bl-67.
- Press the following points on the legs, and tap if sore: Sp-6, Sp-9, St-36, GB-39, GB-34, and Kid-7.

Exercises

The following ankle exercises can help chronic ankle pain:

1. ANKLE ROTATION:
   Rotate the ankle by supporting it with one hand and leading your foot in a circular motion with the other. Repeat in both directions ten times.
2. Do exercise Knee Rotation from Knee Pain, as this also gently rotates the ankles.
3. Do exercise Swing Your Bottom from Weak Qi, if possible, as it gently moves the ankle joint.
4. Do Exercises 2, 4, and 6 of the five-element

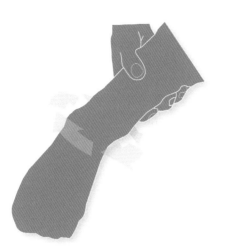

Ankle rotation

stretches. These strengthen the channels that run over the ankle.

Lifestyle advice

- It is important to rest the ankle as much as possible. No amount of bandaging, stretching, and taping to allow you to continue using it will make up for simple rest.
- After exposure to damp or cold conditions, dry and warm the ankle area quickly and thoroughly.
- Ideally, moving the ankle joint through its full pain-free range of motion at least once a day will help to ensure that the qi does not stagnate.
- If the injury is acute, note the advice about putting ice on it in Neck Pain.

Foot and toe pain
Symptoms

Pain or discomfort in the heel, sole, or toes of one or both feet.

Can include or lead to

Osteoarthritis, rheumatoid arthritis, bunions, osynovitis, gout, soft tissue injury, metatarsalgia, plantar fibrositis, plantar fasciitis, and heel spurs.

When to see a doctor

If the symptoms are severe.

Common causes

Living in a damp environment, wading through water, overwork, stress, overuse, a chronic illness, a local traumatic injury, or an improper diet with irregular eating habits.

An explanation

WIND, COLD, AND DAMP IN THE FOOT: Weakness in the feet can allow wind, cold and damp to settle there and block the free flow of blood and qi. This often results in swelling and heaviness, and is worse when cold, damp, or in water.

HEAT IN THE FOOT: With time, heat can develop from wind, cold, and damp in the foot or can come from a hot condition in the body.

The heat burns up the fluids in the channels, tendons, and muscles of the foot, leading to an acute, hot, swollen condition.

STAGNATION OF QI AND BOOD IN THE FOOT: Any trauma to the foot or toes will create a local blockage in the channels and cause pain. This block can continue long after the injury has healed and continue to cause pain. With this condition the pain is often worse when at rest and feels better with movement.

WEAK QI AND BLOOD IN THE BODY: If the body does not have enough qi and blood to maintain itself, it often cannot nourish the body parts farthest away. This can result in stiff, weak feet or toes. Accompanying pain is normally worse after walking and standing, and when tired.

WEAK YIN IN THE BODY: As the body ages, the balance between yin and yang shifts in the Kidneys. For people who develop a weakness in yin, foot and toe pain can occur with a feeling of heat, especially at night.

Dietary factors that can worsen foot or toe pain

Weak qi and blood, and damp, cold, and heat can originate from a poor diet:

- A diet of hot, damp-forming foods, such as processed, junk food high in saturated fats, sugary soft drinks, and alcohol, can lead to damp and heat in the body. This can then sink to the feet. See Damp for more details.
- A recent Canadian study strongly associates sweetened soft drinks with an increased risk of gout (damp and heat in the foot) in men. Researchers looked at tens of thousands of men with no history of gout and monitored them over 12 years. They found that the risk was 85 percent higher among men who drank two or more servings of sweetened soft drinks per day, compared to those who consumed less than one serving per month.[25]
- An excess of dairy products, tropical fruits, concentrated orange juice, and other cold-natured, damp-forming foods cause the Stomach and Spleen to weaken, so that cold and damp collect in the lower joints. See Cold for more details.

Dietary factors that can improve foot and toe pain

Ideally, follow a strengthening diet that allows the Stomach to digest food properly to ensure that the foot can be nourished with qi and blood. See Weak Qi for more details.

Acupressure and massage

ON THE FOOT/FEET (Caution in acute pain):
- Do the Healthy Foot massage in the How Can You Treat Yourself? section.
- Hard-press six points on the sole of the foot, equally spaced from the ball to the start of the heel. The first three are in line with the middle toe, and the other three are in line with the big toe. Repeat the sequence of points three times.
- Thumb-press the inside of the foot. Start from the heel, and thumb-press along the edge of the foot towards the side of the big toe. Knead Sp-3 and any other tender areas.
- Thumb-circle each toe up to the tip, and pull the toe outwards to stretch the joints.
- Thumb-press the Liver and Spleen channels up to the knee for pain on the top or inside of the foot. Knead any sore points.
- Thumb-press the Stomach and Gall Bladder channels for pain on the top or outside of the foot. Knead any sore points.
- Thumb-press the Bladder and Kidney channels for pain on the outside of the foot, the sole, or in the heel. Knead any sore points.

ON THE ARMS: Press TB-5 and LI-11, and knead if sore.

ON THE LEGS: Press Sp-6, GB-34, St-36, and knead if sore.

ON THE HANDS: Press the following points, and knead if sore: LI-4, SI-3, SI-4, Heel Pain, and Kidneys.

ON THE EARS: Press the following points, and knead if sore: Toes, Shen Men, and Muscle Relaxation.

Scraping

Scrape down the lower back and sacral areas. Scrape into the buttocks and the hips.

Tapping

Tap each point up to 30 times.
- Press around the affected area of the foot. Tap any sore areas.
- Also tap Kid-1 on the sole of the foot, Liv-3, and the nail points of the toes and fingers.
  Fingers: Lu-11, Pc-9, He.9, LI-1, TB-1, SI-1.
  Toes: Sp-1, Liv-1, St-45, GB-44, Bl-67.

Exercises

The following foot exercises can help chronic foot or toe pain.

1. Do the Ankle Rotation exercise from Ankle Pain.
2. FOOT SCRUNCH:
- Begin seated, with your legs shoulders' width apart.
- Five rolled-up socks should be prepared and positioned next to your right foot.
- Each pair of socks needs to be moved from the right side to the left side with the toes of your right foot.
- Once completed, the socks can be pushed to the outside of your left foot, and then the process is repeated with the other foot.
- The sequence can be repeated up to five times.

Lifestyle advice

- For pain originating from cold, damp conditions, it is very important to keep the feet warm and dry.
- If possible, avoid exercising very much while you have pain. If the tendons are undernourished, they will easily tire and begin to hurt.
- If the injury is acute, note the advice about putting ice on it in Neck Pain.

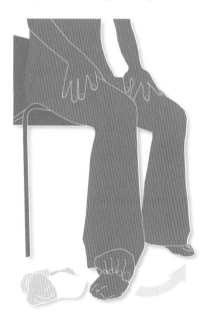

Foot scrunch

3. Do Exercises 2, 4, and 6 of the five-element stretches to strengthen the foot channels.

Chapter 25
氣 # Conditions Affecting Men

Prostate Problems
Symptoms

Pain or discomfort in the perineum and lower back, increased frequency of urination (especially noticeable at night), poor urine flow, pain on urination, and a bloated abdomen.

Can include or lead to

Prostatitis, prostatic hypertrophy, urinary retention, and prostate cancer.

When to see a doctor

If the symptoms are severe.

Common causes

Lack of exercise; a diet of hot-natured, damp-forming foods; emotional stress; or exposure to the weather.

An explanation

DAMP IN THE LOWER ABDOMEN: This is of due to a diet of rich, damp-forming food that weakens the Stomach and Spleen and causes an accumulation of damp to sink in the body. It can be accompanied by a heavy, dragging feeling and bloating, and also either a feeling of heat or cold. In most cases, damp combines with heat, and if left untreated, can burn up yin and cause deep-seated imbalances.

STAGNATION OF QI IN THE BODY: Emotional stress causes muscles and tendons to tense up and creates blockages in the smooth movement of qi around the body. Without exercise, this blockage can lodge in the lower abdomen area.

WEAKNESS OF QI AND BLOOD IN THE BODY: An overall weakness in qi often means that the body is not being properly nourished. In particular, the Spleen should raise qi, but when it is weak, it can sink to the lower half of the body, where, in men, the balance of yin and yang in the Kidneys can have a direct weakening effect on the prostate.

Dietary factors that can worsen prostate problems

- Dairy products and processed foods containing high levels of bad fats, such as donuts, chocolate, biscuits, cakes, and other deep-fried foods, produce damp in the body. See Damp for more details.
- Heat-producing foods, such as red meat, particularly lamb; oily fish, such as tuna, mackerel, salmon, herrings, sardines, and pilchards; and drinks containing caffeine or saccharin, such as coffee, fizzy soft drinks, fruit juice and alcohol, especially beer. See Heat for more details.

Dietary factors that can improve prostate problems

In general a simple, bland diet will strengthen the Stomach and Spleen. See Weak Qi for more details. Beneficial foods include:
- FRUIT: pomegranate, raspberries, blackberries, papayas, cherries, watermelon, and grapefruit.

- VEGETABLES: tomatoes (cooked), carrots (cooked), red or green peppers, cabbage, turnip, cauliflower, broccoli and Brussels sprouts.
- LEGUMES, SEEDS, AND NUTS: pumpkin seeds, Brazil nuts, and lentils.
- GRAINS: rice and quinoa.
- MEAT: chicken and white fish.
- DRINKS: Green tea
- OTHERS: miso, soy sauce, and seaweed (especially kelp).

Acupressure and massage

ON THE FRONT:
- Palm-circle with slight pressure in a sweeping, clockwise, circular motion around the belly button.
- Do the ABDOMEN CIRCLE massage in Feeling Bloated.
- Hard-press Ren-3, Ren-4, and Ren-6 on the lower abdomen.

ON THE BACK: Thumb-press along the Bladder channel either side of the spine. Knead any sore points, including Bl-17, Bl-20, Bl-23, Bl-25, Bl-26, and any sore points on the sacrum.

ON THE LEGS:
- Thumb-press the Liver channel, up to the knee, and knead any sore points, in particular Liv-5.
- Thumb press the Spleen Channel up to the knee and knead any sore points, especially Sp-6 and Sp-9.
- Press St-36 and GB-34, and knead if sore.

ON THE HANDS: Press and knead the following points, if sore: Reproductive Organs area and Kidneys.

ON THE FEET: Press and knead the following points, if sore: Liv-1, Liv-3, Reproductive Organs, Prostate Glands, Kidneys, Bladder, and Liver.

ON THE EARS: Press and knead the following points, if sore: Urethra, Kidneys, Testes, Prostate, Liver, Bladder, Endocrine, and Shen Men.

Scraping

Scrape down the whole back, from the shoulders to the sacral area. Also scrape into the buttocks and hips.

Tapping

Tap each point up to 30 times. You may need an assistant for the back area.

- Feel down the back muscles either side of the spine, and tap any sore points.
- Tap any sore points in the sacral area.
- Press and gently tap any sore points in the abdominal area.
- Tap any sore points along the Liver and Spleen channels in the lower leg and foot, in particular Liv-3, Sp-6, and Sp-9.

Exercises

1. Do Exercises 4 and 6 of the five-element stretches to strengthen the channels in the pelvic area.
2. Do exercises Bend Your Hip and Swing Your Waist from Weak Qi, as both of these help to reduce stagnation in the lower abdomen.
3. Do exercise Body Twist from Constipation to encourage movement of qi in the prostate area.

Lifestyle advice

To prevent stagnation of qi in the lower abdomen, it is very important to take regular exercise, which will stretch and twist the muscles in this area.

Sexual Dysfunction
Symptoms

Low sex drive, inability to sustain an erection, and premature ejaculation.

Can include or lead to

Infertility, impotence, and sexual neurosis.

When to see a doctor

If symptoms are severe.

Common causes

Overwork;, emotional stress; anxiety; depression; old age; drug side effects; a chronic disease; or excessive sexual activity.

An explanation

STAGNATION OF CHI IN THE BODY: Stress and unexpressed emotions can often inhibit the Liver's ability to smoothly send qi around the body. This results in stagnation, both physical – pain and discomfort – and/or emotional, in the form of depression. The Liver channel runs through the groin area, and stagnation can easily slow down or dull the sexual organs.

DAMP AND HEAT IN THE LOWER ABDOMEN: Damp can be the result of an improper diet, which slows down digestion and increases the accumulation of fluids. This damp is heavy and can sink into the lower body and block qi. The blockage can then develop heat. It may often present like an infection but be unresponsive to antibiotics.

WEAK YIN IN THE KIDNEYS: Normal sexual performance requires unhindered interaction between Fire and Water. Like the ignition on a car, Fire shoots down from the Heart and sparks the Kidneys to life. If Kidney yin is weak, there will be too much heat and not enough fluids in the lower abdomen. This pattern interrupts normal sexual functioning.

Dietary factors that can worsen sexual dysfunction

- Overeating and irregular meal times aggravate stagnation.
- Hot, spicy foods and processed, oily, damp-forming foods, such as pizzas, hamburgers, and fast food aggravate damp. See Damp and Qi Stagnation for more details.

Dietary factors that can improve sexual dysfunction

- Smoked fish, oysters, lobster, salmon, shrimp, tuna, lentils, oats, millet, black soya beans, walnuts, chives, and black sesame seeds nourish underlying Kidney weakness.
- Aduki beans, fennel seeds, radishes, watercress, and barley can be very useful in reducing damp. See Damp for more details.
- For hot conditions, cool foods like lettuce, tofu, grapefruit, asparagus, and lemons can be beneficial. See Heat for more details.
- Stagnation can be improved by adding spices such as cardamom, turmeric, cloves, and coriander. See Qi Stagnation for more details.,

Acupressure and massage

ON THE FRONT: Hard-press Ren-3 and Ren-4 on the lower abdomen.

ON THE LEGS: Thumb-press along the Spleen channel, and knead any sore points, especially Sp-6 and Sp-9. Press and knead St-36, if sore.

ON THE BACK: Thumb-press down the back muscles either side of the spine. Knead any sore, tight points, in particular Bl-23 and the sacral area.

ON THE HANDS: Thumb-press up the little finger side of the hand from the wrist. Knead the area below the little finger joint. This is the Reproductive area.

ON THE FEET: Do the Healthy Foot massage in the How Can You Treat Yourself? section. Hard press Kid-1, Kid-3 and Liv-2, if sore.

Press the following points and knead if sore: SI-3, Mingmen, Liver, and Kidney areas.

ON THE EARS: Press the following points, and knead if sore: External Genitals, Brain, Kidneys, Endocrine, and Liver.

Scraping

Scrape down the whole back, from the shoulders to the sacral area. Also scrape into the buttocks and hips.

Tapping

Tap each point up to 30 times. You may need an assistant for the back area.

- Tap on any sore points on the sacrum and down the front and sides of the thigh.
- Press Liv-3, GB-40, and Kid-7 on the legs/feet, and tap if sore.
- Tap down the muscles either side of the spine, especially at the following points: BL-18, Bl-20, Bl-23, and any sore points in the sacral area.
- Gently tap Ren-3 on the lower abdomen.

Exercises

1. Do Exercises 2, 4, and 6 of the five-element stretches to strengthen the Kidneys, Liver, and Spleen.
2. Do exercises Bend Your Hip and Swing Your Waist from Weak Qi, as both of these help reduce stagnation in the lower abdomen.
3. Do exercise Body Twist from Constipation.

Lifestyle advice

- Stop smoking! Numerous studies have shown a link between smoking and sexual dysfunction. A review of studies published in the United States between 1980 and 2001 found that 40 percent of impotent men were smokers, compared with 28 percent of men in the general population.[26]
- While exercise is to be encouraged, some forms of exercise may be a factor in sexual dysfunction. Cycling, for example, if done for more than three hours a week, is thought to lead to something called pudendal nerve entrapment, caused by contact of the perineum with the saddle.[27] If you are a keen cycler and have sexual dysfunction perhaps try a bicycle-free trial period.

Chapter 26
氣 Conditions Affecting Women

Premenstrual Syndrome
Symptoms

Pre-period irritability; depression; changeable moods; swollen breasts, hands, face, or feet; bloating and abdominal pain; nausea; chest tightness; lack of concentration, constipation; or diarrhoea.

When to see a doctor

If the symptoms are severe.

Common causes

Emotional stress, especially when emotions are repressed; a diet of too many hot-natured, damp-forming foods; overwork; lack of exercise; bad posture; or excessive sexual activity.

An explanation

STAGNATION OF QI IN THE BODY: On a monthly basis, qi and blood are redirected down to the uterus to prepare for menstruation. The Liver ensures that this process happens smoothly and without any problems. If, however, the Liver has been affected by emotional stress, it cannot prevent obstructions in this flow. As a result, qi and blood can get clogged up and cause muscle tension, pain, and discomfort.

If qi becomes stuck in the body, it can also limit how the normal range of emotions and feelings are felt. As a result, it can become very difficult to snap out of feeling depressed or irritable.

WEAK QI AND BLOOD IN THE BODY: If there is not enough qi and blood to spare in the menstrual process, both can easily become obstructed. If so, there can be a tendency to be depressed and tearful, with accompanying tiredness and backache.

Dietary factors that can worsen premenstrual syndrome

- Overeating, eating too fast, eating too late at night, eating at irregular times. These cause a sluggish digestion that will stagnate qi.
- Oily, fatty food and processed foods, including foods high in saturated fats, such as red meat, junk food and dairy products. See Qi Stagnation for more details.

Dietary factors that can improve premenstrual syndrome

- Ideally, follow a simple, strengthening diet that builds qi and prevents stagnation. See Weak Qi for more details.
- Beetroot, spinach, and sardines strengthen blood. See Weak Blood for more details.
- Spices and apple cider vinegar can help move stagnation. See Stagnation of Qi for more details.
- Brazilian research published in 2011 suggests that essential fatty acids may be helpful for the symptoms of premenstrual syndrome. In the study, women who received pills containing a few grams of essential fatty acids reported an improvement in symptoms such as sore breasts and depression.[28] Essential fatty acids in the form

of soybean oil, safflower oil, walnuts, sunflower, sesame, and pumpkin seeds, flaxseed, fatty fish such as tuna and mackerel, and dark green vegetables may therefore have a useful qi-moving quality in PMS.

Acupressure and massage

ON THE FRONT:

- Rub in a circular motion around the belly button with your palm until warm.
- Do the ABDOMEN CIRCLE massage in Feeling Bloated.
- ABDOMEN LINE: Hard-press six equally spaced points with the thumb or fingers on both sides of the stomach muscles. The first two above your belly button, the second two in line with your belly button, and the third two below.
- Rub the abdomen as in 1.

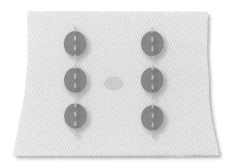

ON THE LEGS:

- Thumb-press the Liver and Gall Bladder channels up to the knee, and knead any sore points, including GB-34 and GB-41.
- Thumb-press the Spleen and Stomach Channels up to the knee, and knead any sore points, including St-40, Sp-6, and St-36.

ON THE BACK: Thumb-press along the Bladder channel either side of the spine. Knead any sore points, including Bl-18, Bl-20, and Bl-23.

ON THE HANDS: Do the Healthy Hand massage in the

How Can You Treat Yourself? section. Press Reproductive area, LI-4, and He-7, and knead if sore.

ON THE FEET: Do the Healthy Foot massage in the How Can You Treat Yourself? section. Hard-press Kid-3 and Kid-6 on the ankle. Also press the following points, and knead if sore: Liv-3, Liver, Kidneys, and Gall Bladder.

ON THE EARS: Press the following points, and knead if sore: Uterus, Ovaries, Liver, and Shen Men.

Scraping

Scrape down the neck and across the shoulders, then down the muscles either side of the spine, to the sacral area and the top of the hips. Pay particular attention to the area between the shoulder blades and spine and the mid-back.

Tapping

Tap each point up to 30 times. You may need an assistant for the back area.

- Feel around the neck and shoulder area, and tap any tender points in the muscles.
- Feel down the back muscles on either side of the spine, and tap any sore points.
- Tap any sore points in the sacral area.
- Follow the Liver and Gall Bladder channels along the upper and lower legs to the feet. Tap any tender points, especially Liv-3, GB-34, GB-39, and GB-40.
- Follow the Spleen channel up to just below the groin, and tap any sore points, especially Sp-6, Sp-8, and Sp-10.

Exercises

1. Do Exercises 1–6 of the five-element stretches. Particularly focus on Exercise 6, as this helps to circulate qi in the Liver and Gall Bladder.
2. Do exercise Bend Your Hip from Weak Qi.

Abdomen line massage

Lifestyle advice

- Regular gentle exercise like swimming, aerobics or jogging can reduce stagnation considerably. It must however be regular and not just when you feel any symptoms.
- Correct posture can also help reduce qi stagnation, especially in work situations. When seated, the ideal height for a work surface is about two inches below your bent elbow. Your back and feet should be well supported, with your forearms and upper legs resting parallel to the floor. Hunching, for example, which restricts the movement of qi in the chest, is to be avoided, wherever possible.

Heavy Periods

Symptoms

A period that initially gushes with blood and that requires frequent changes of sanitary protection. It can continue for a prolonged time.

Can include or lead to

Fibroids, endometriosis, and menopausal problems.

When to see a doctor

If the symptoms are severe.

Common causes

Strong emotional issues, such as resentment, anger, and worry; an improper, irregular diet; a diet with too many hot-natured, spicy foods; overexercise; post-surgery; or post-childbirth conditions.

An explanation

WEAK QI IN THE SPLEEN: The Spleen has many functions in Oriental medicine: one of them has to do with the control of blood. If Spleen qi becomes too weak, often because of an improper diet, it no longer has the power to hold the blood in the blood vessels. The result is that blood quite literally leaks out. In this case, the accompanying blood would normally be pale, and there would be other signs of weak qi, such as tiredness and a pale complexion.

HEAT IN THE BLOOD: If there is too much heat in the blood it spills over, much like boiling water in an unattended cooking pot. Signs of this condition would be bright or dark-red thick blood and headaches, restlessness, and thirst. This could also be caused by diet (too many hot-natured, greasy foods) or a long-term condition of yin weakness, which has switched to heat.

STAGNATION OF QI AND BLOOD: This is a common condition in people with unresolved emotional issues and depression. Stagnation of qi and blood can form a blockage, much like a dam. When fresh blood enters the uterus, the level of the blood rises above the height of the dam and overtops it and the flow cannot be controlled. This condition would normally show as dark, thick blood, with clots and strong pain.

Dietary factors that can worsen heavy periods

- Cold or cool-natured, raw foods damage the digestive process, weaken the Stomach and Spleen, and lead to an inability to control blood flow. See Cold for more details.
- Overeating; alcohol; oily, fatty food; and junk and processed foods may damage the Liver and lead to stagnant qi. See Qi Stagnation for more details.
- Hot-natured, spicy foods such as red meat, coffee, and alcohol will cause more heat. See Heat for more examples.

Dietary factors that can improve heavy periods

- An overall strengthening diet to maintain the Stomach and Spleen will help all conditions but particularly help retain blood circulating in the blood vessels. See Weak Qi for more details.
- Parsnips, fennel, leek, oats, quinoa, aduki beans, pine nuts, black beans, kelp, and other seaweeds strengthen qi and blood capacity.
- Mung beans, aubergines (eggplants), spinach, celery, cucumber, and seaweed can help cool heat in the blood.

Acupressure and massage

ON THE HEAD: Finger-press from Yintang, between the eyes, up to Du-20, at the top of the head. Press and knead any sore points.

ON THE FRONT: Finger-press down the centre line of the abdomen, and knead any sore points, including Ren-12 and Ren-6.

ON THE BACK: Thumb-press down the muscles either side of the spine. Knead any sore points, especially Bl-17, Bl-20, and Bl-23.

ON THE ARMS: Press LI-11, and knead if sore.

ON THE LEGS: Thumb-press up the Spleen channel to the groin. Knead any sore points, including Sp 6 and Sp-10. Hard-press Sp-8, as this can help to stop bleeding.

ON THE FEET: Press and knead Sp-1 and Liv-1 (with a fingernail), as well as Liv-3 and Kid-2. Also knead Liver, Reproductive Organs, Uterus, Groin, and Hips.

ON THE HANDS: Press the following points, and knead if sore: Stop Bleeding, Reproductive area, Spleen, Sanjiao, Perineum, Kidneys, Liver, and Ming Men.

ON THE EARS: Press the following points, and knead if sore: Uterus, Ovaries, Abdomen, Liver, and Spleen.

Scraping

Scrape down the neck and across the shoulders, then down the muscles either side of the spine, as far as the sacral area and the top of the hips. If there is a lot of stagnation, the colour of the dots may be deep red or purple.

Tapping

Tap each point up to 30 times. You may need an assistant for the back area.

- Feel down the back muscles on either side of the spine and tap any sore points.
- Tap any sore points in the sacral area.
- Follow the Spleen channel up to the hip, and tap any tender points, especially Sp-6, Sp-8, Sp-10, and a point two finger widths above Sp-10.
- Tap the following points if sore: Liv-3 and Liv-4 on the foot, GB-34 on the leg, and LI-11 and the arm.

Exercises

Do Exercises 2, 4, and 6 of the five-element stretches. These help harmonize the Spleen, Liver, and Kidney.

Lifestyle advice

- With conditions of weak qi, it is very important to rest and not to stand for long periods. Prolonged standing may make the condition worse.
- Regular gentle exercise for all conditions can be beneficial, but especially for conditions of stagnation.

Period Pain
Symptoms

Abdominal and or back pain before, during, or after a period.

Can include or lead to

Dysmenorrhoea, pelvic inflammation, uterine fibroids, and endometriosis.

When to see a doctor

If the symptoms are severe or accompanied with heavy bleeding.

Common causes

Emotional stress; overwork; an inappropriate diet; exposure to the elements; or excessive sexual activity.

An explanation

STAGNATION OF QI: If qi and blood become blocked during the menstrual cycle, the buildup of pressure causes pain. This can often happen after emotional stress, as the flow of qi becomes affected and clogs up.

    The pain in qi stagnation is often severe, on one or both sides of the lower abdomen, prior to the onset of a menstrual period. Dark, purple blood clots and swollen, painful breasts often accompany this condition, and the painful area is normally worse with pressure.

    If the condition involves stagnation of blood, the pain is usually more of the fixed, stabbing variety a few days before the start of the period. It is often located in the central part of the abdomen, the blood shows as dark, purple clots, and it can be worse at night.

DAMP AND COLD IN THE UTERUS: Cold and damp can enter the uterus from exposure to the cold, commonly from wearing inadequate clothing or sitting on a cold surface. The resulting pain is normally cramping, before or during a period, and there is usually a low quantity of blood. It can feel better with heat (and worse with cold).

DAMP AND HEAT IN THE UTERUS: Long-term cold or stagnation can gradually transform into heat. This can result in heavy, dark-coloured blood, discharges, small clots and a strong burning sensation.

WEAK QI AND BLOOD IN THE BODY: Inadequate qi and blood to support the menstrual cycle can result in duller pain, which is better with pressure and heat and occurs during or after the period. It can be accompanied by low blood loss and tiredness.

FALSE HEAT IN THE LIVER AND KIDNEYS: Heat that originates from yin weakness often does not present with the severe symptoms of many of the other conditions. In this case, a burning sensation is involved, and the pain usually comes a few days after the period. The difference here is that the heat and subsequent pain results from weakness in the body.

Dietary factors that can worsen period pain

- Raw, cold-natured foods, such as bananas, lettuce and cucumbers, aggravate a cold condition. So can citrus fruits, such as grapefruits and lemons, due to their cooling nature. See Cold for more details.
- Red meat, dairy products, eggs, sweet, sugary foods, and other heat-forming foods aggravate a heat condition. See Heat for more details.
- Fatty meat, concentrated fruit juice, bread, milk, and other damp-forming foods aggravate a damp condition. See Damp for more details.

Dietary factors that can improve period pain

- For all conditions it is important to strengthen the underlying weakness with simple, nutritious foods. See Weak Qi and Weak Blood for more details.
- Oats, black beans, dill, caraway, basil, and black peppercorn. oats, black beans, dill, caraway, basil, black peppercorns, and other warming foods improve cold conditions. See Cold for more details on this.

- Spinach, lettuce, celery, carrots, mung beans, tofu, parsley, and other cooling foods improve heat conditions. See Heat for more details.
- Pumpkin, radishes, lemons, and other drying foods improve damp conditions. See Damp for more details.

Acupressure and massage

ON THE FRONT:
- Rub in a circular motion around the belly button with your palm until warm.
- Do the ABDOMEN CIRCLE massage in Feeling Bloated.
- Do the ABDOMEN LINE massage in Premenstrual Tension.
  Return to rubbing the abdomen.
- An alternative to the above: Press and knead Ren-

> CAUTION: Abdominal massages can be of great benefit for period pain, but they should be discontinued during the period itself.

6, Ren-4, Ren-3, and Liv-14, if sore.
ON THE BACK: Rub the lower back up and down with an open palm, either side of the spine. Press and knead Bl-18, Bl-20, and Bl-23, especially if the pain is after the period. Press and knead the sacral area with the knuckles of a clenched fist.
ON THE LEGS:
- If the pain is before or during the period: Thumb-press the Spleen, Stomach, and Liver channels up to the knee. Knead Liv-5, Sp-6, Sp-8, Sp-9, Sp-10, St-36, and St-40, if sore.
- If the pain is pre-period: Sp-8 and Liv-3 (on the foot) are especially useful.
- If the pain is during a period: St-36, Sp-10, and Sp-6 are especially useful.
ON THE HANDS: Press the following points and knead if sore: LI-4, Ming Men, Sanjiao, and Reproductive Organs.

ON THE FEET: Thumb-press along the Kidney channel. Notice that it moves in a circular pattern below the outside ankle. Press Kid-3, Kid-5, Kid-6, if sore. Also knead Uterus, Reproductive Organs, Groin, Hips, Liver, and Kidneys.
ON THE EARS: Press the following points, and knead if sore: Uterus, Ovaries, Liver, Kidneys, Abdomen, Point Zero, and Shen Men.

Scraping

Scrape down the neck and across the shoulders, then down the muscles either side of the spine, as far as the sacral area and the top of the hips. The dots can often be deep red or purple.

Tapping

Tap each point up to 30 times. You may need an assistant for the sacral area. Ideally, treat before the start of the period. Use the following points:

- Follow the Spleen channel up to the groin area and tap on any sore points, in particular Sp-6, Sp-8, and an extra point two finger widths above Sp-10.
- Follow the Liver channel along the lower and upper leg, and tap any tender points. Start with Liv-3 on the foot.
- Tap around the sacral area, if sore.

Exercises

The following exercises can help to move blood and qi in the lower abdomen.

1. AIR CYCLING
While lying on your back, lift your legs high into the air. Then bend your knees and slowly simulate riding a bicycle in the air with your legs. Put your hands at your waist to support your back. Do this for a minute or until tired, then rest.

Air cycling

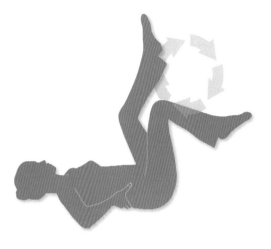

Leg circle

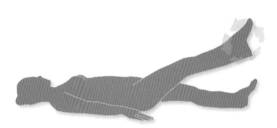

2. LEG CIRCLES
Lie face up, with both legs straight. Raise one leg, and make a circle in the air with the foot. The leg should remain straight, and the movement should come from the hip joint. The circle should begin small but increase in size. Continue for 20 rotations, if you can, then repeat with the other leg. Repeat the sequence several times.
3. Do the exercise Body Twist in the Constipation section.
4. Do Exercises 2, 4, and 6 of the five-element stretches, which help improve the circulation of qi in the Spleen, Liver, and Kidneys.

Lifestyle advice

• Keep the body as warm and dry as possible, and avoid regularly swimming in cold water.

• Heat helps qi and blood circulate better, so applying something warm to the abdomen can relieve pain. This could be a hot water bottle, a heated pad, or even your pet cat.

Light or No Periods
Symptoms

Light bleeding during periods that is of short duration (two days or under), or periods absent altogether.

Can include or lead to

Amenorrhea, polycystic ovarian syndrome, anorexia nervosa, endometriosis, and menopause.

When to see a doctor

If accompanied by abdominal pain.

Common causes

Emotional stress, especially when repressed: overexercise; inappropriate diet; competitive work atmosphere; chronic illness; overwork; long-term use of oral contraceptives; or pregnancy.

An explanation

WEAK BLOOD IN THE BODY: The absence of periods can be because of weak qi and blood, arising from insufficient life force to pump it around the body. This can be accompanied by other signs of weak blood, such as dizziness, insomnia, and heart palpitations.
STAGNATION OF QI AND BLOOD IN THE BODY: Qi and blood can become stuck and prevented from moving freely from the uterus. If the blood stagnates there can be pain. The blood is usually dark with clots.

DAMP AND PHLEGM: Sometimes blocks are created by sticky damp or phlegm built up in the abdomen, either from an improper diet or from exposure to cold. This condition is more likely to occur in someone who is overweight and can be accompanied by discharge and heaviness.

WEAK QI IN THE KIDNEYS: Sometimes the balance of yin and yang in the Kidneys has swung too much in one direction. Weak Kidney yang can mean there is not enough yang energy to move the blood. It can be accompanied by lower back and knee pain.

Dietary factors that can worsen light or missing periods

Overeating or undereating regularly, and a diet containing lots of red meat, dairy products, and raw fruit and vegetables, can aggravate stagnation.

- Raw and frozen foods or foods that taste bitter and sour have properties that interfere with the circulation of blood and cause weak blood. See the Bitter and Sour lists for more details.
- Dairy products, processed, fatty foods high in bad fats, and other raw, cold-natured, and damp-forming foods aggravate damp and cold conditions. See Damp and Phlegm for more details.

Dietary factors that can improve light or missing periods

- Dark, leafy greens, carrots, aubergines (eggplants), chives, turmeric, nutmeg, garlic, and chamomile tea improve stagnation associated with damp and phlegm conditions. See Qi Stagnation and Blood Stagnation for more details.
- Egg yolk; almonds; dried fruit such as figs, currants, and apricots; spinach; oats; fish; and high-quality red meat build up weak blood and qi. See Weak Blood for more details.

- Barley, rye, pumpkin, button mushrooms, and aduki beans improve conditions of damp and phlegm. See Damp and Phlegm for more details.

Acupressure and massage

ON THE FRONT:
- Palm circle with slight pressure in a clockwise direction around the belly button.
- Do the ABDOMEN CIRCLE massage in Feeling Bloated.
- Press and knead Ren-12, Ren-6, and Ren-4.
- Rub in a circular motion around Ren-4 with the palm to create warmth.

ON THE BACK:
- Rub the lower back from side to side with the palm to create warmth.
- Press and knead with the knuckles of a clenched fist at Du-3, Du-4, Bl-18, Bl-20, Bl-23, and any sore points in the sacral area.

ON THE LEGS: Hard-press St-36, Liv-8, Sp-10, and Sp-6.

ON THE FEET:
- Do the Healthy Foot massage in the How Can You Treat Yourself? section.
- Thumb-press along the Kidney and Bladder channels on the foot. Hard press Bl-61 and Kid-5, and thumb-press over the ankle joint from one to the other.
- Also knead Reproductive Organs and Uterus area.

ON THE HANDS: Press the following points, and knead if sore: LI-4, Reproductive Organs, Mingmen, Kidney, and Liver area.

ON THE EARS: Press the following points and knead if tender: Uterus, Ovaries, Endocrine, Liver and Kidneys.

Scraping

Scrape down the neck and across the shoulders, then down the muscles either side of the spine, as far as the sacral area and the top of the hips. If the problem is one of weakness, scrape lightly.

Tapping

Tap each point up to 30 times. You may need an assistant for the back area.

- Feel down the muscles of the back on either side of the spine and tap any sore points.
- Tap any sore points in the sacral/hip area.
- Follow the Stomach channel up to the hip and tap any sore points, especially St-36, St-40 and the thigh points.
- Follow the Spleen channel up to the groin and tap any sore points, especially Sp-6, Sp-9, and Sp-10.
- Tap Kid-3 on the foot, Kid-7 and Liv-8 on the leg if tender.

Exercises

The exercises in the Period Pain section will also be helpful here.

Lifestyle advice

- For all conditions, it is important to do regular gentle exercise to encourage the movement of qi and blood.
- It is also important to keep your legs and feet warm and dry as much as possible. Watch where you sit, especially when outside.

Menopausal Discomfort
Symptoms

Hot flushes, tiredness, irritability, insomnia, aching joints, vaginal irritation, irregular bleeding, palpita-

tions, sweating at night, headaches, stiff shoulders, depression, lower back pain, low libido, bone and muscle pain.

Can include or lead to

The onset of menopause.

When to see a doctor

If there are severe mental or emotional symptoms.

Common causes

Emotional stress; worry, anxiety; an improper diet and eating habits; overwork; a chronic illness; or multiple pregnancies.

An explanation

The changes in menopause often reflect the imbalances that existed before the onset of menopause. If the imbalances are minor, the symptoms will be, too. However, imbalances of many years' standing do tend to lead to stronger symptoms as a woman goes through menopause, and Oriental medicine can help to prevent or relieve some of the more unpleasant symptoms.

WEAK YIN IN THE KIDNEYS: The Kidneys hold our stores of qi, and it is here, at the very source of life, that an imbalance either way can trigger symptoms. While both yin and yang can be weak, the most common condition is that the yin in the Kidney, which has been chipped away slowly over the years, gets so weak that is can no longer contain yang. Yang then rises from the Kidneys, bringing heat with it.

WEAK QI AND BLOOD IN THE HEART: Insufficient Kidney yin has other knock-on effects at menopause. One of these is the relationship between Fire and

Water. In nature, their relationship is very obvious: to put out a fire, you need to pour water over it. If there is not enough water because the source of the water has dried up, the fire will get hotter and spread.

In the body, the Kidneys represent Water and the Heart represents Fire, and the balance between the two can often be the source of heat. Resultant symptoms include palpitations, insomnia, and sweating at night.

WEAK YIN IN THE LIVER: The yin imbalance in the Kidneys can also affect the Liver and cause common Liver yin weakness symptoms, such as dizziness, irritability, and dryness.

Dietary factors that can worsen menopausal discomfort

- Overconsumption of coffee, hot chocolate, caffeinated soft drinks, and alcohol can all cause heat and agitation.
- Avoid roasting, deep-frying and other warm methods of cooking.
- Warming bitter and pungent foods, such as chilli, basil, cinnamon, cloves, ginger, prawns, shrimps, can weaken Yin. See Weak Yin for more details.

Dietary factors that can improve menopausal discomfort

- A generally strengthening diet benefits Kidney qi and yin. See Weak Qi and Weak Yin for more details.
- Oats, aduki beans, kidney beans, asparagus, eggs, sweet potato, walnuts, raspberries, quinoa, shrimp, lobster, mussels, and parsley strengthen the Kidneys.

Acupressure and massage

ON THE HEAD: Finger-press from the midpoint of the hairline, following the hairline to the ear. Knead any sore points, especially Du-24.

ON THE FEET AND LEGS:

- Thumb-press the Kidney channel up to the knee. Hard-press on Kid-3 and Kid-6 on the foot and any other tender points.
- Thumb-press the Spleen channel up to the knee, and knead any sore points, especially Sp-6.
- Hard-press Liv-8 on the leg.

ON THE FRONT: Finger press down the middle of the breastbone and then to the belly button. Knead any sore points, especially Ren-15.

Hard-press Ren-6 and Ren-4 below the belly button.

ON THE BACK: Thumb- or finger-press down the back muscles in the lower back either side of the spine. Knead any tightness or sore areas, especially Bl-23 and Bl-52.

ON THE HANDS: Press the following points, and knead if tender: Essence, Reproductive area, Head area, Insomnia area, Fatigue, and Hypertension areas.

ON THE EARS: Press the following points, and knead if tender: Ovaries, Uterus, Endocrine, Shen Men, Kidneys, and Liver.

Scraping

Scrape down the neck and across the shoulders, then down the muscles either side of the spine, as far as the sacral area and the top of the hips.

Tapping

Tap each point up to 30 times. You may need an assistant the back area.

- Tap down the muscles of the back either side of the spine. Check Bl-15 and Bl-18, and tap if sore.
- Tap Kid-6 on the ankle, and Sp-6 and St-36 on the legs.

Exercises

Do Exercises 3–6 of the five-element stretches to strengthen the Kidneys, Heart, and Liver.

Lifestyle advice

Symptoms associated with menopause vary from woman to woman. However, it is very common to come across women who have been diagnosed with a certain condition on the basis of a slight abnormality on a medical test, been medicated, then developed a more complicated condition.

It is standard in mainstream medicine to diagnose a woman at menopause with a "hormonal imbalance," and many women are encouraged to have pharmaceutical hormone replacement therapy (HRT), despite sometimes not even showing symptoms. The argument is usually made that it will protect against heart disease and osteoporosis.

Recently the dangers of long-term use of synthetic HRT have led to the popularity of bioidentical HRT, which is thought to have less long-term side effects as it has the same molecular structure as the hormones produced naturally within the body.

A much better approach is to see menopause as a natural process. After all, a woman's body is supposed to stop ovulating and reduce its oestrogen levels once it reaches a certain age. It has been designed to do this. From an Oriental medicine viewpoint, both Kidney yin and Kidney yang should naturally decline, or they will simply run out.

Rather than keeping these oestrogen levels artificially high, thereby forcing the body to use up more Kidney qi, a woman should be supporting the balance of yin and yang in her changing body by making shifts in lifestyle, work, diet, exercise, and general state of mind to support what is a natural and powerful passage in her life. Doing this offers a much safer and effective way of protecting a menopausal woman against heart disease and osteoporosis.

- If you are using synthetic or bio-identical HRT, you need to be aware that while your hormones are being regulated by this treatment, your Kidneys are not being strengthened, and you need to take measures (diet and lifestyle) to preserve Kidney qi to prevent potential health problems in the future.
- Negative lifestyle factors can no longer be ignored at menopause. It is, after all, a transition from yang to yin, and leading a yang lifestyle should be replaced by more of a yin one. This should involve less overworking, more slowing down, and more rest than before.
- Regular gentle exercise is also very important at menopause, to strengthen the Kidneys. Do not exercise later in the day, though, as this can draw on your yin stores and make menopausal symptoms worse.
- Some factors, such as smoking, have been shown to bring on early menopause in women. According to research in Turkey, the likelihood of this happening correlates with the number of cigarettes a woman smokes daily: women who smoke more than 10 cigarettes a day have an increased risk of going into menopause early.[29] This means that the heat generated in their Lungs severely weakened their stores of yin.

Chapter 26
氣 Conditions Affecting the Whole Body

High Blood Pressure
Symptoms

Headaches, dizziness, palpitations, sleep problems, numbness, pins and needles, pressure in the head, tinnitus.

NOTE: Blood pressure readings normally have two sets of numbers. The first number is the systolic rate (referring to the contraction of the heart muscle), and the second is the diastolic (referring to the relaxation of the heart muscle).

Blood pressure is considered to be normal when the reading reads within the range of 90–120/60–80. Blood pressure is considered to be higher than normal when it reads 120–140/80–90. High blood pressure is categorized as any reading above 140+/90+. Note, however, that this should be an average of several blood pressure readings at different times and on different days.

Can include or lead to

Hypertension, stroke, peripheral arterial disease, cardiac insufficiency.

When to see a doctor

If the symptoms are severe.

Common causes

Emotional stress; overthinking; work stress; overwork; a diet of too many hot-natured, spicy, greasy foods; too much alcohol; smoking; or old age.

An explanation

WEAK YIN AND RISING YANG: High blood pressure normally has a strong component of yin weakness. Any long-standing heat in the body can gradually burn up the yin stores, which are located in the Kidneys. This can affect other organs, especially the Liver, and cause imbalances in both organs.

Once the levels of yin in both the Kidneys and Liver have reached a low enough point, strong signs of yang appear from the Liver, as it is no longer controlled by the strength of Liver yin. Hyperactive yang can rise in the body, go straight to the head, and cause a rise in speed and blood pressure. Often accompanying this imbalance is weakness in the area below the belly button, and the chest can feel warm. For some people with this condition, any fluctuations in blood pressure cause stress and worry, and there can be almost an obsession in maintaining a constant blood pressure.

WEAK YANG: Sometimes the opposite pattern is present. If Kidney yang weakens, damp can accumulate and prevent the movement of yang. Without yang, the blood vessels will remain tense, and the smooth flow of blood can then be restricted.

STAGNATION OF QI AND BLOOD: When the Liver gets disturbed by emotions, it ceases to maintain the smooth flow of qi around the body. This can lead to emotional stagnation in the form of depression and physical discomfort and pain. Any long-standing stagnation will build up heat, and this heat can rise in the body and disturb blood flow.

Dietary factors that can worsen high blood pressure

- Hot-natured, spicy, and warm foods, such as ginger, cinnamon, and lamb, fuel the fire. See Heat for more information.
- Too much table salt can thicken the blood and raise blood pressure. It is the same with processed, packaged food and junk food. A British report claims that as much as 75 percent of the salt we eat is surreptitiously hidden in our food. One takeaway pizza, for example, was found to contain an entire day's recommended allowance of salt (the report found one that was more salty than sea water!).[30] See the Salty Foods list for more details on salty food.
- Coffee and alcohol can dry up yin and blood over time. See Weak Yin for more details.
- Caffeinated drinks, such as coffee, tea, fizzy soft drinks, and energy drinks, also agitate yang and can adversely affect blood pressure.

Dietary factors that can improve high blood pressure

- Sour foods, such as citrus fruit, can be beneficial to the liver and so to blood flow. See the list of Sour Foods for more details.
- Apples, pears, oranges, wheat, mung beans, spinach, green tea, and milk help bring down rising yang qi. See Yang Rising for more details.
- Crab, octopus, blueberries, lemons, dandelion, spinach, celery, tomatoes, water chestnuts, and green tea help keep qi moving smoothly. See Qi Stagnation for more details.
- Duck, pork, chicken, grapes, spinach, celery, tomatoes, black soya beans, pine nuts, black sesame seeds, and sunflower seeds improve yin and blood. See Weak Yin and Weak Blood for more details.

Acupressure and massage

ON THE HEAD: Press Yintang, Taiyang, Du-20, GB-20, and press outwards towards the ear.

ON THE FRONT:
- Rub in a circular motion around the belly button with your palm until warm.
- Do the ABDOMEN CIRCLE massage in Feeling Bloated.
- Do the ABDOMEN LINE massage in Premenstrual Tension.

ON THE ARMS: Hard-press LI-11 and PC-6, if sore.

ON THE BACK: Knead GB-21 and the area around it.

ON THE LEGS: Thumb-press along the Liver, Stomach, and Spleen channels, and knead any sore points, especially St-36 and Sp-6.

ON THE HANDS: Press the following points, and knead if sore: PC-9, SI-3, Liver, Shixuan (on the tips of the fingers), Reduce Blood Pressure, Head area, Hypertension area, and Dizziness area.

ON THE FEET: Do the Healthy Foot massage in the How Can You Treat Yourself? section. Press and knead Kid-1, Liv-3, Adrenal, Liver, Kidneys and Heart.

ON THE EARS: Press the following points, and knead if sore: Hypertension, Heart, Liver, and Shen Men.

Scraping

Scrape down the neck and across the shoulder muscles. Also scrape down the upper back, especially in the area between the shoulder blades.

Tapping

Tap each point up to 30 times. You may need an assistant for the back area.

- Tap down the neck and across the shoulder muscles. Feel for any tight, sore points.
- Feel down the back muscles either side of the spine, and tap any sore points.

- Tap down the Huatuojiaji points on either side of the spine. These points are either side of the gaps in the vertebrae. Find a vertebra, drop down into the gap, and the point lies to the side of this, slightly away from the spine. Caution: Tap close to but be careful not to tap actually on the spine.

Exercises

Do Exercises 3–6 of the five-element stretches. This can strengthen the Heart, Kidneys, and Liver.

Lifestyle advice

In the USA, studies have clearly linked dietary changes and exercise with a reduction in blood pressure. It is very important, therefore, to take regular exercise in combination with any dietary changes made above.[31]

Low Blood Pressure
Symptoms

Tiredness, dizziness, difficulty in getting up in the mornings, fainting, lack of appetite, tinnitus, cold hands and feet, diarrhoea, and palpitations. Unlike high blood pressure, low blood pressure is not usually defined by a specific blood pressure number, but purely on signs and symptoms.

Can include or lead to

Hypotension, idiopathic orthostatic hypotension, heart disease, and Shy-Drager syndrome.

When to see a doctor

If there are severe symptoms.

Common causes

An inappropriate diet; a shock or accident; being overweight; a constitutional imbalance; heavy bleeding; or side effects of medications.

An explanation

WEAK YANG AND COLD: Low blood pressure happens when yang is unable to move upwards and outwards to warm the body and move the blood. This yang weakness often originates in the Spleen, particularly if the tiredness worsens after meal times and there is difficulty finding the energy to speak.

The Spleen should transform the food we eat into energy and send energized blood as far as the four limbs, but when weakened by an improper diet or worry and stress it no longer has the power. This can result in circulatory symptoms such as cold hands and feet, a lack of strength and dizziness, as not enough clear qi can travel to the head.

The resulting cold condition can also create stiff and sore muscles as they contract more than usual.

Dietary factors that can worsen low blood pressure

- Coffee is very drying and can have a weakening effect on blood.
- Too many cold and cool-natured foods, such as salads, raw foods, dairy products, and fruit juice, slow down digestion. See Cold for more details.

Dietary factors that can improve low blood pressure

- Eating regularly is very important, especially breakfast, which should be substantial. Food should be stewed, grilled, or lightly fried.
- In general, follow a strengthening diet consisting of lots of easy-to-digest grains and sweet-natured foods that promote digestion: duck, chicken, beef,

salmon, tuna, eel, cherries, peaches, fennel, carrots, dates, short-grain rice, corn, millet, oats, chili, ginger, garlic, pepper, cinnamon, chestnuts, and walnuts.
*   A little of the following salty food can help raise Kidney qi and yang: venison, lamb, mussels, oysters, sardines, raisins, cherries, corn, honey, and fennel.

Acupressure and massage

ON THE HEAD:
*   Put both hands on your head, with your fingers bent and separate. Press and massage the whole head for a few minutes.
*   Raise your chin slightly. Put your left palm on the right side of your neck. Knead and rub from your jaw to your clavicle several times. Then swap sides and repeat.
*   Rest the fingers of both hands on the midline of your forehead, and finger-knead outwards to your temples. Repeat this several times.
*   Press Taiyang with your middle and index fingers, first gently and then stronger. Press for five seconds, and repeat several times.

ON THE LEGS: Thumb-press the Stomach and Spleen channels, as far as the knee. Knead any sore points, especially St-36 and Sp-6.

ON THE HANDS: Press the following points, and knead if sore: LI-4, LI-10, LI-11, Raise Blood Pressure, Dizziness area, and Insomnia area.

ON THE FEET: Press the following points, and knead if sore: Spleen, Pancreas, Liver, Heart, and Kidneys.

ON THE EARS: Press the following points, and knead if sore: Blood Pressure, Heart, Shen Men, and Point Zero.

Scraping

Scrape down the neck, across the shoulders, and down the whole back.

Tapping

Tap each point up to 30 times. You may need an assistant for the back area.
*   Tap any stiffness or soreness in the neck and shoulder areas. In particular Bl-10 and GB-20 on the neck and GB-21 on the shoulders.
*   Feel down the back on either side of the spine, and tap any sore points, especially Bl-20, Bl-21, and Bl-22.

Exercises

Do Exercise 4 of the five-element stretches to strengthen the Kidneys.

Lifestyle advice

*   Some medications, such as beta-blockers (often prescribed for heart conditions) and antidepressants, can cause low blood pressure as a side effect.
*   Be aware of how you move if you suffer from hypotension. There is very little yang energy inside, so actions such as standing up should be done gradually.

Hyperthyroidism
Symptoms

Swelling of the thyroid gland, palpitations, tiredness, sweating easily, agitated, increased appetite yet weight loss, diarrhoea, and possibly protruding in one or both eyes.

Can include or lead to

Graves' disease, thyrotoxicosis, and autoimmune disease.

When to see a doctor

If there are severe symptoms.

Common causes

Emotional stress, especially frustration; a shock; or an inappropriate diet.

An explanation

The condition of hyperthyroidism is one of heat rising to the thyroid glands in the neck. It can occur with the following patterns:

STAGNATION OF QI IN THE BODY: Qi can become stuck due to sustained emotional stress or overwork, and over time will heat up the Liver. This simmering heat can slowly burn off fluids and moisture and damage the level of yin.

WEAK KIDNEY YIN WITH HEAT: When Kidney yin becomes weak, it can no longer be the counterbalance for Kidney yang. The increased agitation of yang causes heat to move upwards. In both of these conditions, the heat can rise to the heart and overheat heart qi, causing palpitations. It can also rise to the Stomach and cause hunger, and to the Spleen, causing tiredness.

The swelling in the thyroid is a progression of this pattern, as qi rises through the body and settles where both branches of the Kidney and Liver channels run through the neck. The subsequent weight loss that sometimes accompanies this condition is often due to the burning up of fluids from heat and sweating.

Dietary factors that can worsen hyperthyroidism

- Hot-natured, pungent foods, such as hot spices, alcohol, and coffee, can be too drying and overly stimulating. See the Hot and Pungent food lists for more details.
- Too many uncooked, chilled foods, saturated oils and fats, and dairy products such as milk and cheese aggravate fatigue and damp. See Damp for more details.

Dietary factors that can help hyperthyroidism

- Foods that strengthen yin can be beneficial. See Weak Yin for more details. Note: Be cautious about eating too many heavy yin foods, such as dairy products, as they can be very damp-forming.
- Oats, aduki beans, kidney beans, asparagus, eggs, sweet potato, walnuts, raspberries, quinoa, shrimp, lobster, mussels, and parsley specifically build Kidney qi.

Acupressure and massage

ON THE ARMS:
- Thumb-press along the Triple Burner channel, up to the face. Knead any sore points.
- Thumb-press along the Small Intestine channel, up to the neck. Knead any sore points.

ON THE LEGS: Press the following points, and knead if sore: St-36, St-40, Sp-6, Kid-7, and GB-34.

ON THE FEET: Thumb-press the Kidney channel on the foot (note that it circles around the ankle). Knead any sore points, in particular Kid-2. Also press the following points, and knead if sore: Liv-3, Thyroid, Kidneys, Liver, Stomach, and Spleen.

ON THE HANDS: Press the following points, and knead if sore: Thyroid, Throat, Kidneys, Heart, Sanjiao, and Liver.

ON THE EARS: Press the following points, and knead if sore: Thyroid, Neck, Liver, Spleen, Kidneys, Endocrine, and Sympathetic.

Scraping

Scrape across the shoulders to the top of the arms, then down the muscles of the back on either side of the spine.

Tapping

Tap each point up to 30 times. You may need an assistant for the back area.

- Feel down the back muscles on either side of the spine, and tap any sore points.
- Tap Kid-2 and Liv-3 on the foot and Kid-7 and GB-34 on the leg.

Exercises

Do Exercises 3, 4, and 6 of the five-element stretches. These can strengthen the Heart, Kidneys, and Liver.

Lifestyle advice

- Relaxation is very important, as is the removal of any sources of stress and tension.
- Avoid vigorous exercise; activities such as walking, qi gong or tai chi are preferable.

Hypothyroidism

Symptoms

Feeling cold, weight gain, fatigue, constipation, joint stiffness, and an enlarged neck or the presence of a goitre.

Can include or lead to

Hashimoto's disease, thyroiditis, lymphadenoid goitre, autoimmune endocrine disorders, including diabetes mellitus, Addison's disease, Grave's disease, hypoparathyroidism, hypopituitarism, and vitiligo.

When to see a doctor

If there are severe symptoms.

Common causes

Emotional stress; overworry; anxiety; an inappropriate diet and eating habits; an overly yang lifestyle; overuse of antibiotics; a constitutional weakness; or old age.

An explanation

In conventional terms, this condition involves the underactivity of thyroid gland function and normally requires thyroid hormone replacement therapy in the form of thyroxine. In Oriental medicine terms, the condition of hypothyroidism is essentially one of sustained weakness of yang in the body, and it can occur with the following patterns:

WEAK SPLEEN AND KIDNEY YANG: The Spleen extracts nutritive qi from the food we eat and sends it around the body. When there is not enough yang to do this effectively, the parts of the body farthest away, the hands and feet, receive less than they should and can frequently feel cold. Less yang also means less movement in the intestine and a greater tendency to constipation. As you need strong yang to function in your day-to-day life, you can also get tired easily.

STAGNATION OF QI IN THE BODY: The Liver guides qi around the body and ensures that it flows smoothly, but strong emotional stress, inappropriate dietary habits, overwork, or a lack of strong yang can cause it to stop working correctly. Symptoms of stagnation usually appear in areas directly related to the Liver or around the two Wood channels (the Liver and Gall Bladder). The thyroid gland area is one of these areas (a branch of the Liver channel goes through the neck), and a very visual manifestation of this is a large lump known as a goitre.

ACCUMULATION OF DAMP AND PHLEGM: A weak digestive system cannot process food well and tends to accumulate and store damp. With the addition of a little heat, over time this can harden and turn into phlegm, resulting in palpable lumps in the throat or the feeling of phlegm at the back of the throat. As the origin of this condition usually lies in weak Spleen yang, it is essential to adjust your diet to remedy this imbalance.

Dietary factors that can worsen hyperthyroidism

Overconsumption of bad oils and fats, processed, sugary foods, raw fruits and vegetables and dairy products such as milk and cheese weaken the Spleen and Stomach. See Damp for more details.

Dietary factors that can help hyperthyroidism

- A simple, bland diet that is easy for the Stomach and Spleen to digest is ideal. See Weak Qi for more details.
- Warming foods, such as cooked grains and soups, sweet potatoes, chestnuts, and walnuts, can help yang, but be cautious if there are symptoms of stagnation or heat, as too much of these can be counterproductive. See Weak Yang for more details.
- Warm spices, such as cloves, black peppercorn, ginger, cardamom, rosemary, turmeric, nutmeg, and black pepper, will both help yang and also move any stagnation. But again be cautious if you have heat symptoms.
- Foods that reduce damp and phlegm, such as aduki beans, onions, lemons (and their peel), radishes, olive oil, and garlic, can help digestion. See Damp and Phlegm for more details.

Acupressure and massage

ON THE BACK: Thumb-press down the back muscles either side of the spine, and hard-press Bl-13, Bl-20, Bl-23, and Du-4.

ON THE FRONT: Hard-press Ren-6, Ren-12, and Ren-17 on the centre line of the body.

ON THE LEGS: Press the following points, and knead if sore: St-36, St-40, Sp-6, Kid-7, and GB-34.

ON THE FEET: Thumb-press the Kidney channel on the foot (note that it circles around the ankle). Knead any sore points, in particular Kid-2. Also press the following points, and knead if sore: Liv-3, Thyroid, Kidneys, Liver, Stomach, and Spleen. Also do the Healthy Foot massage in the How Can You Treat Yourself? section.

ON THE HANDS: Do the Healthy Hand massage in the How Can You Treat Yourself? section. Press the following points, and knead if sore: Thyroid, Throat, Kidneys, Heart, Sanjiao, and Liver.

ON THE EARS: Do the Healthy Ear massage in the How Can You Treat Yourself? section. Press the following points, and knead if sore: Thyroid, Neck, Liver, Spleen, Kidneys, Endocrine, and Sympathetic.

Scraping

Scrape across the shoulders to the top of the arms, then down the muscles of the back on either side of the spine.

Tapping

Tap each point up to 30 times. You may need an assistant for the back area.

- Feel down the back muscles on either side of the spine, and tap any sore points.
- Tap at regular intervals down the middle of the body from the bottom of the breastbone over the belly button and up to where the pubic bone begins.
- Tap Kid-2 and Liv-3 on the foot and Kid-7 and GB-34 on the leg.

Exercises

Follow Exercises 1–6 of the five-element stretches. Ideally, do the sequence daily and without exertion.

Lifestyle advice

In Oriental medicine there is a strong (and often sudden) emotional component to this condition, especially when there is swelling in the thyroid gland. Resolving this underlying emotional aspect, whatever it may be, could help in the management of the condition.

Painful or Aching Joints
Symptoms

Pain or discomfort of the joints and the muscles and tendons around them; swelling; limitation in movement; bony lumps; redness; and numbness.

Can include or lead to

Osteoarthritis, rheumatoid arthritis, osteoporosis, and fibromyalgia.

When to see a doctor

If the symptoms are severe and getting worse.

Common causes

Overuse; exposure to the elements; overexercise; accidents; emotional stress, especially when repressed; or an improper diet.

An explanation

In many cases of joint pain, the main source of discomfort is one of five conditions. They can be distinguished by the distinctive symptoms each produces:

WIND: The pain seems to move from joint to joint.

DAMP: The pain is fixed and often accompanied by numbness, Swelling, and heaviness. It can worsen in damp, rainy weather.

HEAT: The joint may feel hot to the touch and be swollen and inflamed. The pain is usually severe.

COLD: The pain is fixed in one joint and is very painful. It may also worsen in cold weather.

PHLEGM: The joint may be swollen with bony lumps and deformities.

Underlying these conditions, there is normally a weakness of qi and blood that needs to be redressed.

Dietary factors that can worsen painful joints

- In general, a strengthening diet will support digestion. See Weak Qi for more details.
- Cold foods, such as raw vegetables, fruit, and cold drinks, aggravate cold conditions. See Cold for more details.
- Dairy products, concentrated fruit juices, and other damp-forming foods aggravate damp and phlegm. See Damp and Phlegm for more details.
- Seafood, such as shrimp, prawns, lobster, and crab, and spinach and mushrooms aggravate wind.
- Lamb, beef, alcohol, and hot spices aggravate heat in the body. See Heat for more details.

Dietary factors that can improve painful joints

- Meat, ginger, eggs, garlic, and alcoholic spirits such as brandy (but only in small amounts) can be helpful. See Cold for more details.
- Chicken, rice, and carrots nourish the blood and help wind conditions. See Weak Blood for more details.

Acupressure and massage

For specific details see the section related to the corresponding pain area:

Shoulder: p. 147

Elbow: p. 185

Wrist: p. 187

Hand and fingers: p. 189

Back: p. 179

Knee: p. 191

Ankle: p. 193

Foot and toes: p. 195

Scraping

Many parts of the body can be scraped to release ten-

> NOTE: Be aware of the cautions in the Scraping introduction, such as not to scrape over bone and skin conditions. In general, scrape over fleshy, muscular areas and downwards or outwards from the centre of the body.

sion in the muscles and tendons and increase the flow of blood and qi to the area.

Tapping

Tap each point up to 30 times. An assistant may be needed for the back area.

- In general: palpate GB-21, Bl-18, Bl-20, Bl-23, and Bl-52 on the back, Sp-10 and Sp-6 on the leg, and Kid-3 on the foot, and tap if tender.
- Specific joints: gently tap in a circular motion around the joint. Tap at a distance of 1 inch for small joints and 2 inches for larger joints. If the Tapping is painful, increase the distance.

Exercises

Choose from Exercises 1-6 of the five-element stretches and many of the specific exercises in each section, according to symptoms and the location of the channels and the joint. See the relevant section for more details.

Lifestyle advice

- Regular gentle exercise is essential to keep the joints supple.
- If the pain is from an acute, not a chronic, injury, note the advice about putting ice on it in Neck Pain.

Fatigue

Symptoms

Tiredness, lack of concentration, heaviness, depression, and aching muscles.

Can include or lead to

Chronic fatigue syndrome, myalgic encephalomyelitis, Addison's disease, hypoadrenia, hypothyroidism, glandular fever, and narcolepsy.

When to see a doctor

If the symptoms are severe.

Common causes

Stress; overwork; irregular eating patterns; an improper diet; overeating; constitutionally weak; anxiety; worry; overthinking; long-term illness; trauma or shock; or overuse of antibiotics.

An explanation

STAGNATION OF QI IN THE BODY: Stagnant qi in the Liver prevents qi from moving around and nourishing the body. The most common cause of this is emotional repression or stress. A clear indicator of stagnant qi being involved is feeling better after doing exercise, as the exercise moved the qi.

WEAK QI IN THE SPLEEN: The Spleen is very important in all cases of fatigue. For example, the Spleen is involved in sending qi to the arms and legs, and these will become heavier and more difficult to move if qi is weak.

DAMP IN THE MUSCLES: When deficient in qi, both the Stomach and Spleen are unable to process food properly and tend to store dampness. This is heavy and sticky and can weigh you down, thereby increasing fatigue. Indications of damp in the body include a feeling of heaviness, especially after eating or in the morning, and sometimes a strong desire to lie down.

TRAPPED WIND AND HEAT: Wind entering the body may cause symptoms, such as a cold for example. If not cleared properly, it can go deeper into the layers of the body, where it can remain for a long time and transform into heat. The heat will eventually burn outwards and come to the surface, causing sudden weakness and hot feverish symptoms.

Dietary factors that can worsen fatigue

- Eating too much, too quickly, or irregularly, especially while not being in a relaxed state, will create stagnation.
- Damp-forming foods, such as fatty, oily foods; processed foods that are highly sweetened; dairy products; bananas; and fatty meat such as lamb slow down the body. See Damp for more details.

Dietary factors that can improve fatigue

- The Stomach and Spleen need to be nourished with a simple diet of easily digestible, freshly cooked food. See Weak Qi for more details.
- Pears, cherries, grapes, and other warming and drying foods help counteract fatigue with damp conditions. See Damp for more details.
- Aubergines (eggplants), sunflower seeds, celery, bananas, and rabbit help counteract fatigue with conditions of internal wind.

Acupressure and massage

ON THE FRONT: Hard-press any sore points on the centre line of the abdomen, including Ren-6, Ren-9, and Ren-12. Check Liv-13 and Liv-14 for soreness, and knead.

ON THE BACK: Thumb- or finger-press down the muscles either side of the spine. Knead any sore points, especially Bl-20 and Bl-21.

ON THE ARMS: Hard-press LI-11 and TB-5, if sore.

ON THE LEGS:

- Thumb-press along the Spleen channel, as far as the knee, and knead any sore points, especially Sp-6 and Sp-9. Press and knead St-36 and GB-34, if sore.
- Thumb press along the Kidney channel, as far as the knee, and knead any sore points

ON THE HANDS: Do the Healthy Hand massage in the How Can You Treat Yourself? section. Knead the channel areas at the finger tips, Essence, and Stomach, Spleen, and Large Intestine areas.

ON THE FEET: Do the Healthy Foot massage in the How Can You Treat Yourself? section. Also press the following points, and knead if sore: Lungs, Heart, Spleen, Stomach, Duodenum, and Kidneys.

ON THE EARS: Press the following points, and knead if sore: Vitality point, Brain, Adrenal gland, Point Zero, and Shen Men.

Scraping

Scrape gently across both shoulders and down the muscles of the back either side of the spine. Avoid using too much pressure or force when scraping, especially if the receiver is weak or frail.

Tapping

Tap each point up to 30 times. You may need an assistant for the back area.

- Feel down the back muscles either side of the spine, and tap any sore points.
- Tap along the shoulder muscles, then down the main muscles of the upper arm and forearms, include LI-11 on the arm and LI-4 on the hand.
- Tap at regular intervals down the middle of the body, from the bottom of the breastbone, over the belly button, and down to where the pubic bone begins.
- Tap along the thigh muscles, then down the calf muscles, both at the front and back. Include St-36 and any sore points along the Spleen Channel.

Exercises

1. Do Exercises 2 and 6 of the five-element stretches to strengthen the Earth and Wood organs.
2. Do exercise Body Twist from the Constipation section.

Lifestyle advice

- Light physical exercise is very important in order to keep qi circulating well. It is, however, equally important not to do too much. The end result should be a feeling of more energy and rejuvenation not further tiredness or exhaustion.
- Learning to pace yourself on a daily basis is one of the most important aspects of managing a fatigue condition.

Diabetes

Symptoms (see below for an explanation of the groupings):

Usually a combination of the following, although the key symptoms are in bold:

- UPPER: **Thirst** and copious drinking, dry mouth and tongue, mouth ulcers, lack of appetite, and a red tongue tip.
- MIDDLE: Increase in appetite, **weight loss**, restless, stomach discomfort, sweating, constipation, thirst, and **weakness**.
- LOWER: **Frequent and profuse urination**, dry mouth and tongue, dizziness, blurred vision, red cheeks, hunger but poor appetite, lower back and knee pain, and weakness.

Can include or lead to

Type 1 or Type 2 diabetes mellitus, gestational diabetes, atheroma, infections, arteriosclerosis, ketoacidosis, peripheral neuropathy, and retinal damage.

When to see a doctor

If the symptoms are severe, rising blood sugar levels, hypoglycaemic episodes (dizziness, fainting or seizures) and the presence of ketones in urination.

Common causes

In the case of Type 2 diabetes, lifestyle is the culprit: an improper diet of too many processed, fried, oily foods (bad fats) or hot-natured and spicy foods; smoking; overconsumption of alcohol; emotional stress, especially when emotions are repressed; overworry; overweight; lack of exercise; old age; or too much sexual activity. Type 1 is usually more related to constitutional weakness, although lifestyle factors can be a factor.

An explanation

Diabetes is a massive worldwide health problem. In the USA alone, diabetes affects 25.8 million people, and an astonishing 7 million of these are thought to be undiagnosed.[32]

In conventional terms, a diagnosis of diabetes mainly consists of either being insulin dependent (Type 1), requiring regular injections of insulin, or non-insulin dependent (Type 2), which tends to appear later in life and requires lifestyle changes and medication.

Traditionally, Oriental medicine views diabetes in general as a condition of heat and dryness (known in ancient times as Wasting and Thirsting Disease), specifically affecting the upper, middle, or lower organs.

UPPER: Heat in the Lungs
MIDDLE: Heat in the Stomach
LOWER: Weak Kidney yin

The general condition that is known as Wasting and Thirsting disease in Oriental medicine, or diabetes in conventional medicine, can be diagnosed with or without presenting symptoms. As a result, while many of the above symptoms may be present, sometimes they have not reached that stage yet, and instead resemble more a weakness in digestion and stagnation of qi (See Qi Stagnation for more details).

WEAK QI IN THE STOMACH AND SPLEEN: The general pattern that can lead to diabetes often has its origins in a weak Stomach and digestion. This could be constitutional and associated more with Type 1 diabetes, or due to a habitually poor diet, lack of exercise, and a general yin-type lifestyle associated with Type 2, although more and more incidences of Type 1 in both young people and adults are due to the latter.

DRYNESS AND HEAT IN THE STOMACH: As the Stomach gets weaker and more sluggish, heat builds up, drying up body fluids and creating intense hunger and thirst. This condition is normally associated with eating a lot and being overweight.

DRYNESS AND HEAT IN THE LUNGS: The heat burning in the Stomach can also rise to the Lungs and consume body fluids. In a regular smoker, the Lungs are often already weak and dry, so the condition will be exaggerated. This condition is normally associated with the desire to drink lots of liquids.

STAGNATION OF LIVER QI: Emotional stress can lead to blockages in the flow of qi around the body. Over time, these blockages create heat, which can rise and burn up the body fluids of the Stomach and Lungs.

WEAK YIN IN THE KIDNEYS: Any heat in the Stomach, Lungs, or Liver that consumes body fluids will have a knock-on effect on the Kidneys. Kidney yin can weaken considerably, and the resulting hyperactivity of yang can create more heat and rising fire. This condition is normally associated with both drinking and urinating a lot.

The blood sugar-regulating hormone insulin, which must be injected daily by some diabetics, particularly those with Type 1 (insulin-dependent) diabetes, is very cooling and moisturizing to the body. The Oriental medicine view, though, is that it can damage the Stomach and Spleen further and cause the buildup of damp, bloating, and digestive symptoms. These should be remedied by changes in diet.

Dietary factors that can worsen diabetes

- Overeating, large meals, and irregular eating habits weaken digestion and increase stagnation.
- Eating a lot of greasy, fatty food with high levels of bad fats, such as processed and dairy products and poor-quality vegetable oils; meat; nuts; refined sugar and sugar products; overly salty or spicy foods; alcohol; caffeine; and cigarettes weakens the Stomach and Lungs.

Dietary factors that can improve or prevent the onset of diabetes

- The Stomach and Spleen function best with regularity, so eating at the same time every day and not skipping meals will help to optimize digestive qi.
- Slow-burning, high-fiber complex carbohydrate foods, such as whole grains, fruits, and vegetables, are usually recommended for people diagnosed with diabetes. The theory is that these are broken down into blood sugar, or glucose, slowly and steadily in the body and prevent unpleasant blood sugar spikes that exhaust insulin supplies and break down the body. In fact, the recommended diet for diabetes is remarkably similar to the standard healthy diet in Oriental medicine (high in unrefined carbohydrates, low in protein and bad fats), which appears frequently in this book to strengthen weak Stomach and Spleen qi. See Weak Qi for more details.
- As the digestive organs are severely weakened in people with diabetes, it makes sense that the Stomach and Spleen cannot function properly with large meals. Small frequent meals will help them to process food better and stimulate the production of the blood sugar–controlling hormone insulin, which is normally faulty in Type 1 diabetics and depleted by lifestyle choices in Type 2.
- For conditions of dryness and heat in the Stomach, cooling and moistening foods, such as rice, avocado, cucumber, watercress, tofu, and yogurt, can help. Eat them in moderation only, though, as too many can weaken digestion. See Heat for more details.
- Foods such as garlic, radishes, the peel of oranges and tangerines, and carrots move qi and can reduce stagnation in the Liver. See Qi Stagnation for more details.
- Strengthening foods for Kidney yin include black beans, kidney beans, black sesame seeds, and pork. See Weak Yin for more details.

- The following foods can help regulate blood sugar and the level of fluids in the body:
  FRUIT: plums, pears, blueberries, avocados, and any fruit with a sour taste, such as lemons, limes, strawberries, and grapefruit.
  VEGETABLES: carrots, radishes, turnips, spinach, asparagus and dark leafy greens.
  GRAINS: rice, oats, and whole wheat.
  BEANS: chickpeas, (garbanzo) and mung beans.

Acupressure and massage

ON THE FRONT:
- Palm-circle with slight pressure in a clockwise direction around the belly button.
- Do the ABDOMEN CIRCLE massage in Feeling Bloated.
  Press and knead Ren-12, Ren-6, and Ren-4.
- Rub in a circular motion with the palm around Ren-4 to create warmth.

ON THE HEAD: Hard-press Ren-23 and Ren-24.

ON THE LEGS:
- Thumb-press along the Stomach and Spleen channels, as far as the knee. Knead any sore points, especially Sp-6 and Sp-9, and hard press St-36 and Kid-7.

ON THE BACK: Thumb-press down the Bladder channels on the back, and knead any sore points, including Bl-13, Bl-15, Bl-18, Bl-20, Bl-21, Bl-23, and Weiguanxiashu.

ON THE FEET: Hard press Kid-3. Also press the following points, and knead if sore: Liv-3, St-44, and the Kidneys, Liver, Stomach, Lungs, and Pancreas areas.

ON THE HAND: Press the following points, and knead if sore: Lu-10, Lungs, Spleen, and Kidneys areas.

ON THE EAR: Press the following points, and knead if sore: Pancreas, Stomach, Kidneys, Lungs, Sanjiao, and Shen Men.

Scraping

Scrape down the back muscles either side of the spine to the top of the buttocks. In particular, scrape along the muscles at the side of the scapula, the mid back nearer the spine, and the lumbosacral area across to the hips.

Tapping

Tap each point up to 30 times. You may need an assistant for the back area.

- Tap down the back muscles either side of the spine, including any of the following, if sore: Bl-13, Bl-15, Bl-18, Bl-20, Bl-21, Bl-23, Weiguanxiashu, and also the Huatuojiaji points, as described in High Blood Pressure.
- Tap any sore points on or near Kid-3 at the ankle, Sp-6, Kid-7 and St-36 on the legs, and Lu-9 on the wrist.

Exercises

Exercises 1, 2, 4, and 6 of the five-element stretches will strengthen the Lungs, Stomach, and Kidneys.

Lifestyle advice

- If you have developed the symptoms of Wasting and Thirsting disease, or diabetes, your body is telling you to stop and take stock of your health.
- You should regulate not only your diet and eating habits but also your sleeping times, levels of stress, and exercise regime.
- Regular gentle exercise – at least 30 minutes a day, five days a week – can increase the circulation of blood and qi and help lower blood sugar levels.
- Losing weight is essential. US Research has shown that weight loss in combination with exercise is more effective than medication in preventing or delaying the development of Type 2 diabetes.[33]

Obesity and Weight Loss
Symptoms

Overweight, excessive or no appetite, low energy, sleep problems, a bland taste in the mouth, scanty or no periods, impotence, chest and abdominal pain, dizziness, and palpitations.

Can include or lead to

Cushing's syndrome; orthopedic problems, such as back or joint pain; osteoarthritis; hypertension; diabetes; and heart disease.

When to see a doctor

If very or morbidly obese.

Common causes

Lack of exercise; improper diet and eating habits; overeating; constitutional tendency; emotional stress; a medical condition, such as diabetes; or a glandular malfunction.

An explanation

Obesity can be graded by measuring body mass index (BMI). To find your BMI requires simply dividing your weight (kg) by your height (m). The result can be classified below:

WHO class	BMI (g/m)
Underweight	Below 18.5
Normal range	18.5–24.9
Overweight	25–29.9
Obese	30–35
Very obese	35–40
Morbidly obese	40 and above

A recent study in The Lancet offers a grim reminder of what carrying excess bodyfat does to health. According to the study, people with a BMI of 30–35 can expect to die 2–4 years earlier, and people with a BMI of 40–45 will live 8–10 years less than someone of normal weight. The study goes on to list the causes of early death, including heart disease, stroke, diabetes, liver disease, kidney disease, cancer, and lung disease.[34]

Obesity is a medical condition that is becoming all too common, and for many people arises from a lack of understanding about how the body functions.

WEAK QI IN THE STOMACH AND SPLEEN: After eating, the digestive organs (the Stomach and Spleen) are hard at work transforming the food into qi and sending it where needed around the body. When these two organs become weak, the whole process gets clogged up and runs inefficiently. Stomach and Spleen often become weak due to a combination of bad eating habits and a poor diet of damp-forming, fatty foods.

DAMP IN THE BODY: When the body is unable to process food properly, it often leads to an accumulation of damp, which will then further impair the functioning of the Stomach and Spleen. The damp then builds up in the form of fat, which is stored around the body.

In addition, the lack of qi going to the arms and legs can create an additional weakness and fatigue. Imagine the Stomach and Spleen as a garden where occasional light drizzle allows plants and flowers to grow abundantly. When someone is overweight, the garden has become water-logged and mud has replaced the grass. Not much can grow well in this environment.

Symptoms such as discomfort in the stomach area, body heaviness, and scanty urine are often associated with this condition.

STAGNATION OF QI IN THE BODY: The Liver can easily be affected by emotional stress, which prevents it from doing its job of safeguarding the smooth flow of qi around the body. Stagnation of qi then devel-

ops, along with the stagnation of blood and body fluids. The body fluids collect and congeal into damp and phlegm, which further blocks the smooth flow of fluids.

This condition normally has an emotional component to it and can be accompanied by a tight and phlegmy chest and a bitter taste in the mouth.

HEAT IN THE STOMACH: Stagnation over time will create heat. When the heat is in the Stomach, it can manifest as insatiable hunger and subsequent overeating. Any attempt to reduce weight needs to take into account the weakness of the Stomach and Spleen, qi stagnation, and the presence of damp and phlegm. If not, at best the weight reduction, if any, may be only temporary. The way to do this is to follow simple guidelines in eating habits and exercise.

Dietary factors that can worsen obesity

- Raw foods can put a strain on a weak Stomach and Spleen by forcing them to work harder in digestion. Raw food should therefore be avoided unless the cooling nature of raw food is needed in conditions of heat.

- Dairy products can be damp-forming in the body, especially when it is weak, as they are often too rich in nutrients for the Stomach to digest well. This can encourage some people's bodies to do the exact opposite of losing weight. See Damp for more details.

- Highly processed, artificially sweetened foods. These are deficient in the nutrients needed to make strong Stomach qi.

- Man-made hydrogenated fats and cheap refined vegetable oils. These contain too many damaging fats – common in manufactured margarine spreads and frying oils in restaurants and supermarkets – which lead to damp and heat in the body.

- Very sweet fruits, such as figs, dates, and dried fruit. These contain concentrated sugars that do not aid weight loss.

- Bananas, avocados, and coconuts. These are damp-forming fruits and prevent weight loss.
- Meat is very nutritious, and for this reason should be eaten in moderation or it will lead to stagnation of the digestive system and weak Stomach and Spleen qi. It is important, therefore, to dramatically reduce the amount of meat consumed if you want to lose weight.
- Salt should be used very sparingly.

Dietary factors that can improve obesity

- Regular meal times. The Stomach and Spleen need regularity to function well.
- An ideal diet is a strengthening diet of cooked foods in the form of soups or stews that are easy to digest, including vegetables, whole grains, and legumes, and only a small amount of good quality meat (less than ten percent).
- Emphasize bitter and sour foods. Choose from the following list of useful foods:

GRAINS: Rye, amaranth, quinoa, and oats are bitter, and therefore drying and beneficial to digestion. Corn also helps to expel fluids, so can be useful in reducing body fat.

FRUIT: Emphasize bitter fruits, such as lemons and grapefruits. Eat apples, plums, peaches, berries, oranges, and pears in moderation.

VEGETABLES: Lettuce, celery, asparagus, scallions, and other bitter vegetables, and turnips, radishes, and other pungent vegetables.

HERBS AND SPICES: Pungent spices, such as cumin, ginger, cloves, cayenne, fennel, peppermint, chamomile, and white pepper. (Be cautious about eating too many of these herbs and spices if also suffering from a heat condition.)

DRINK: Chinese green tea.

OTHER: Dairy products made from goat or sheep's milk are a viable alternative to cow's milk products. Use cold-pressed extra-virgin olive oil or unrefined sesame oil as an alternative to oils high in bad fatty acids.

Acupressure and massage

ON THE FRONT:

- Rub in a circular motion around the belly button with your palm.
- Do the ABDOMEN CIRCLE massage in Feeling Bloated. Finger-press and knead Ren-12, St-21, and St-25. Press Liv-14, and knead if sore.

ON THE LEGS: Thumb-press the Stomach, Spleen, Liver, and Gall Bladder channels as far as the knee, and knead any sore points, especially St-36, St-40, Sp-10, Sp-9, Sp-6, Liv-4, GB-34, and GB-40.

ON THE BACK: Press and knead any sore points on the Bladder channel, including Bl-18, Bl-19, Bl-20, Bl-21, and Bl-23.

ON THE ARMS: Thumb-press the Large Intestine channel, and knead any sore points, including LI-10, and LI-11.

ON THE HANDS: Press the following points, and knead if sore: LI-4, Spleen, Liver, Stomach, Spleen, and Large Intestine area.

ON THE FEET: Press and knead the middle area of the soles of the feet, including the Stomach, Small Intestine, Duodenum, Spleen, and Liver areas. Also St-44, Liv-3, and Sp-3, if sore.

ON THE EARS: Press the following points, and knead if sore: Appetite Control, Spleen, Stomach, Liver, Esophagus, Point Zero, and Shen Men.

Scraping

Scrape across the shoulder muscles and down the back muscles, either side of the spine. Pay particular attention to the mid-back area.

Tapping

Tap each point up to 30 times. You may need an assistant for the back area.

- Feel across the shoulder muscles, and tap any sore points, including GB-21 at the top of the shoulder muscle.
- Feel down the back muscles either side of the spine, and tap any sore points, including Bl-18, Bl-20, and Bl-21.
- Tap at regular intervals down the midline of the front of the body, from the top of the breastbone, down the abdomen, to where the pubic bone begins.
- Tap along the thigh muscles, including Sp-10, and then down the calf muscles. Also tap Sp-6 and St-36 on the leg, and Liv-3 on the foot, if sore.

Exercises

1. Do Exercises 1–6 of the five-element stretches to generally harmonize and strengthen the body.
2. Do these specific exercises for losing weight:

TWIST AND ROLL THE BODY:
- Lie face up with your knees bent up to your chest and both arms stretched out to the side level with your shoulders.
- Breathing in and, keeping your shoulders tightly on the ground, turn your buttocks slowly to one side. Try to bring both knees to the ground, and meanwhile turn your head to the opposite side and breathe out.
- Slowly twist back, breathe in, and repeat on the other side.

RAISE THE PELVIS:
- Lie face up, with both arms relaxed at your sides.
- Bend your knees, keeping your feet on the ground.
- Breathe in, contract the buttock muscles, and raise the buttocks slowly to make the whole back lift off the ground supported by the shoulders.
- Hold for a few seconds, then breathe out, and slowly return to lying flat.
- Repeat five times or until tired.

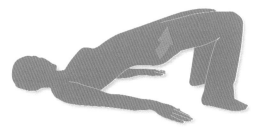

(top right) Raise the pelvis

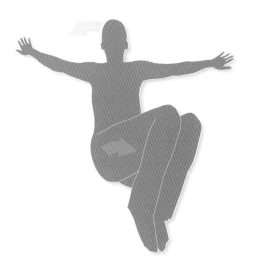

(left) Twist and roll your body

(bottom right) Dry swimming

DRY SWIMMING:
- Lie face down, arms bent, and palms flat pushing downwards.
- Lift both legs at the same time slightly. Contract your buttock muscles, and move your legs up and down as a fish might swim.

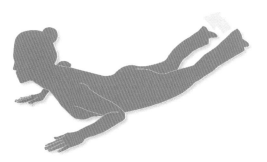

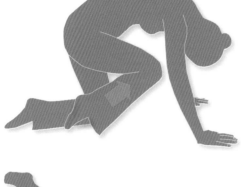

Kick in an arched position: knee lift

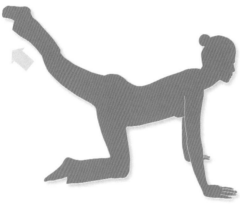

Kick in an arched position: kick and stretch

KICK IN AN ARCHED POSITION:

- Begin on all fours and breathe in.
- Keep your back perpendicular with the ground, and hang your head down so you can see your knees. Then lift one knee towards your forehead.
- Breathe out and contract your buttock muscles. Then lift your head up and stretch out your right leg backwards at the same time.
- Repeat this several times. The movement should be quick and continuous.
- Repeat with the other leg.

Lifestyle advice

Moderate, regular exercise is essential to any change in diet. Without it, long-term change can be difficult. The aim should be to gradually build up to two hours of moderate-intensity activity per week, doing activities like brisk walking, doubles tennis, bike riding (avoiding hills), and water aerobics.

Chapter 28
氣 Skin Conditions

Acne
Symptoms

Red spots on the face, neck, chest, and upper back; blisters filled with pus; and post-inflammatory scarring.

Can include or lead to

Acne vulgaris.

When to see a doctor

If the symptoms are severe.

Common causes

Strong emotional stress; living in a damp environment; irregular eating habits; or an improper diet of greasy; damp; and heat-forming foods.

An explanation

HEAT: Acne is a very visible manifestation of internal heat in the body. The redder it is, the more heat is being generated from within. Often pubescent changes in young teenagers can release much of this heat, which can come from a variety of internal sources.

The Lungs have a major influence over the skin and often too much heat in the Lungs can cause lesions on the forehead and nose area.

Lesions around the mouth, in front of the ears, in the corners of the forehead, and on the chest and upper back are more likely to be caused by heat in the Stomach. This can often be as a result of a highly processed, junk food diet, with too many fried and oily foods. It can often be accompanied by an almost insatiable hunger, a craving for spicy or oily foods, and thirst.

DAMP AND PHLEGM: The pus that often accompanies the lesions is quite literally damp and phlegm and, if the Stomach and Spleen have been damaged by an inappropriate diet, there is usually an excess of these substances rising with the heat. This gets lodged in the space between the skin and muscles and oozes its way out.

STAGNATION OF BLOOD: If the condition is particularly severe, with deep, inflamed spots and possible scarring, the heat has transformed into "toxic" heat, and the blood has become stuck.

Dietary factors that can worsen acne

Hot-natured, spicy, and damp-forming foods. See the Heat and Damp Foods sections for more details. In particular, overconsuming deep-fried foods, citrus fruits, oysters, herring, grilled or smoked fish, and shrimp, meat, artificial sweeteners, coffee, and alcohol.

Dietary factors that can improve acne

- A simple diet strengthens the digestive organs. See Weak Qi for more details.
- The following foods can also help with soothing the inflammation and removing damp:

FRUIT: pears.

VEGETABLES: cucumbers, celery, carrots, squash, pumpkin, leafy greens, such as spinach and watercress.

LEGUMES, SEEDS, AND NUTS: Mung beans and aduki beans.

DRINKS: green tea and goat's milk.

OTHER: seaweed.

Acupressure and massage

ON THE BACK: Thumb-press down the Bladder channels, and knead any sore points, especially Bl-13 and Bl-17.

ON THE ARMS: Press on and around TB-6 and LI-11. Knead if sore.

ON THE LEGS:

- Thumb-press the Spleen channel as far as the top of the thigh. Knead any sore points, especially Sp-6, Sp-9, and Sp-10.
- Thumb-press the Stomach channel, as far as the knee. Knead any sore points, especially St-40 and St-36.

ON THE HANDS: Press the following points, and knead if sore: Head area, LI-4, Pc-9, Stop Itching, Stomach, Spleen, Large Intestine area, Lungs, and Chest.

ON THE FEET: Press the following points, and knead if sore: Liver, Stomach, Spleen, Lungs, and Large Intestine.

ON THE EARS: Press the following points, and knead if sore: Face, Skin Disorder, Lungs, Large Intestine, and Shen Men.

Scraping

Scraping can be very useful in removing the stagnation of qi and blood at the skin surface. Scrape across the shoulders and down the back, either side of the spine.

CAUTION: Avoid Scraping on or near skin conditions.

Tapping

Tap each point up to 30 times. You may need an assistant for the back area.

- Follow the midline of the breastbone (the Ren channel), and gently tap any sore points.
- Tap down the arm muscles to the wrist, then tap LI-4 on the hand and the nail points of the fingers: Lu-11, Pc-9, He-9, LI-1, TB-1, and SI-1.
- Feel across the shoulder muscles, and tap on any tense, tender areas of muscle (avoid Tapping directly on any inflamed areas).
- Tap down the muscles in the back at regular intervals, doing both sides before moving downwards. Feel for any sore points as you go but avoid any areas of skin inflammation.
- Tap down the main thigh muscles and the calf muscles.
- At the feet tap Liv-3, Kid-1, and the nail points of the toes: Sp-1, Liv-1, Bl-67, GB-44, and St-45.

CAUTION: Do not tap directly over the skin condition area.

Exercises

Do Exercises 1, 2, and 6 of the five-element stretches to strengthen the Lungs, Spleen, and Liver.

Lifestyle advice

- Apply aloe vera gel to the affected area, as it has a cold, bitter, and antitoxic quality. This makes it a very useful anti-inflammatory and antibacterial, and it can help in tissue repairs. Lemon juice also can have a similar effect.
- Avoid a lifestyle that is going to generate internal heat. Staying up late, sitting in front of a computer or TV screen for long hours, irregular eating hours, and eating too many junk and processed foods (basically, the average life of a teenager!) all should

be minimized.

- Avoid extended periods of exposure to the sun, such as sunbathing, as this can aggravate acne.

Eczema
Symptoms

Scaly, itchy rash. with blisters, dry skin, crusted skin coating, and inflamed and broken skin. Often affecting the skin creases at the elbow, wrist, and back of the knee.

Can include or lead to

Atopic eczema and dermatitis.

When to see a doctor

If the symptoms are severe.

Common causes

Overwork, emotional stress; a diet of hot-natured; damp-forming foods; exposure to the elements; vaccinations; or allergies.

An explanation

Research in the UK has found a steady rise in the diagnosis of eczema, noting a huge 42 percent rise in cases between 2001 and 2005.[35] The main issue with eczema is that its causes are not normally to be found on the skin but in what is happening inside.

WEAK QI IN THE LUNGS AND SPLEEN: The condition of the Lungs is directly related to the state of the skin. An underlying weakness in Lung qi accompanies most cases of eczema. In many eczema conditions, this is combined with a weakness in the Spleen, often connected to an improper diet. This could be due to the Stomach not being ready to handle rich foods at a young age, due to a diet of

processed, damp-forming foods. This pattern can of result in dull pale red or brown lesions.

WEAK BLOOD IN THE BODY: If the blood is not being nourished correctly, it cannot then moisten and nourish the skin. This can often lead to dry thicker skin accompanied by pale red lesions. This too could be diet related. More details can be found in the Weak Blood section.

WIND AND HEAT IN THE BODY: The redness and itchiness on the surface of the skin is caused by heat burning underneath. This is usually heat rising from yin weakness and spreading out to the yang channels, which run close to the surface of the body. It could also come from stagnation of qi, caused by emotional stress, such as feelings of being annoyed or frustrated.

Wind often appears when the blood becomes energetically weak and can combine with heat to cause dryness, severe itching, scaling, and a tendency to move from place to place in the body.

DAMP AND HEAT IN THE BODY: If the Spleen is weak, it can accumulate damp. This damp can make the digestive process sluggish, and in turn it generates heat. The heat can often combine with the damp under the skin, causing red, itchy, moist lesions, small blisters with clear or yellow fluid, and yellowish scabs and crusts.

Dietary factors that can worsen eczema

- Red meat, alcohol, and hot-natured and damp-forming foods encourage damp-heat. See Heat and Damp for more details.
- Chicken, shrimp, lobster, clams, mussels, and peanuts send yang outwards to the surface and cause heat to build up below the skin.
- Coffee, black tea, pungent spices, salt, and bitter foods are drying. See the Bitter food list.
- Some foods like apricots are too moistening and can provoke eczema.

Dietary factors that can improve eczema

- A simple diet nourishes both qi and blood. See Weak Qi for more details.
- Radishes, pumpkin, and rye help remove damp conditions. See Damp for more details.
- Carrots, radishes, spinach, celery, tomatoes, mung beans, wheat, and green tea help remove heat. See Heat for more details.
- Pears, kiwis, bananas (cooked), watermelons, soya beans, pine nuts, wheat, honey, tofu, pear juice, and soya milk help moisten dry skin.
- Cherries, plums, grapes, liver, beef, octopus, pine nuts, black sesame seeds, and eggs help strengthen blood. See Weak Blood for more details.

Acupressure and massage

ON THE BACK: Press GB-20 and Du-14, and knead if sore. Then press and knead down the back muscles either side of the spine, especially Bl-13, Bl-17, Bl-19, Bl-20, and Bl-21.

ON THE ARMS: Thumb-press up the Large Intestine and Triple Burner channels, and knead any sore points, especially LI-11 and TB-5.

ON THE LEGS:

- Thumb-press along the Spleen channel from the foot to Sp-10, just above the knee. Knead any sore points along the way, especially Sp-6 and Sp-9.
- Hard-press St-36.

ON THE FEET: Press the following points, and knead if sore: Liv-2, Liv-3, GB-43, Kid-6, Lungs, and Chest area.

ON THE HANDS: Press the following points, and knead if sore: LI-4, Spleen, Lungs, Lu-11, Stop itching, Spleen, Chest and Respiration, and the corresponding areas of the body.

ON THE EARS: Press the following points, and knead if sore: the corresponding body area, Skin Disorder, Lungs, Liver, Kidneys, and Shen Men.

CAUTION: Be careful to avoid any points or areas on or very close to any skin condition.

Scraping

Scrape down the neck, across the shoulders, and down the muscles of the upper back either side of the spine.

CAUTION: Care must be taken if there are any spots on the back not to scrape over them. A finger must be placed over the spot while Scraping that area. Also avoid Scraping on or near to any red or inflamed areas.

Tapping

Tap each point up to 30 times. You may need an assistant for the back area.

- Feel down the back muscles either side of the spine, and tap any sore points, including Bl-12, Bl-13, and Bl-17–23.
- Tap down the arm muscles towards the wrist, including LI-11, TB-5, and LI-4 on the hand.
- Tap at regular intervals down the midline of the body, down the breastbone, over the belly button, and down to where the pubic bone begins.
- Feel along the thigh muscles and tap any sore points, including GB-31 and Sp-10, then down the calf muscles. Also tap Sp-6, St-36, and GB-41 on the leg.

Exercises

Do Exercises 1–6 of the five-element stretches to strengthen digestion and respiration, and to help expel wind and damp.

Lifestyle advice

- Some form of relaxation is essential when the eczema worsens with stress. This could be anything from yoga or tai chi to playing golf or painting.
- Regular gentle exercise, such as walking, swimming, and cycling, can also help. However, try to avoid temperature extremes and any physical activity that will involve sweating a lot. When exercising wear lightweight and airy clothing over any affected areas to avoid this – ideally, cotton fabrics.
- Soaps and shampoos should be organic and chemical-free, and Epsom Salts and oils can replace regular bath and shower gels.
- Warm water is usually preferable over hot for bathing and showering.

Urticaria (Hives)
Symptoms

Commonly known as hives, urticaria often causes a red itchy rash, round swollen areas on the skin, and swollen lips and eyes. The symptoms can come and go.

Can include or lead to

Dermatographia.

When to see a doctor

If symptoms are severe.

Common causes

Exposure to cold weather; an irregular lifestyle; emotional stress; or an improper diet of hot-natured; greasy food.

An explanation

Urticaria is surprisingly common. As many as 15–24 percent of people in the United States will experience acute urticaria at some point in their lives.[36] Few sufferers are usually aware that the problem lies more on what is happening internally than externally.

DAMP IN THE BODY: Damp accumulates in the body, usually via the Stomach and Spleen, and is often directly related to diet. An inappropriate diet of processed, fried, or fatty foods can weaken digestion and cause excess damp to be stored.

This damp can then block or slow down normal functioning and lead to heat and poor circulation of qi to the skin. This condition is often accompanied by a red patchy rash and stomach and abdominal pain, low energy, poor appetite, constipation or diarrhoea, nausea, or vomiting.

WIND AND HEAT OR COLD IN THE BODY: Wind can sometimes get stuck within the body after a cold, an infection, a windy day, or when the body's defences are low.

If cold is predominant, there can be a white patchy rash that improves with heat and worsens with cold and wind. This is more common in the winter months.

If heat is predominant, it will feel worse with cold, be more of a red patchy rash, and be more common in the summer.

WEAKNESS OF QI AND BLOOD IN THE BODY: When qi and blood are weak, often from doing too much, the rash often appears and disappears rapidly and is periodic in nature. It is often worse when tired or overworked and is often accompanied by low energy levels.

CHANNEL DISHARMONY: With this condition, a rash often occurs several days before a period and disappears soon afterwards. This is because the balance between the two main channels responsible for the correct functioning of menstruation (known as the Ren and Chong channels) are not working in harmony. It is usually part of a pattern including painful and irregular periods.

Dietary factors that can worsen urticaria

- Pungent, hot-natured, and drying foods with a bitter taste, such as coffee, black tea, acrid spices, and too much salt. See the Pungent and Hot food lists.

Dietary factors that can improve urticaria

- Cool, cold-natured, and sour foods, such as yogurt, tangerines, strawberries, cranberries, and grapefruit, will reduce the heat. See the Cool, Cold, and Sour food lists for more details.
- Carrots, radishes, and tomatoes help with conditions of wind and heat.
- Bananas (cooked), pears (especially juice), kiwis, watermelons, soya beans, wheat, pine nuts, soya milk, yogurt, and honey help moisten hot, dry conditions.
- For conditions of weak qi and blood, foods should be included to strengthen the body and should preferably be boiled or steamed. See Weak Qi for more details.
- Cherries, plums, grapes, chicken, liver, beef, octopus, black sesame seeds, and eggs help strengthen blood. See Weak Blood for more details.

Acupressure and massage

ON THE BACK: Press GB-20 and Du-16, and knead if sore, then thumb press down the Bladder channels, either side of the spine.

ON THE ARMS: Thumb-press along the Large Intestine channel, from the hand to the elbow. Press and knead LI-11, if sore. Also press Pc-6, TB-5, and Lu-7 and knead, if sore.

ON THE LEGS: Thumb-press along the Spleen channel up to Sp-10, above the knee. Knead Sp-4, Sp-6, and Sp-9, if sore. Press GB-31, GB-41, St-36, and Kid-6, and knead if sore.

ON THE HANDS: Press the following points, and knead if sore: Stop itching, LI-4, Pc-8, SI-1, TB-3, Chest and Respiration, and Spleen area.

ON THE EARS: Press the following points, and knead if sore: the corresponding body area, Skin Disorder, Lungs, Liver, Spleen, Stomach, and Shen Men.

Scraping

Scrape down the neck, across the shoulders, and down the muscles of the upper back either side of the spine.

> CAUTION: Keep in mind that any scraping must not be done on or near any skin conditions.

Tapping

Tap each point up to 30 times. You may need an assistant for the back area.

- Feel down the back muscles either side of the spine, and tap any sore points, including Bl-12, Bl-13, and Bl-17–23.
- Tap LI-11 and any sore points down the forearm muscle.
- Tap at regular intervals down the middle of the body, from the bottom of the breastbone over the belly button and down to where the pubic bone begins.
- Tap along the thigh muscles including, Sp-10, then down the calf muscles. Also check Sp-6 and St-36 on the legs.

Exercises

Do Exercises 1–6 of the five-element stretches to generally harmonize and strengthen the body.

Lifestyle advice

For relief of the itchiness, the affected area can be rubbed with sliced cucumber.

氣 Further reading

This section suggests books for you to read if you would like to learn more. Most are very technical and written for practitioners. It also serves as an ad hoc bibliography.

Chinese medicine, in general

Flaws, Bob. The Treatment of Modern Western Medical Diseases with Chinese Medicine. Boulder, Colorado: Blue Poppy Press, 2001.

Kaptchuk, Ted. J. Chinese Medicine: The Web That Has No Weaver. London: Rider, 1990.

Maciocia, Giovanni. The Foundations of Chinese Medicine: A Comprehensive Text for Acupuncturists and Herbalists. New York : Churchill Livingstone, 1989.

Maciocia, Giovanni. The Practice of Chinese Medicine: The Treatment of Diseases with Acupuncture and Chinese Herbs. New York: Churchill Livingstone, 1994.

Sun, Peilin. The Treatment of Pain with Chinese Herbs and Acupuncture. New York: Churchill Livingstone, 2002.

MaClean, Will and Lyttleton, Jane. Clinical Handbook of Internal Medicine: The Treatment of Disease with Traditional Chinese Medicine. Vol.1. Sydney, Australia: University of Western Sydney, 1998.

MaClean, Will and Lyttleton, Jane. Clinical Handbook of Internal Medicine: The Treatment of Disease with Traditional Chinese Medicine. Vol.2. Sydney, Australia: University of Western Sydney, 2002.

Japanese acupuncture techniques

Birch, Stephen and Junko Ida: Japanese Acupuncture: A Clinical Guide. Brookline, NY: Paradigm Publications, 1998.

Ikeda, Masakazu. The Practice of Japanese Acupuncture and Moxibustion. Seattle: Eastland Press, 2005.

Manaka, Yoshio: Chasing the Dragon's Tail. Brookline, NY: Paradigm Publications, 1995.

Food and nutrition

Flaws, Bob. The Tao of Healthy Eating: Dietary Wisdom According to Traditional Chinese Medicine. Boulder, CO: Blue Poppy Press, 1998.

Kastner, Joerg. Chinese nutritional Therapy: Dietetics in Traditional Chinese Medicine. New York: Thieme, 2008.

Leggett, Daverick. Helping Ourselves: A Guide to Traditional Chinese Food Energetics. UK: Meridian Press, 1997.

Leggett, Daverick. Recipes for Self-Healing. UK: Meridian Press, 1999.

Pitchford, Paul. Healing with Whole Foods: Asian Traditions and Modern Nutrition. Berkeley, CA: North Atlantic Books, 2002.

Microsystems

Jinlin, Qiao. Hand Acupuncture Therapy. Beijing, China: Foreign Languages Press, 2006.

Oleson, Terry. Auriculotherapy Manual: Chinese and Western Systems of Ear Acupuncture. New York: Churchill Livingstone, 2003.

Shaozhi, Li and Xiaohong, Tan. Chinese Threapeutic Methods Of Acupoints. Beijing, China: Human Science and Biology Press, 2005.

Wang, Yajuan. Micro-Acupuncture in Practice. New York: Churchill Livingstone, 2009.

Scraping

Nielson, Arya. Gua Sha: A Traditional Technique for Modern Practice. New York: Churchill Livingstone, 2002.

Exercises

Hashimoto, Keizo. Sotai Natural Exercise. Chico, CA: George Ohsawa Macrobiotic Foundation, 2010.

Hesheng, Li. Self-Therapies for Common Diseases. Beijing, China: Foreign Languages Press, 2001.

Useful sources of information

For information about where to buy a hammer/needle set, videos on how to do many of the techniques in this book, and to contact the author, go to www.oriental-medicine.org.

氣 Endnotes

1. Dynamic spread of happiness in a large social network: longitudinal analysis over 20 years in the Framingham Heart Study. *British Medical Journal* Dec 4, 2008; 337: a2338.
2. Keeping the young-elderly healthy: is it too late to improve our health through nutrition? *American Journal of Clinical Nutrition* Nov 2007; 86(5): 1572S–6S.
3. Improvement in chewing activity reduces energy intake in one meal and modulates plasma gut hormone concentrations in obese and lean young Chinese men. *American Journal of Clinical Nutrition* July 20, 2011, doi: 10.3945/ajcn.111.015164.
4. The joint impact on being overweight of self-reported behaviours of eating quickly and eating until full: cross-sectional survey. *British Medical Journal* Oct 21, 2008; 337: a2002.
5. Anatomy of health effects of Mediterranean diet: Greek EPIC prospective cohort study. *British Medical Journal* Jun 23, 2009; 338: b2337.
6. Combined impact of lifestyle factors on mortality: prospective cohort study in US women. *British Medical Journal* Sep 16, 2008; 337: a1440.
7. Sleep duration and all-cause mortality: a systematic review and meta-analysis of prospective studies. *Sleep.* May 1, 2010; 33(5): 585–92.
8. Sedentary time and cardio-metabolic biomarkers in US adults: NHANES 2003–06. *European Heart Journal* Mar 2011; 32(5): 590–7.
9. The Effect of *Gua Sha* Treatment on the Microcirculation of Surface Tissue: A Pilot Study in Healthy Subjects. *Journal of Science and Healing* doi: 10.1016/j.explore.2007.06.001.
10. More details of this can be found in Dr. Manaka's book, *Chasing the Dragon's Tail* (see Further Reading). In it Manaka details the following metronome frequencies:

Ren channel	104	Du Channel	104
Lung	126	Large intestine	108
Spleen	132	Stomach	132
Heart	126	Small intestine	120
Kidney	120	Bladder	112
Pericardium	176	Triple burner	152
Liver	108	Gall bladder	120

11. Does participating in physical activity in outdoor natural environments have a greater effect on physical and mental wellbeing than physical activity indoors? A systematic review. *Environmental Science and Technology* Mar 1, 2011; 45(5): 1761–72.
12. Dietary pattern and depressive symptoms in middle age. *British Journal of Psychiatry,* Nov 2009; 195(5): 408–13.
13. Coronary Heart Disease Statistics 2010 Edition. *British Heart Foundation Health Promotion Research Group.* Oxford, 2010: 77.
14. Virtanen M., S.A. Stansfeld, R. Fuhrer, J.E. Ferrie, M. Kivima. Overtime Work as a Predictor of Major Depressive Episode: A 5-Year Follow-Up of the Whitehall II Study. *PLoS One* 2012; 7(1): e30719.
15. Janson C. et al. The European Community Respiratory Health Survey: what are the main results so far? *European Respiratory Journal.* 2001; 18:598–611.
16. The Diagnosis and Management of Rhinitis: An Updated Practice Parameter. Joint Task Force on Practice Parameters. *Journal of Allergy Clinical Immunology* 2008; 122: S1-S84.
17. Nathan, R.A. The burden of allergic rhinitis.

Allergy Asthma Proceedings 2007; 28:3-9.

18. Platts-Mills T.A.E. & L.J. Rosenwasser. Chronic sinusitis consensus and the way forward. *Journal of Allergy Clinical Immunology* 2004; 114: 1359–1361.

19. Patel S., R. Henderson, L. Bradley, B. Galloway, L. Hunter. Effect of visual display unit use on blink rate and tear stability. *Optom Vis Sci.* Nov 1991; 68(11): 888-92.

20. Upper respiratory tract infection is reduced in physically fit and active adults. *British Journal of Sports Medicine* Nov 1, 2010.

21. Effect of honey, dextromethorphan, and no treatment on nocturnal cough and sleep quality for coughing children and their parents. *Archives of Pediatrics and Adolescent Medicine* Dec 2007; 161(12): 1140–6).

22. Braman, Sidney S. The Global Burden of Asthma. *Chest* July 2006 130:1 suppl 4S-12S; doi: 10.1378/chest.130.1_suppl.4S.

23. Association of duration of television viewing in early childhood with the subsequent development of asthma. *Thorax.* Apr 2009; 64(4): 321–5.

24. Borrelli, F., R. Capasso, G. Aviello, et al. Effectiveness and safety of ginger in the treatment of pregnancy-induced nausea and vomiting. *Obstetrics & Gynecology* 2005; 105(4), 849-856.

25. Soft drinks, fructose consumption, and the risk of gout in men: prospective cohort study. *British Medical Journal* Feb 9, 2008; 336(7639): 309–12.

26. Tengs, T.O. & N.D. Osgood. The link between smoking and impotence: two decades of evidence. *Preventive Medicine* 2001; 32(6): 447–452.

27. Hackett, G., P. Kell, D. Ralph, et al. British Society for Sexual Medicine guidelines on the management of erectile dysfunction. *Journal of Sexual Medicine* 2008; 5(8), 1841–1865.

28. Filho Rocha et al. Essential fatty acids for premenstrual syndrome and their effect on pro-

lactin and total cholesterol levels: a randomized, double blind, placebo-controlled study. *Reproductive Health* 2011 8:2. doi: 10.1186/1742-4755-8-2.

29. Saraç F., K. Oztekin, G. Celebi. Early menopause association with employment, smoking, divorced marital status and low leptin levels. *Gynecological Endocrinology* 2010. [Epub ahead of print]

30. Salt Awareness Week survey reveals high levels of salt in takeaway pizzas. *CASH*, March 26 2012.

31. Blumenthal J.A., M.A. Babyak, A. Hinderliter, et al. Effects of the DASH diet alone and in combination with exercise and weight loss on blood pressure and cardiovascular biomarkers in men and women with high blood pressure: the ENCORE study. *Archives of Internal Medicine* January 2010; 170 (2): 126–35.

32. Centers for Disease Control and Prevention. National Diabetes Fact Sheet: national estimates and general information on diabetes and pre diabetes in the United States, 2011. Atlanta, GA: U.S. Department of Health and Human Services, Centers for Disease Control and Prevention, 2011.

33. Knowler W.C. et al. Diabetes Prevention Program Research Group. Reduction in the incidence of type 2 diabetes with lifestyle intervention or metformin. N Engl J Med. Feb 7, 2002; 346(6): 393–403.

34. Body-mass index and cause-specific mortality in 900 000 adults: collaborative analyses of 57 prospective studies. *The Lancet.* March 28, 2009; 373(9669): 1083–96.

35. Simpson C.R., J. Newton, J. Hippisley-Cox, A. Sheikh. Trends in the epidemiology and prescribing of medication for eczema in England. *Journal of the Royal Society of Medicine* 2009; 102: 108–117.

36. Urticaria: Part 1. *Annals of Allergy, Asthma and Immunology* 2000; 85: 525–531.

氣 Index

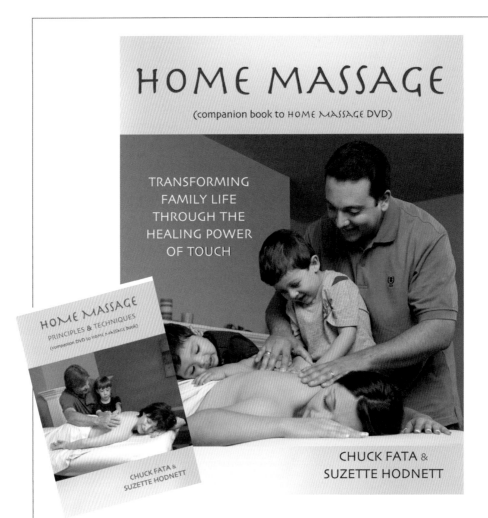

Home Massage
by Suzette Hodnett & Chuck Fata

The innate healing power of touch helps to reduce stress, improves the immune system and brings closer connection with loved ones. Designed for the non-professional with simple step-by-step instructions, this practical manual teaches the principles that make learning massage easy and fun. Also included are ideas for bringing home massage into daily life and how to use these principles to share massage with infants, children, adolescents, spouses, and the elderly.

ISBN 978-1-84409-559-9

Also available: *Home Massage: Principles and Techniques* (DVD) by the same authors
ISBN 978-1-84409-562-9